The Health Equity Case Studies Handbook

20 Delivery Systems, Health Plans, Community Organizations, and 9 Executive Interviews

Peter Boland, PhD

The Health Equity Case Studies Handbook:
20 Delivery Systems, Insurance Plans, Community Organizations, and 9 Executive Interviews

Peter Boland, PhD
Berkeley, CA
Peter@Bolandhealthcare.com

Ordering Information:
Special discounts are available on quantity purchases by corporations, associations, educational institutions, and others. For details, contact Peter Boland, PhD above.

Printed in the United States of America

First Edition
Softcover ISBN 979-8-89898-212-6
Ebook ISBN 979-8-89898-211-9

LCCN: 2025945506

Publisher
Winsome Entertainment Group LLC
Murray, UT

Acknowledgments

Numerous healthcare professionals around the country made this handbook possible. I am indebted to their willingness to take time from demanding schedules and day-to-day responsibilities to share what they learned about implementing initiatives based on health equity principles and objectives.

These organizations embodied "doing the right thing for the right reason" by making healthcare services more accessible to a broad range of communities based on what mattered most about health and how to meet local priorities. Their stories demonstrate the power of collaboration and the necessity of building trust as a prerequisite for partnering with local communities on a broad range of social care needs and place-based health improvement.

Many health-related leaders offered invaluable program advice, shared their personal journey, and documented how their organizations developed the necessary skills and tenacity to deliver what can be summed up as whole person care. The latter is a hallmark of health equity initiatives.

These individuals made significant contributions to this case studies handbook by sharing how their organizations went about designing and implementing unique approaches to furthering health equity in their communities:

Justina Acevedo-Cross, Karen Albright, Emily Anderson, Julia Andrieni, David Barley, Barbara Baumgardner, Michelle Beidelshies, Emily Berman, Gina Bericchia, Elizabeth Bradley, Eric Burnmeister, Ashley Carroll, Dave Chase, Shannon Duval, Jenny Erickson, Kevin Fiori, Neva Francis, Charise Fong, Michelle Fong, Robert Galvin, Gabrielle Gardner, Ean Gleeson, Boaz Goan, Lowell Goodman, Maria Grajski, Romi Hall, Thomas Hawkins, Zuhur Hilary, Ann Somers Hogg, Jazmin Holdway, Nick Jones, Maulik Joshi, Micah Kahn, Michael Keany, Erin Kelly, David Kibbee, George Kleb, Larissa Kick, Erin Kongshaug, Sunil Kripalani, Anita Kumar, Norman Lancit, Annie Ledbury, Brian Li, Wes Lo, Jan Lowery, John Lumpkin, Kyle Marshall, Amy McHugh, Elizabeth Miller, Angela Mingo, Adam Moneypenny, Melissa Monbouquette, Susan Oweli, Amanda Parsons, Ashley Perry, Peter Pronovost, Sara Redding, Mike Reilly, William Ries, Francesca Rinaldo, Jan Runa, Aurora Santana, Amanda Schoenberg, Barman Sheikh, Charlie Shields, Debra Sisco, Mark Smith, Nadeja Steager, Lori Taft, Katie Thompson, Bryan Trujillo, Debbie Well-Powell, Gretchen West, Joshua Wilking, Trenor Williams, Keeley Yednock, Emily Yu, Michelle Zambrano, Lorena Zamgrano, and Moses Zapien.

I am especially indebted to my publisher Juliet Clark at Winsome Publishing, and my editor Kathy Dunho. Each guided me through this multi-platform approach in the hopes that with a better understanding of health equity, more right things can be done for the right reasons.

Content

Case Study Highlights of Executive Initiatives v

Introduction 1

Delivery Systems 7

Chapter 1. Boston Medical Center 9

Chapter 2. Nationwide Children's Hospital 28

Chapter 3. University Hospitals, Cleveland

Executive Interview: Peter Pronovost, MD 49

Chapter 4. CommonSpirit Health 57

Chapter 5. Presbyterian Health 110

Chapter 6. Houston Methodist Hospital 139

Chapter 7. Cleveland Clinic, Executive Interview:

Elizabeth Bradley, MD and Michelle Beidelshies, PhD 173

Chapter 8. Vanderbilt University Medical Center 183

Chapter 9. Essentia Health 196

Chapter 10. Christensen Institute. Executive Interview:

Ann Somers Hogg 216

Chapter 11. Montefiore Health System 237

Chapter 12. University Hospital, Kansas City 267

Health Plans and Self-Funded Employer Plan 289

Chapter 13. Blue Cross Blue Shield of Massachusetts 291

Chapter 14. Blue Cross Blue Shield of Massachusetts: Consumer Health Research 311

Chapter 15: Executive Interview: Robert Galvin, MD 327
Chapter 16. Blue Cross Blue Shield of Minnesota 340
Chapter 17. Wisdo Health. Executive Interview: Boaz Goan......349
Chapter 18. Blue Cross Blue Shield of North Carolina 363
Chapter 19. Socially Determined. Executive Interview:
Trenor Williams, MD 390
Chapter 20. Geisinger Health Plan..404
Chapter 21. SCAN Health. Executive Interview:
Francesca Rinaldo, MD 432
Chapter 22. UMPC Health Plan...441
Chapter 23. Health Rosetta. Executive Interview:
Dave Chase 467

Community-Based Organizations *495*
Chapter 24. Pathways Community Hub Institute 497
Chapter 25. Bon Secours. Executive Interview:
George Kleb 531
Chapter 26. The BUILD Health Challenge (Des Moines).....547
Chapter 27. The BUILD Health Challenge: San Pablo
Area Development Collaborative (Oakland) 566
Chapter 28. Women, Infants and Children
Program (New York)..591
Chapter 29. Hawaii Community Foundation.........................606

Case Study Highlights of Equity Initiatives

The health equity initiatives presented in the *Health Equity Case Studies Handbook* highlight various building blocks of equity strategies. These examples reflect how different organizations are collaborating with communities and earning trust as full partners with a shared objective.

There is growing proof-of-concept that validates health equity principles and policies and how they lead to better care, better health, and the potential for greater health resiliency in the population.

With a renewed sense of urgency, we can learn the lessons of COVID and look ahead to solutions already put into practice in local communities. The case studies and executive interviews outlined below reflect the breadth of initiatives working to improve the health and well-being of individuals, communities, and states. Health equity programs serve as working models, and in these examples, we can see the hope of a healthier future for all.

Neighborhood Revitalization

Nationwide Children's Hospital Case Study. Columbus, Ohio

To break the intergenerational cycle of poverty and discrimination, the hospital began to treat the neighborhood as the patient. This initiative integrates education, health resources, workforce development, community safety, and strong partnerships to develop affordable housing as a catalyst for transformation. The objective is overall improvement.

Hospital System Equity Roadmap

CommonSpirit Health Case Study. Chicago, Illinois

CommonSpirit Health's Total Health Roadmap is a framework of thinking and action to address emerging accountabilities for patient outcomes influenced by social determinants to renew the role of healthcare delivery systems to increase community capacity to shape outcomes, engage in multi-sector collaboration, and make health equity a shared vision and value. This approach shifts ROI calculation from clinical outcomes to a new emphasis on improving community outcomes based on outreach activities and closing care gaps that contribute to health disparities.

Zero Defects Strategy

Peter Pronovost, MD, PhD, Executive Interview. University Hospitals. Cleveland, Ohio

The initiative focuses on eliminating all low-value behaviors with incentives based on four principles: align around a common purpose and definition of value, create a common framework and analytical platform for measuring defects and a management system to reduce defects, design incentives around a common purpose for all stakeholders, and ensure that patients can be traced. This strategy reduced member costs by 9 percent over twelve months. Such savings could fund a hospital system's upstream community health investments.

Outcomes-Based Payment

Pathways Community Hub/Pathways Community Hub Institute Case Study (Parts 1-3). Toledo, Ohio
Pathways employs a risk-reduction model incorporating evidence-based and best-practices intervention for high-risk individuals. Outreach includes support for the whole family. Home visits build trust in the community and better outcomes, which lead to performance-based payment to Community Health Workers to implement care coordination. Payment is tied to completed pathways.

Employer Health Savings Dividend

Dan Chase Executive Interview. Health Rosetta. Seattle, Washington
Health Rosetta principles apply to self-insurance models that reduce expense and improve outcomes based on financial precepts of employee retirement plans. Health Rosetta principles include open networks with no financial penalties, health profiles with individual preferences, incentives for advanced primary care, independent oversight of plan management, and transparent information on pharmacy

benefits. Spending is controlled with employee incentives to approved visits, value-based physicians, and specialists. The savings dividend can be used to address SDOH or return savings to participating employees.

Food as Medicine

Boston Medical Center Case Study. Boston, Massachusetts The first hospital to pioneer providing healthy food to medically underserved people with nutrition-related illnesses, distributing over one million pounds of food each year. Its three-pronged "food as medicine" model includes a preventive food pantry, rooftop farm, and a teaching kitchen. Food programs are aligned with specific chronic conditions.

Health Status Improvement

Geisinger Health Plan Case Study. Danville, Pennsylvania The health plan looked at Social Determinants of Health (e.g., diet and exercise) to understand why so little progress was made in treating type 2 diabetes. The Fresh Food Farmacy program was initiated to determine if "food as medicine" would impact type 2 diabetes treatment. Clinical results showed a decrease of 40 percent in the risk of death or serious complications. There was an 80 percent reduction in cost for pilot patients (yearly cost of $240,000 per member was decreased to $48,000 per member) with an average of $8,000-$12,000 for each percentage point reduction in patients' HbA1c level. Most patients also lost 10-50 pounds during the program.

Shared Medical Appointments

Elizabeth Bradley, MD and Michelle Beidelschies, PhD, Executive Interview. Cleveland Clinic. Cleveland, Ohio

Nutrition and lifestyle-based interventions incorporate exercise and movement, sleep, stress resilience, and social relationships to prevent and mitigate chronic disease. A shared medical appointments system was designed to provide better care through a small and more integrated multi-disciplinary team of caregivers. It provided more opportunities for interaction with team members and for patient education than individual appointments.

Culture of Health

Presbyterian Health Case Study. Albuquerque, New Mexico

The program integrates four beliefs: health as a shared value, cross-sector collaborations, stronger integration of health services and systems, and healthier more equitable communities. Community health interventions must be clearly stated, easy to read, and understood by patients and members. Interventions must promote equity to be sustainable.

Affordable Healthy Homes

Healthy Homes Des Moines Case Study. Des Moines, Iowa

The program changes substandard housing for children at risk for respiratory conditions such as asthma, allergies, and COPD. Home inspectors assess homes for asthma triggers like lead, allergens, and pests, and home repair is coordinated between health inspectors and contractors. Families receive household cleaning supplies, HEPA vacuum cleaners, and access to Community Health Workers and nurses specializing in asthma.

Healthy Neighborhoods

George Kleb Executive Interview. Bon Secours Baltimore Community Works. Baltimore, Maryland
Healthy neighborhoods are cocreated rather than focusing only on correcting illness conditions like diabetes, asthma, and cardiovascular and metabolic conditions. Up to 1 percent of its investment portfolio is committed to community sustainability initiatives for ten years. The focus is healthy housing, open spaces, early childhood education, safe streets, and employment opportunities. For each dollar invested, $1.30 to $1.99 accrues.

Value-Based Care

Houston Methodist Case Study. Houston, Texas
The Medicare Shared Savings Program, part of a broader strategy to prepare the organization for value-based care, aims to improve quality of care, reduce hospital admissions and readmissions, decrease post-acute facility and home health utilization, and lower total cost of care. Coordinated Care ACO admissions decreased 16 percent, all-cause thirty-day readmissions by 15 percent, and avoidable ER visits by 21 percent during COVID by implementing virtual visits.

Social Risk Screening Tools

Montefiore Medical Center Case Study. Bronx, New York

Social needs screening was implemented across twenty-one primary care locations to identify and match community services to impact patient and population health. The tool was available in eight languages and balanced the breadth of SDOH domains with brevity of questions for feasibility. Setting firm criteria up front drove consensus on choice of screening questions. Collecting the right data leads to solutions. Seventy-five percent of patients screened positive for one or more issues.

Health Literacy Screening

Vanderbilt University Medical Center Case Study. Nashville, Tennessee

A health literacy screening tool with three standard questions is administered to inpatients and outpatients. Increased literacy is associated with higher rates of preventative care, better disease control, and lower mortality rates. Twenty percent of hospital patients and 10 percent primary care patients have low health literacy. This provides a roadmap to address SDOH.

Innovation and Health Value Proposition

Ann Somers Hogg, MSPH, Executive Interview. Christensen Institute. Richmond, Virginia

Innovative business models that address drivers of health are most effective when paid through value-based arrangements like global capitation arrangements or partnerships with upside and downside risk. Atrium Health aligned social impact goals to existing success measures in preparation for value-based payment. Advocate Aurora invested in consumer health and wellness programs as a diversified revenue stream that required an asset-light approach. The Health Impact Index tracks performance of participating portfolio companies.

Root Cause System-Level Change

Essentia Health Case Study. Duluth, Minnesota

The organization is working to develop community partnerships to further care transformation. By working across multiple levels of impact—individual, organizational, and community—Essentia Health is analyzing the broader context around poverty and inequity in the community. The focus is on identifying root causes and resource gaps, along with improving communication and coordination among services and resource providers.

Cultural Health Navigation

University Hospital Case Study. Kansas City, Missouri

Cultural Health Navigators are a hybrid of Medical Interpreter and Community Health Workers that bridge the cultural and language barriers of immigrant populations and assist with navigating the healthcare system. They address social needs and connect patients with primary and specialty care, secure insurance and financial aid, and convey the patient "voice" to hospital administrators and medical personnel in the system.

Provider Contract Incentives

Blue Cross Blue Shield of Massachusetts Case Study. Boston, Massachusetts

The company's corporate citizenship mission is focused on eliminating physical and social barriers to health equity. This requires implementing sustainable strategies on three drivers of inequity: food justice, environmental justice, and racial justice. This rests on linking financial incentives in provider contracts to improving racial inequalities in care. The Foundation is addressing measurable change on behalf of residents, community organizations, and providers.

Healthy Living Investment

Blue Cross Blue Shield of Massachusetts Consumer Health Research Case Study. Boston, Massachusetts

Focus groups of customers were conducted to better understand the challenges employees face trying to keep healthy. The most pervasive issue was the extent of "surprise costs" and navigating the healthcare system. Employees did not understand why out-of-pocket expenses were so high, what to do about it, and who to turn to. The next most important issue was cultural: how to find a "comfortable" physician who listens well and accepts new patients.

Managed Regulation Threat

Robert Galvin, MD, Executive Interview. Blackstone Senior Advisor. Fairfield, Connecticut

Some form of managed regulation may be necessary at the federal and state level to deal with the magnitude of health expenditures within the decade, including the bolus of life sciences breakthroughs coming through the system. Furthermore, the "quality industrial complex" has too little to show in the way of inpatient hospital improvement or metrics that patients and providers find useful. Quality terminology and mandates are too confusing. It is time for an overhaul and to begin again with a clean slate about what constitutes quality and how to measure it.

Tobacco Cessation and Prevention Strategy

Blue Cross Blue Shield of Minnesota Case Study. Saint Paul, Minnesota

The mission of the Center for Prevention is to transform communities by increasing access to healthy, affordable, culturally relevant food and to eliminate the use of commercial tobacco. The health plan's approach to population management focuses on clinical issues such as poverty and environmental factors to impact wellness and improve health status. The Fresh Food Farmacy was initiated to determine if "food as medicine" would impact type 2 diabetes treatment.

Social Sector Partnerships

Blue Cross and Blue Shield of North Carolina Case Study. Durham, North Carolina

More than half the population has an unmet need relating to social, economic, or environmental factors. Food insecurity is the most reported unmet social need. Multi-sector health partnerships are needed to sufficiently scale "upstream" health-related interventions in underserved communities. Training under-represented health professionals is critical to addressing gaps in rural healthcare.

Individual-Level Social Risk Factors

Trenor Williams, MD, Executive Interview. Socially Determined. Washington, DC

Health plans want to know what social risk looks like for every individual at a member level combined with traditional healthcare data—disease, cost, utilization, and quality measurement data. With this information, they can integrate social risk data and identify cohorts of individuals who share specific characteristics (e.g., diabetes, financial strain, transportation barriers). After identifying groups of individuals who share certain clinical and social characteristics, health plans can design and deploy focused interventions to better address them.

Elder Chronic Care Prevention

Francesca Rinaldo, MD, Executive Interview. SCAN Health Plan. Long Beach, California

SCAN's mission is to keep seniors healthy and independent, which serves as an ethical foundation to address and solve problems. The goal is to create services that fill the gaps in care across the healthcare value chain. The health plan's benefit design and clinical interventions are designed to prevent disease. Financial incentives focus on preventive care because upfront interventions mean fewer expensive and unnecessary acute care services, like emergency department trips or extended hospital stays.

Holistic Outcomes Approach

UPMC Health Plan Case Study. Pittsburgh, Pennsylvania

The Center for Social Impact addresses initiatives on Social Determinants of Health well beyond utilization and costs. They should align with corporate and social responsibility, enhance charitable giving, and show how health-related social needs are impacted. These factors guide business and investment opportunities. Initiatives focus on employment and workforce development, housing, homelessness, food insecurity, intellectual disabilities and autism, STEM programs, behavioral health, social isolation and dementia, LGBTQ+, gun violence, health equity regarding cancer and other chronic diseases, and access to care.

Patient Feedback-Based Solutions

Women, Infants and Children Program Case Study. New York, New York

First person feedback is far more insightful and persuasive than ordinary enrollment trend information. Hospital leaders are far more receptive to data on what is occurring on the ground than reports from program directors detached from what is happening to patients and CHWs in the community. State administrators are similarly persuaded by first-person accounts and recommendations on practical ways to improve enrollment data. The combination of qualitative data from first person feedback, alongside more quantitative data, provides a level of detail and insight required for effective program administration.

Asset-Based Development

The BUILD Health Challenge: San Pablo Area Development Collaborative Case Study. Oakland, California

Involvement of 500 community leaders was the core asset to mobilize for improving health status of local residents. The area-wide initiative, anchored by a transportation corridor, focused on social, environmental, and economic factors that most influence health. The project implemented four main priorities: preserving culture, centering community power and voice, collaboration across sectors, and affordable housing.

Trust-Based Philanthropy

Hawaii Community Foundation Case Study. Honolulu, Hawai

As the steward of more than 1,000 funds, the Foundation listened to community feedback on the first year of the CHANGE grantmaking program. The CHANGE framework covered six sectors: Community and Economy, Health and Wellness, Arts and Culture, Natural Environment, Government and Civics, and Education. Constructive feedback from the community led to designing a new approach that builds more equitable relationships with nonprofits through multi-year, unrestricted funding that gives flexibility and freedom to nonprofits to carry out their missions in the best way. Paperwork is simplified to reduce time and labor burden with only four questions asked. More capacity is thereby developed to effectively address complex local and state challenges.

Peer Counseling Digital Support

Boaz Goan Executive Interview. Wisdo Health. New York, New York

Wisdo Health addresses the impact of loneliness, social isolation, and other drivers of mental health on medical costs and employee engagement. Employers spend $14 billion a year on additional workdays lost to loneliness. The peer support platform methodology reduces inpatient and ER visits, decreases costs to the mental health system, and improves quality of life for members. Providing connection with people who have similar lived experiences ("been in one's shoes") as health plan members is the key.

Additional full length Executive Interviews are featured in the companion publication *More Health. Less Healthcare: Doing the Right Thing for the Right Reason at the Right Price* (2026).

Disparities and Inequality Dashboard

Maulik Joshi, DrPH, Executive Interview. Meritus Health. Annapolis, Maryland

Leadership in Equity and Disparities Council's six goals are each measured by decreased disparities in care outcomes, increased diversity of leadership and workforce, increased staff awareness and knowledge of multicultural and observances, improved staff level comfort with asking about racial differences, and measure community perception of diversity.

Accountability and Moral Hazard

Mark Smith, MD, Executive Interview. Clinical Professor of Medicine, UCSF. Oakland, California

Sooner or later, healthcare leaders will face difficult decisions they have to make—to their business models and income expectations—no matter how reluctantly. It will be preferable to price setting and regulation. That is what they court by continuing to resist the inevitable. Furthermore, in our desire to inject social determinates of health into healthcare, we might give health systems a role in deciding access to those scarce resources—not based on some publicly agreed-upon criteria but based on what serves the health system best.

Introduction

Health Equity: A Mandate for Change and Better Health for All

In the United States and around the world, discussions of health focus on access to medical care, new advances in treatment, and cost. Yet abundant evidence confirms that our health is shaped far more by where we live, our financial security, the communities that surround us, and countless policies that sit upstream of the clinic. In short, social, economic, and environmental factors account for the majority of health outcomes—while clinical care alone addresses only a fraction of what really determines a person's well-being.

Despite decades of research and reform, glaring health inequities persist. Race, ethnicity, income, education, and geography continue to predict the burden of chronic disease, the likelihood of surviving health crises, and life expectancy. The COVID-19 pandemic exposed and intensified these inequities, but they were with us long before—and will remain unless systems change at scale.

A Growing Movement for Solutions

In recent years, health systems, payers, community organizers, and bold leaders across the country have stepped forward to ask: What can we do differently? Can hospitals, health plans, and community-based organizations work beyond their traditional boundaries? Are there models for sustainable, measurable progress in health equity that other regions, clinicians, and policymakers can adopt?

The Health Equity Case Studies Handbook is a response to this urgent need for practical, proven answers. Across more than twenty chapters, this handbook spotlights organizations, delivery systems, health plans, and community partnerships pioneering new approaches to bridge the chasm between what is—and what should be.

From Theory to Transformation—Stories That Lead the Way

The chapters that follow are grounded in experience. Each case study confronts complex local disparities and offers designed, implemented, and measured programs that make a tangible difference. Some stories show how healthcare providers can integrate social determinants into routine care and close resource gaps for vulnerable populations. Others highlight partnerships between hospitals and civic leaders that invest in affordable housing, expand career pathways, stabilize neighborhoods, and support families for decades, not just months.

You will find models for:

- Screening and addressing food insecurity and housing instability as integral parts of care
- Building comprehensive community wellness initiatives beyond the hospital's four walls
- Financing and scaling programs to ensure long-term sustainability
- Centering patient and community voices to design relevant, inclusive solutions
- Measuring what works—not just by clinical metrics, but by gains in empowerment, self-sufficiency, and opportunity

Why Case Studies?

There is no single template for achieving health equity. Context matters—rural or urban, large system or community clinic, local economic and political realities, historical trauma, and local assets. By presenting the how and why behind each initiative—successes, barriers, pivots, and lessons learned—this handbook empowers readers to both replicate and adapt proven strategies for their own communities.

Who Is This For?

This book is intended for a wide audience:

- Healthcare leaders seeking to make the business case for social health investments

- Community organizations hoping to scale impact or partner with larger institutions
- Clinicians who want to equip themselves and their teams with upstream solutions
- Policymakers and payers building accountability for equity into measurement, payment, and policy
- Researchers and students exploring the cutting edge of population health
- Funders and social impact investors seeking systemic, measurable returns on equity initiatives

How This Book Is Organized

Each chapter presents a stand-alone case, with a consistent structure: background and context, problem definition, program design and partnerships, implementation challenges and success factors, key results and metrics, sustainability and business case, and lessons learned. Select chapters feature executive interviews, commentary, and practical tools such as screening questions, sample workflows, and evaluation frameworks.

At the close of each section, "Key Takeaways" capture actionable insights—distilled advice for leaders and changemakers striving toward health equity in their own context.

A Call to Leadership and Action

If there is one central lesson across all these stories, it is this: Achieving health equity requires more than goodwill or one-time grants. It requires leadership, sustained investment, courageous partnerships, rigorous data, a willingness to learn and adapt, and a relentless focus on the systems and policies that shape opportunity.

Change is hard, but the collective wisdom and innovations shared in these pages offer both a roadmap and encouragement for the journey ahead.

The Health Equity Case Studies Handbook sparks new conversations, deeper collaborations, and bold action—so that every person and community, regardless of zip code or background, has a fair and just chance at a healthy, thriving life.

Peter Boland

Delivery Systems

Chapter 1

Boston Medical Center Case Study and Executive Interview

Introduction

Boston Medical Center is the principal teaching affiliate of Boston University School of Medicine and the largest safety net hospital in New England. More than half its patients come from underserved populations such as low-income and elderly. More than 32 percent of patients do not speak English as a primary language. Medical care and services are offered in more than 250 languages.

Boston Medical Center Health System is a $6 billion integrated healthcare system with 880 physicians and 1,756 nurses. It provides dozens of social health-related services and invests in underserved communities in Greater Boston.

Initiatives

Food

The medical center was the first hospital in the country to provide healthy food to medically underserved people with nutrition-related illnesses, most often due to poverty and living in urban food deserts. More than one million pounds of food is distributed every year. Three healthy food programs make up a three-pronged "food as medicine" model: preventive food pantry, rooftop farm, and the teaching kitchen.

Preventive Food Pantry was begun in 2001 to address nutrition-related illness for low-income patients. Boston Medical Center had been providing food to families long before that unofficially. Desperate to help her food insecure patients, BMC pediatrician and founder of the pediatric Grow Clinic, Dr. Deborah Frank started the "food pantry" from her desk drawer, keeping a stash of canned vegetables on hand for young families who needed it most. Over time, this operation grew and developed into the hospital-wide food pantry.

The pantry fills a therapeutic gap by linking physicians and nutritionists to patients. Primary care providers screen patients and then write prescriptions for supplemental food to promote recovery and better health. Culinary medicine incorporates food and nutrition to prevent and treat diseases.

Patients can visit the food pantry every two weeks and receive four days' worth of food for their household, up to twice a month. Each month, thousands of patients and their families use the program, half of whom are children. The pantry manager is a registered dietetic technician who determines what food corresponds to a patient's dietary needs as prescribed by the physician. The pantry is most often frequented by patients with chronic conditions such as cancer, HIV/AIDS, hypertension, diabetes, and heart disease. Staff are fluent in four languages to assist refugee and immigrant patients.

Outpatient Adult Nutrition

Counseling with a Registered Dietitian Nutritionist for adult patients is available for a variety of nutrition and medical problems, including:

- Cancer
- Diabetes
- Food Allergies/Intolerances
- Gastrointestinal Disorders
- Healthy Eating/Wellness
- Heart Disease
- HIV/AIDS
- Home Tube Feeds
- Malnutrition
- Pregnancy
- Renal Disease/Transplant
- Sports Nutrition
- Vegetarian/Vegan Diets
- Weight Management

Counseling with a registered dietitian nutritionist for pediatric and adolescent patients is likewise available for a variety of nutrition and medical problems, including:

- Diabetes/Endocrine
- Failure to Thrive
- Food Allergies/Intolerances
- Formula
- Gastrointestinal Disorders
- Healthy Eating
- Ketogenic Diet
- Malnutrition
- Picky Eating/ARFID
- Preventive Cardiology
- Tube Feeds
- Vegetarian/Vegan Diets
- Weight Management
- Outpatient Pediatric Nutrition

Specialized pediatric nutrition clinics include:

- Grow Clinic for poor growth
- Nutrition and Fitness for Life Program for obesity treatment
- Feeding Team Clinic for feeding difficulties

Boston Medical Center also offers community-based nutritional classes with a different focus each month such as cooking for picky eaters, and recovery from substance abuse disorders. First-year medical students can attend cooking and nutrition classes and virtual classes on how to communicate with patients about nutrition while considering cultural and socioeconomic diet factors.

Rooftop Farm is 2,700 square feet of plantable space on top of the medical center's power plant. It produces 5,000-7,000 pounds of healthy vegetables each year (twenty-five varieties), which are then transported to the Preventive Food Pantry, used as ingredients for inpatient hospital trays, and in medical center cafeterias. The farm's resident bees help the produce pollinate while providing local honey. The rooftop farm reduced carbon emissions by 50 percent and, with the addition of a solar farm, Boston Medical Center is now among the greenest hospitals in the country.

Teaching Kitchen allows patients to prepare healthy meals at a low cost. Three hundred classes a year are free for more than 2,000 patients and staff, and open daily for drop-in sessions and recipes. Classes serve individuals at community centers like Boston Healthcare for the Homeless and the substance use treatment Hope House. Classes are dedicated to patients with specific medical diagnoses.

The Teaching Kitchen's focus is on incorporating dietary recommendations with medical interventions in hospital clinics. For example, the bariatric weight loss surgery class is a required step before the clinical portion. Quarterly intensive interventions are provided to pregnant women with diabetes. Monthly classes for kids with barriers to eating are led by a multidisciplinary team, including a speech pathologist, psychologist, and a dietitian.

Cultural awareness is addressed in all areas of the program. Patients can exchange certain items for alternatives at the Food Pantry to support autonomy over what patients bring home based on what they are most comfortable with. The same choice is provided by the Teaching Kitchen with recipes, allowing patients to have a choice in what they prepare.

"We support choices that relate to a patient's culture as well as choices that reflect socioeconomic backgrounds. We don't always know what's affordable to most families, so we try to be extremely conscious of that," explains Olivia Weinstein, RD, the Culinary Nutrition Director.

Participants learn about healthy meal preparation and how to make sustainable nutritional changes in diet. All the food is sourced from the Food Pantry and Rooftop Garden Farm.

Online classes cover cancer and sickle cell support, bariatric surgery preparation, employee wellness (including recipes from parts of the world with the largest number of centennials), and kids' kitchen, which includes how to make healthy meals and snacks.

Social Determinants

Boston Medical Center is also where numerous other social determinants-related activities began. Many of these efforts are highlighted below.

Screening

A Social Determinants of Health screener was developed for primary care patients to better identify and address patients' unmet social needs. Clinician researchers developed an electronic health record-based model (THRIVE) that facilitates an automatic print-out of referral information for resources based at the hospital and in the community when the patient asks for help with a need identified in the screener.

The one-page screener, available in six languages, is filled out in the waiting room prior to an appointment. Patients are asked to answer questions related to eight Social Determinants of Health domains: homelessness and housing insecurity, food insecurity, inability to afford medications, lack of transportation to medical appointments, utilities, caregiving, unemployment, and educational aspirations. It also asked patients if they wanted assistance with any of the needs identified on the THRIVE screening tool.

Responses are then entered into the patient's EHR by a medical assistant. When a patient requests assistance with an unmet need, referral guides are automatically printed with information about resources available to them both at BMC and in the community. The EHR also prompts the provider to address any issues raised by the patient in the screener during the visit.

During the initial study period in 2017, which involved 1,696 patients, 26 percent responded positively to one or more social needs: employment was 12 percent, food insecurity 11 percent, and medication affordability 11 percent.

BMC now screens all patients with THRIVE in all ambulatory primary care clinics, including family medicine, pediatrics, obstetrics and gynecology, and general internal medicine. Twenty-eight percent report having at least one need and 19 percent request help with at least one need. Housing, food, and education are the most prevalent health-related social needs of BMC patients.

Children's HealthWatch

Children's HealthWatch was founded in 1998 by Dr. Deborah Frank and pediatric colleagues to develop research and analysis on child health and development. This included the impact of economic hardship on food insecurity and poor nutrition, unstable housing, and inability to afford adequate household energy. It draws upon a network of pediatricians, public health researchers, and child health experts in Boston, Baltimore, Philadelphia, Minneapolis, and Little Rock. The goal is to inform policies that alleviate economic hardship, promote health among families with young children, and advance healthy equity.

As an example of applied research, Children's Health Watch led a study of the Housing Prescription as Health program, which helped 736 families experiencing homelessness and housing instability in Boston during 2016-2019. The randomized trial showed that coordination of services that address housing, financial, legal, social, and health needs improves health outcomes when compared with siloed approaches. The intervention reduced the share of children with fair or poor health by 32 percent in the first six months of the study.

Children's Health Watch research focuses on five inter-related areas:

- **Nutritional Assistance:** Food and nutrition assistance programs are a cornerstone of health for low-income families.
- **Affordable Housing:** Affordable housing options support healthy child development, which means not falling behind on rent, doubling up in over-crowded units, or moving frequently.
- **Energy Assistance:** Healthy child development includes consistent utility services with adequate heat in winter and cooling in summer.
- **Healthcare Access:** Families with special-need children often require financial support to pay medical bills and to fill prescriptions, as well as basic living needs such as food, rent, childcare, and utility bills.
- **Anti-Poverty Policies:** Economic hardships for families with young children require program assistance (and policy solutions) that address under-nutrition, affordable housing, utility and energy shutoffs.

Each of these topics is the subject of ongoing interdisciplinary research at Children's HealthWatch.

Additional initiatives that support child health are profiled below.

Medical Legal Partnership (MLP) ensures basic patients' needs for vulnerable populations such as children, elderly, patients with cancer, pregnant women, and formerly incarcerated individuals. The program integrates legal expertise with clinicians and social workers to address structural problems at the root of health inequities. The services result in fewer hospital admissions, higher medical adherence, and reduced stress levels.

Elders Living at Home (ELAP) has addressed homelessness for twenty-five years, affecting the lives of 2,500 people. Since 2012, ELAP has provided intensive case management to older adults at imminent risk of losing housing and becoming homeless. Ninety percent of clients have been able to retain their housing in conjunction with the assistance of MLP staff.

Financial Wellness program helps people apply for health coverage, access low cost or no-cost medications, obtain food and groceries, pay utility bills, file tax returns, and secure refunds. These interventions reduce financial stress and toxic stress, which impact physical and emotional health for children and adults in impoverished situations.

Patient Financial Assistance is provided to low-income uninsured patients with incomes up to 300 percent of the federal poverty level.

StreetCred was established to offer free tax assistance to families receiving pediatric care at the medical center. The objective is to improve family health status through poverty reduction and achieving greater financial stability. IRS-certified tax preparers help patients apply for tax credits and maximize refunds. Since 2016, more than $8.3 million has been returned to more than 2,700 families. The service has expanded to include financial coaching and enrollment in 529 college savings accounts, which the state funds with fifty dollars if opened during the first year of life.

HIV Drug Assistance is a comprehensive program for people living with HIV and without access to HIV-related medications or health insurance. More than half of enrollees come from communities of color, and three-quarters have incomes less than 200 percent of the federal poverty level ($12,760).

Violence Intervention Advocacy Program (VIAP) was founded in 2006 and provides specialized services to victims of violence, using two Violence Intervention Advocates (Community Health Workers) who provide counseling, triage, and referral services for victims of violence brought to BMC Emergency Department. VIAP provides services to more than 400 victims a year, with a nearly equal number of gunshot and stabbing victims. VIAP provides victims and their families with direct services and referrals to outside services, including crisis intervention and stabilization, housing and transportation, legal assistance, education, vocational and life skills development, mental health, employment, and health and wellness. VIAP model has been disseminated to two other hospitals in Massachusetts.

Project ASSERT (Alcohol & Substance Abuse Services, Education, and Referral to Treatment) was established in 1998, and has been an ongoing component of safety-net services in BMC's Emergency Department. As members of the ASSERT team, Health Promotion Advocates consult and collaborate with hospital staff to offer ED patients alcohol and drug screening, brief intervention, and referrals to health and social resources such as substance abuse treatment and primary care services.

Project ASSERT also educates patients at risk for opioid overdoses and distributes more than 2,000 naloxone rescue kits to ED patients, family, and friends each year. ASSERT has more than 4,000 ED and 225 inpatient consults annually. Twelve hundred patients receive referrals each year to outpatient Narcotics Anonymous/Alcoholics Anonymous, behavioral health services, and shelters annually. More than 200 patients receive a primary care appointment through the project every year.

Immigration status affects a host of factors for patients in need of housing, legal services, social work, primary care, perinatal care, behavioral health, and chronic stress. Boston Medical Center addresses the social and medical needs of immigrants, refugees, and asylum seekers in its specialty clinics with multilingual staff (Spanish, French, Haitian, and Creole).

Clinical and social health services are coordinated through the hospital's Immigrant and Refugee Health Center, which functions as a single point of entry for medical, mental health, and social services for patients arriving from more than twenty countries.

Boston Center for Refugee Health and Human Rights offers comprehensive outpatient care, social services, and legal referrals to 375 individuals from more than forty countries in thirty languages each year. Whole person care is stressed in a culturally sensitive environment that recognizes many patients have survived torture and related trauma.

Affordable housing was supported by a three-year $5 million award from Morgan Stanley to pay for occupational support services for 1,000 people in Mattapan, Dorchester, and Roxbury.

The goal is funding living-wage jobs for 500 people, including at hospitals and biotech companies, while creating 100 affordable housing units.

Child Witness to Violence Project is a therapeutic, advocacy, and outreach effort that focuses on children who are hidden victims of domestic and community violence and other trauma-related events. The project involves identifying young children who witness acts of significant violence and providing developmentally appropriate counseling for them and their families.

Additional programs for children and families include:

- Kids Fund targets basic emergency needs like a mattress or specialty baby formula for malnutrition.
- Baby Steps provides developmental evaluation and nutritional assessments for children leaving the hospital.
- Child Life Program helps families manage stresses associated with hospitalization and focuses on children's individual developmental and emotional needs.
- Community Violence Response Team provides case management and individual and family counseling to survivors of violence and family members impacted by violence at no cost.
- Good Grief Program trains adult professionals to support families and children under stress with coping skills to better manage the impact of an illness, a difficult diagnosis, death, and divorce.
- Grow Clinic is dedicated to families with failure-to-

thrive infants and children. Social workers are available to visit with parents wherever the patient is fed, including day care and school.

- Helmet Program works in collaboration with city agencies to provide low-cost helmets to patients and anyone in Boston.
- Nutrition and Fitness for Life supports children and families dealing with obesity through community-centered obesity prevention and treatment.
- SPARK Center helps Boston's highest-risk children with therapeutic, medically specialized programs for children of all ages.
- Vital Village Network, established by Dr. Renee Boyton-Jarrett, facilitates collaborative learning and leadership opportunities among residents and communities with an emphasis on enhancing families and communities to prevent and mitigate adversities.
- Windows Falls Prevention is an injury prevention program that supplements the city's "Kids Can't Fly" campaign. It provides education on window safety and provides home inspections through the injury prevention program at Boston Medical Center.

Health Equity

Health Equity Rounds is a longitudinal, case-based conference series and curriculum. It was developed by pediatric trainees to address how implicit bias, race, and structural racism factor into healthcare.

The program is based on the belief that medical education has the power to improve health equity. Participants are encouraged to be change agents in their communities.

Summary

Boston Medical Center is committed to promoting a wide range of Social Determinants of Health programs and initiatives in underserved neighborhoods. Its early focus on food insecurity and children's health-related research has been a hallmark for decades.

Key Takeaways

- Food and nutrition are central to the health of low-income families (food as medicine).
- Food programs should be closely aligned with clinical diagnoses of patients.
- Financial wellness counseling reduces stress, which impacts physical and emotional health in impoverished situations.
- Sustainable livelihoods are required to break generational cycles of poverty and poor health.
- Anchor institutions like hospitals must support community-led decision-making and power sharing.

Executive Comments

Megan Sandel, MD, MPH, is a pediatrician at Boston Medical Center and the Principal Investigator for The Boston Opportunity System (BOS) Collaborative.

Institutions need to change, not people.

What is the approach and focus of BOS?

The BOS Collaborative is a partnership between the City of Boston, large city hospitals, including BMC, Boston Children's Hospital, Brigham and Women's Hospital, and community organizations Dudley Street Neighborhood Initiatives and Jewish Vocational Services. An initial investment of $5 million was made by JP Morgan Advancing Cities Grant.

It's a community-driven approach to open pathways to employment and affordable housing options in historically disinvested communities.

The focus is the Fairmont Corridor, a rail line running through Dorchester, Mattapan, and Hyde Park where half the households earn less than $40,000 a year. That's way below the Boston median income of $74,000. The poverty in these neighborhoods is a direct result of generations of disinvestment and historical trauma.

What is the clinical rationale for this initiative?

Our doctors are used to treating illnesses caused by living in low-income ZIP codes like these. Respiratory attacks are triggered by inadequate housing. Obesity results from a lack of fresh food options. Crippling depression comes from the stress of raising a family on minimum wage with no chance of earning more. These factors aren't related to a person's biology, but they severely impact health trajectories and life expectancy—and perpetuate a generational cycle of poverty and poor health.

Current programs and subsidies are only designed to fill gaps temporarily rather than advance families toward sustainable livelihoods. To move toward sustainable advancements in health equity, health systems must address the disinvestment in communities of color and work to change systems that make economic opportunities, including living wage jobs, inaccessible for so many.

What is the relationship between inequity and where people live?

Place is where we concentrate inequity in this country. It's places and neighborhoods where systems don't work and where policies perpetuate inequity. Place-based investing, place-based hiring, and place-based small business procurement is a part of our healthcare anchor mission.

We must undo decades of racism in these zip codes to get there.

What is BOS's main goal?

The Collaborative's goal is to radically reinvent the city's job ecosystem by supporting people interested in new opportunities through skills training and hiring procedures, ultimately helping launch them into new careers within the city's anchor institutions. Much of the work is offering holistic support so people can stay healthy and thrive in their new roles.

When people begin to earn money, they hit a ceiling when they are no longer eligible for government programs like SNAP, childcare subsidies, or housing subsidies.

We need to tear down these barriers so people can be successful at every stage in the process.

What is the business opportunity presented by BOS?

The Collaborative is focused on identifying recession-proof career paths that span the city's major industries, including banking, life sciences, tech, and healthcare. This is a huge opportunity for such companies to say "yes" to the communities they have made to hire people of color.

The Collaborative's initial aim is to fill 500 jobs at a family-sustaining wage. We're working on recruiting candidates from these neighborhoods to be trained quickly and hired into the career pipelines that anchor institutions and downtown businesses offer. Jewish Vocational Services is providing the necessary training for many roles and connecting participants across job pipeline programs. Dudley Street Neighborhood Initiative is leveraging

$1 million into more creative investment strategies for tangible neighborhood revitalization.

Will anchor institutions continue to lead this effort?

Our role is to help catalyze this collaborative effort in conjunction with partners. Anchor institutions can wield influence to create change, yet also lean back and let the community lead the way.

It's the institutions that need to change, not people. Community needs to lead. That's the Collaborative's theory of change we try to live every single day.

Chapter 2.

Nationwide Children's Hospital Case

Introduction

Nationwide Children's Hospital is an academic medical center in Columbus with more than 1.6 million patient visits a year and nearly 20,000 inpatient discharges. Nationwide Children's also is affiliated with a pediatric accountable care organization, Partners for Kids®, and carries full financial risk for more than 470,000 children enrolled in Medicaid.

More than fifteen years ago, Columbus' South Side neighborhood, located adjacent to the main campus of Nationwide Children's Hospital, faced many challenges, such as high foreclosure and vacancy rates, along with poor health outcomes.

There was no single intervention that would break the intergenerational cycle of poverty and discrimination. A comprehensive program was called for with a long-term commitment. Otherwise, poverty, lack of education, and employment opportunity would continue to be insurmountable barriers to improving individual and neighborhood health.

If a family could not afford to buy nutritious food and lacked transportation to sources of healthy and affordable food, then the child's health would suffer—even with a large children's hospital in its backyard.

"Nationwide Children's Hospital's goal is to care for children," said Nick Jones, Nationwide Children's Hospital vice president of community wellness. "We know that children's mental and physical health is impacted by their environment. We believe that a zip code should not determine health outcomes. That is why our work must extend beyond the hospital walls into the places where children work, live, and play."

At that time, Nationwide Children's hospital leaders set out to revitalize the neighborhood by joining with a faith-based organization, Community Development for all People (CD4AP), the city of Columbus, community members, and other partners. In 2008, the hospital's Healthy Neighborhoods Healthy Families initiative launched. The initiative targets five impact areas: affordable housing, education, health and wellness, community enrichment, and economic development.

The first goal was to transform three census tracts into a mixed income community through its affordable housing prong. Neighborhood stabilization and neighborhood-level health improvement was the objective. The hospital thought of the entire neighborhood surrounding it as "the patient" and its goal was to treat it holistically. As Rev. John Edgar, previous executive director and pastor emeritus of CD4AP, noted: "It's impactful when the neighborhood itself is viewed as a patient, so the neighborhood can become healthier. Housing is an essential place to begin."

Strategic Focus

The hospital began with housing because a stable, quality home is fundamental to health. Poor housing quality and inadequate conditions—such as the presence of lead, mold, or asbestos, poor air quality, and overcrowding—can contribute to negative health outcomes, including chronic disease and injury, according to the U.S. Department of Health and Human Services Office of Disease Prevention and Health Promotion. Poor housing can expose children to toxins such as mold and lead. The neighborhoods around the hospital are resilient, but many were continuing to deal with the long-term impact of eighty years of redlining, racism, and disinvestment.

Community members also identified housing as a high priority. Nationwide Children's wanted the community to know that it was financially committed to removing barriers to better health, economic opportunity, and educational readiness for children from low-income families. Focusing on families and housing were the visible symbol of this commitment.

Nationwide Children's and CD4AP formed a subsidiary non-profit called Healthy Neighborhoods Healthy Families Realty Collaborative, now called Healthy Homes, owned by CD4AP. Healthy Homes is the affordable housing arm of Healthy Neighborhoods Healthy Families.

Since beginning the Healthy Neighborhoods Healthy Families initiative, the hospital has partnered with the city and community organizations. Since 2008, it has invested $77 million to build 244 affordable rental units, repair 236 homes, and build or renovate 110 new ones on the South Side. This work has focused on three census tracts on the South Side.

By 2015, the neighborhood had become far more desirable and, as a result, higher home values and rents were displacing some homeowners and renters. CD4AP brought together forty community leaders to figure out how South Side could be preserved as a mixed-income community. Many residents were paying more than 50 percent of their income for housing and utilities. A South Side Housing strategy was formed to develop more affordable housing for people with incomes below 80 percent of AMI.

A $15 million loan fund was established for acquisition and construction costs and permanent financing for the majority of the rental units scattered throughout the three census tracts. A loan loss protection guarantee equals 10 percent of the total fund and a blended annual interest rate is set at 3 percent. An annual payment on the principal is 95 percent of the net remaining income once all the expenses (e.g., interest payment on the loan, maintenance, insurance, taxes, capital repair reserve) have been paid in full.

Nationwide Children's and CD4AP secured financing for all rental units to remain affordable. Various partners have raised grant funds to cover 25 percent or more of the development cost for each unit. A number of national and local leaders joined together to make this happen, including J.P. Morgan Chase, the City of Columbus, United Way, Columbus Realtors Foundation, Central Ohio Community Improvement Corporation, and individual donors.

Neighborhood Health Impact

This initiative shows that developing affordable housing, when integrated with education, health resources, workforce development, community safety, and building strong partnerships, can be a catalyst for transforming distressed neighborhoods.

There was a modest reduction in hospital use by children in the targeted zip codes between August 2008 to July 2018 and August 2015 to July 2017. When matched with comparable neighborhoods, the rate of emergency department visits decreased 20.8 percent compared to 16.1 percent the year before. Inpatient admissions decreased by 12.7 percent compared to 12.2 percent the year before. The average length of stay increased 28.9 percent compared to 36.6 percent in the comparison census tracts.

Large-scale changes in neighborhood health outcomes were not expected because broad-based improvements in residential neighborhoods have an indirect impact on healthcare use. The health status of neighborhoods, especially low-income ones, is affected by the cumulative effects of childhood toxic stress, epigenetic changes, and adverse childhood experiences that show up later in life.

From 2008 through 2017, $22.3 million was invested in the three census tracts through the Healthy Homes program: $6.7 million from Nationwide Children's, $5.4 million from the city of Columbus, $1.8 million from United Way of Central Ohio, $7.9 million through home sales, $420,000 from Franklin County Land Bank, and $220,000 from donations.

These high visibility investments signaled the hospital was a good neighbor and committed to making a difference. Buying and renovating residences for individuals and families with low incomes benefits the South Side. The hospital safeguards residents from encroaching gentrification and protects its bond rating and assets from devaluation.

The hospital also worked to become a better neighborhood and built stronger connections in the community as part of this work. In the 1990s, as the hospital grew, community members watched the hospital's construction without receiving clear communication about the hospital's growth plans. Years of relationship building and two-way conversations have made it clear to surrounding neighborhoods that Nationwide Children's is committed to improving and sustaining the entire South Side community.

In addition to community development programs on housing, Healthy Neighborhoods Healthy Families helped launch the Residences at Career Gateway. The project combines fourteen townhouses, forty-four multifamily apartments, and a career development training center. All units are available to individuals with incomes 60 percent below AMI. The project's $12 million development costs was financed through low-income housing tax credit equity.

The economic development prong of Healthy Neighborhoods Healthy Families was a natural extension of investing in sustainable neighborhoods. The hospital realized that to create sustainable housing long-term, it would need to make sure that residents had adequate training and stable employment.

The hospital offers free work readiness training and coaching for residents through monthly classes. The classes prepare residents for interviews and potential careers at Nationwide Children's starting at eighteen dollars an hour. In addition, Nationwide Children's has expanded youth programs to offer summer work experiences and opportunities throughout the school year to introduce youth to careers in healthcare.

Financial Risk

Partners For Kids is an accountable care organization responsible for 470,000 children enrolled in Medicaid in the central, west and southeastern Ohio region that is affiliated with Nationwide Children's Hospital. Partners For Kids is paid on a capitated basis for providing whatever care is necessary each year for enrollees. When children covered under full-risk contracts stay healthy, the hospital saves money.

In this role, Nationwide Children's Hospital and Partners For Kids carry the responsibility for the clinical and financial outcomes for the children under risk contracts. To improve outcomes in a financially sustainable manner, Nationwide Children's invested both upstream and downstream in activities that addressed Social Determinants of Health. This required adding a layer of intervention beyond individual patients to a geographically defined population as well. Care coordination and other support programs were initiated to serve individual patients with challenging clinical and social needs.

Recognizing downstream clinical outcomes would present an ongoing challenge without addressing the upstream nonclinical needs of patients, they began funding upstream initiatives. The financial risk the hospital held became part of the business case for addressing social determinants.

As an example, addressing the social causes of premature births would lower infant mortality rates, thus reducing the cost burden on the hospital while benefiting the community.

A long-term funding strategy was developed to support Nationwide Children's and Partners For Kids initiatives based on three principles:

1. Will it help to make children healthier?
2. Does it match the strategic plan?
3. Is it financially sustainable?

The hospital also worked to make a shift in how impact was measured. Working with partners, Nationwide Children's co-developed ten-year goals to measure and improve the health of every child in Franklin County, not just in the Healthy Neighborhoods Healthy Families area: Pediatric Vital Signs. It uses eight metrics to measure the well-being of all children in the county and then leverages that information to improve overall outcomes. The measures include:

- Infant mortality
- Kindergarten readiness
- High school graduation

- Obesity
- Teenage pregnancy
- Suicide
- All-cause child mortality
- A hybrid measure called preventive services delivery

Comprehensive Initiatives

In addition to Healthy Homes, Nationwide Children's has implemented a number of social health initiatives through other prongs of Healthy Neighborhoods Healthy Families:

- **School-Based Health Services:** Nationwide Children's offers school-based services in its neighborhoods, offering primary care, behavioral health, and asthma therapy directly in the school, along with having its Mobile Care Centers visit sites. For the nine school-based health centers offering primary and behavioral healthcare, Nationwide Children's nurse practitioners work with school nurses to coordinate acute medical treatment for children.
- **SPARK (Supporting Partnerships to Assure Ready Kids):** This is an evidence-based kindergarten readiness program with group-based learning activities for children with an emphasis on assisting parents to be their child's first and best teacher. Typically, between 60-80 students are enrolled during a school year.
- **Mentoring:** Nationwide Children's employees visit schools weekly to offer homework help and advice to students.

- **PlayStreets:** These events promote outdoor play and social interaction in the community. Healthy Neighborhoods Healthy Families partners with community organizations to host PlayStreets events featuring activities that promote health and wellness.
- **Upward Bound Math and Science:** This program aims to increase the number of students who pursue postsecondary education in math and science. Students receive support through the academic year program, including mentoring, tutoring, and Saturday workshops with cultural and career exposure and hands-on learning.
- **Free Tax Clinics:** These clinics allow community members making under $70,000 to file their taxes for free and get all qualifying credits.
- **My Bridge 2 Success:** This free mentoring program for adults is designed to help promote economic stability. A coach works with the participant to set goals and help in achieving those goals. Sample goals could include earning a degree, changing jobs, or sustaining savings.

Nationwide Children's believes that a full-fledged program addressing social determinants is necessary to improve community health status with an investment horizon over a span of decades. Healthy Neighborhoods Healthy Families has pinned its future on its ability to improve the life and livelihood of residents surrounding the hospital as full partners.

To accomplish each of these goals, Nationwide Children's works closely with community navigators, internally and externally.

Internal champions are the driving force behind successful population health strategies and improving Social Determinants of Health in the community. Choosing the right partners is the cornerstone of any successful population health strategy. It means believing in the common mission of wanting more equitable neighborhoods.

Moreover, partners should be co-pilots rather than passengers, including community activists and extenders (i.e., philanthropic organizations). Building relationships, attending community neighborhood meetings, and recruiting their talent is critical for success.

Lessons learned from the South Side helped Healthy Neighborhoods Healthy Families expand into another neighborhood, Linden, in 2020. They formed a resident advisory council to provide feedback on needed programs and services and look to make an impact in that neighborhood.

Conclusion

Nationwide Children's demonstrates that health systems across the country can be a catalyst for change in neighborhoods that have suffered because of racism, redlining, and disinvestment. As anchors in the community and trusted partners, health systems can bring partners together to create thriving, more equitable neighborhoods.

Nationwide Children's started with its own neighborhood and has now expanded into a new neighborhood in need of resources and investment. Improvement in the next neighborhood will take time. The hospital learned the first step is to find the right community partners and build strong relationships with neighborhood residents to understand their unique needs.

Key Takeaways

- Internal champions are key to success.
- Highly visible programs enhance trust.
- Navigators, integrators, and extenders are essential.
- Recruiting committed partners is fundamental.
- Understanding neighborhood needs is critical.

Appendix

Overview: Healthy Neighborhoods Health Families Initiative

Nationwide Children's Hospital, located in Columbus, Ohio, has built one of the United States' most comprehensive initiatives to improve child health beyond traditional healthcare. In cities and rural communities, in schools and neighborhoods, the hospital and its community partners are working to advance the health of Ohio children and their families.

Community engagement and partnerships are critical to understanding how to serve and work with the neighborhood. The hospital has worked to build trusted relationships with neighborhood groups and multiple nonprofit organizations to serve tens of thousands of families each year.

Why is a children's hospital focused on building healthy neighborhoods?

- A zip code helps determine a child's health. The home a child lives in, their access to healthcare, and the economic opportunities available to their families can impact a child's health and wellness throughout their lifetime.
- High-quality housing, a stable family income, safe neighborhoods, and a good education are all factors that influence a child's health and well-being.
- Nationwide Children's Hospital, which has been taking care of children for more than 130 years, explains that its work must extend beyond the hospital walls into the places where children work, live, and play.

About Healthy Neighborhoods Healthy Families

- Nationwide Children's Hospital created the Healthy Neighborhoods Healthy Families initiative in 2008. This initiative fosters community collaboration to create heathy neighborhoods where children can thrive and connect families with other important programs that will help benefit their children's mental and physical health.
- The initiative started in Columbus' South Side neighborhood, which is adjacent to the hospital, fifteen years ago and expanded to include the Linden neighborhood in 2020 after listening to Linden residents about their hopes and their needs.

- The Healthy Neighborhoods Healthy Families initiative targets five impact areas: affordable housing, education, health and wellness, community enrichment and economic development.
- Healthy Neighborhoods Healthy Families initiatives include home ownership, home rentals, and home repairs, job training, community engagement activities, kindergarten readiness, resource referrals, free tax preparation, and a match savings program.

Affordable Housing

Affordable housing is a big community problem that is going to take big community solutions. Nationwide Children's is working with community partners to find solutions through Healthy Homes.

- Healthy Homes is the affordable housing arm of Healthy Neighborhoods Healthy Families and is a joint effort of Nationwide Children's and Community Development for All People.
- Healthy Homes takes a three-pronged approach to safe and affordable housing: rental units, home ownership, and home repair grants for current residents to allow them to stay in their homes.
- Healthy Home builds high-quality homes and sells them at below-market rates—the average Healthy Home in Linden cost $270,000 to develop in 2023 but was sold

at $140,000. A shared equity model with the Central Ohio Community Land Trust keeps homes affordable for decades into the future.

- Healthy Homes began work in 2008 focused on home ownership, but residents soon let the partnership know that families also needed more rental options. Since 2017, Healthy Homes has emphasized developing single-family rental homes and multifamily rental units.
- Healthy Homes has impacted more than 800 homes. Nationwide Children's announced in 2023 a new $50 million fund that will help develop 150 new rental units, oversee 300 home repairs, and lead sixty home ownership projects in Linden. This fund was made possible with low-interest loans from a group of financial institutions and support from the county and city through grant funding and philanthropic contributions.
- Healthy Homes is now the largest children's hospital-backed housing effort in the United States.

Economic Development and Workforce Opportunities

Neighborhood and family health depend on access to good jobs, living wages, and long-term financial stability. Nationwide Children's offers programs to help South Side and Linden residents achieve those goals.

- BOOST offers free monthly career preparation classes in Healthy Neighborhoods Healthy Families for anyone eighteen years and older seeking a job. Many BOOST graduates are offered positions at Nationwide Children's and other local organizations starting at eighteen dollars per hour.

- Nationwide Children's has hired more than 1,300 employees from South Side and Linden.
- The Summer Youth Employment program provides the opportunity for approximately one hundred youth to work at Nationwide Children's each summer to learn about healthcare careers, and to work for eight weeks in a field of their choosing—medical, research, community development, and many others. This workforce pipeline often leads to permanent employment for youth who otherwise would have no exposure to healthcare as a career.
- The My Bridge 2 Success program helps residents of Linden and the South Side who are living near or below the poverty line connect with a Nationwide Children's mentor to set financial goals and create a path for self-sufficiency. Ultimately, Nationwide Children's helps participants set up a bank account and provides funds to reach certain crucial goals, like purchasing a vehicle. More than $50,000 has been matched to help participants find stable housing, pay off debt, and create an emergency savings.
- Nationwide Children's free tax preparation effort is the largest of its kind in the United States run by a healthcare organization, in partnership with the United Way of Central Ohio.

Volunteer tax preparers help families access tax credits and refunds—sometimes totaling thousands of dollars for a single family—free of charge.
Since 2020: 1,661 total returns, $4 million total refunds, $1.4 million Child Tax Credit, $978,000 in Earned Income Tax Credit.

Community Enrichment

- Healthy Neighborhoods Healthy Families is a founding partner of both the All People's Fresh Market on the South Side and the Linden Fresh Market. The South Side market is now the largest point of free food distribution in Ohio. The Linden Market, created in 2021 and run by the Community of Caring Development Foundation, includes a charitable pharmacy, operated by the Charitable Pharmacy of Central Ohio, for people who cannot afford their medications.
- Leadership training programs, including South Side Neighborhood Leadership Academy and Leadership Linden, help give residents tools to strengthen their communities. More than one hundred have completed the six-month South Side course since 2015. Leadership Linden launched in January 2024.
- PlayStreets neighborhood block parties began on the South Side in 2019 and expanded to Linden in 2020. The eleven total events held in 2023 set attendance records with more than 2,230 attendees enjoying free food, activities, and even

a petting zoo. The Linden Fall Festival celebrates all things Linden, with special performances by Linden-McKinley STEM Academy cheerleaders and the school's marching band. More than 800 residents attended the first one.

Education

Nationwide, Children's has implemented several programs, starting before kindergarten, that help youth with school readiness.

- **Screening:** Nationwide Children's is screening three- and four-year-old children for school readiness and linking children who may be at-risk to community resources and supports that are designed to prepare young children to start school ready to learn.
- **Family Visits:** Specially trained educators visit families with young children to help them learn skills they will need in kindergarten through the SPARK program. Ninety-seven percent of children in Nationwide Children's SPARK program test ready for kindergarten.
- **Mentorship:** Nearly 100 Nationwide Children's employees volunteer to mentor children who live and attend the schools near the hospital. They meet weekly to provide homework help, reading support, and guidance.
- **Proud Linden Parent Program:** This is an evidence-based parenting program, modeled after the Chicago Parenting Program, that brings parents together to

talk through their challenges and learn and practice parenting strategies. Run by a pediatric psychologist and a primary care physician, twenty-five have now graduated from the program.

- **Upward Bound Math and Science:** Focusing on high school students who would be the first in their families to attend college, this program provides tutoring, academic advising, SAT and ACT test prep, and other services that enhance the intellectual, social, and cultural development of the student. Nationwide Children's is the only hospital in the United States with its own UBMS—targeted to reaching students at Linden-McKinley STEM Academy, Marion-Franklin High School, and South High School.
- **Be the One:** This initiative at Linden-McKinley STEM Academy serves students who may be at risk for not graduating, often because they have experienced family trauma, homelessness, and other adverse childhood experiences. The program has led to increases in graduation rates, fewer suspensions, less frequently missed classes and other successes.

Health and Wellness

- Since 2015, Nationwide Children's has partnered with Columbus City Schools to run full-service primary care centers in school buildings in the Healthy Neighborhoods Healthy Families zip codes.

These school-based health centers provide the same services that a pediatrician's office can—physicals, ongoing prescriptions, vaccinations—but they focus on children who don't have a healthcare provider.

Nationwide Children's operates a total of seventeen school-based primary care clinics in central Ohio and has partnered with the state of Ohio, healthcare providers, nonprofit funders, school nurses, and school districts across the state to support the development of school-based health programs in thirty-eight mostly Appalachian counties.

- With the City of Columbus, Nationwide Children's reintroduced Safety City for the first time in more than thirty years. Safety City teaches kids about bike safety, firearm safety, and more, dependent on their neighborhood's most common causes of injury. Behavioral health and nutrition elements are included in the program curriculum.

References

John Edgar, "Getting Ahead of Gentrification in the South Side of Columbus," *Shelterforce Magazine*, Spring 2018.

Boyer, K. B. and D. I. Chang. 2017. "Case Study: Nationwide Children's Hospital: An Accountable Care Organization Going Upstream to Address Population Health." NAM Perspectives. Discussion Paper, National Academy of Medicine, Washington, DC. doi: 10.31478/201704.

Deena Chisolm, Claire Jones, Elisabeth Root, Millie Dolce, and Kelly Kelleher. "A Community Development Program and Reduction in High-Cost Health Care Use." *Pediatrics*, July 2020. 146(2) e20194053. DOI.1542/peds.2019-4055

Kelly Kelleher, Jason Reece and Megan Sandel, "The Healthy Neighborhood, Health Families Initiative," *Pediatrics*, September 2018, 142(3) e20180261; DOI: https://doi.org/10.1542/peds.2018-0261

Mark Ferenchik, "Neighborhood around Children's Hospital getting healthier, study shows," *The Columbus Dispatch*, August 3, 2018.

Deena Chisolm, Claire Jones, Elisabeth Root, Millie Dolce and Kelly Kelleher, "A Community Development Program and Reduction in High-Cost Health Care Use." *Pediatrics*, July 2020, e20194053. https://doi.org/10.1542/peds.2019-4053.

Chapter 3.

University Hospitals, Cleveland

Executive interview with Peter Pronovost, MD, PhD, Chief Clinical Transformation and Quality Officer

University Hospitals implemented a "zero defects" strategy that reduced annual per member per year cost by 9 percent over twelve months. The implication is that such levels of savings could adequately fund a hospital system's social health investment program.

Question: What is at stake?

The healthcare system offers few financial incentives for patients to change unhealthy behaviors. Same for physicians. We aren't compensated enough for counseling patients on healthy behaviors and aren't held accountable when we don't counsel patients. As a result, hospitals have much stronger incentives to treat rather than prevent disease.

Twenty-two percent of all healthcare spending is associated with just ten modifiable risk factors ($780 billion annually). If physician and patient incentives were aligned, we could see a 10 percent reduction of costs, ranging from $761 for healthy people to $2,598 for patients with chronic conditions.

Keep in mind that where care is provided makes a huge difference in costs. Seeing a physician in the office is about $150, ER visits run $1,500 per visit, and hospitalizations average $3,000 to $5,000 per day.

Question: What were the main guiding principles?

We focused on eliminating *all* low-value behaviors and incentives, not just the most obvious ones. We established four key principles:

1. Align around a common purpose and definition of value.
2. Create a common framework and analytical platform for measuring—and making transparent—defects in value and a disciplined management system to reduce defects.
3. Craft incentives to fundamentally change the system from one with uncoordinated incentives to one in which multiple stakeholders are incentivized toward the common purpose.
4. Ensure an appropriate population of attributable patients for whom creating this system change and alignment is tractable.

This is a daunting task, but it's doable.

Question: What methodology was used to shift fee-for-service business to a value framework?

We applied the zero defects framework for the 37,000 members in the employee health plan and the 580,000 patients in our ACO, which represents half our patients. When we began this project in 2018, most of the business was fee-for-service medicine, physician incentives were based on relative value units, and senior management executives focused mostly on increasing hospital admissions and ED visits.

Then we shifted direction in late 2018, and the hospital system aligned around improving value, which we defined that as the quality and experience of care divided by the annual cost of care.

Question: What were the key operating principles?

It was a fundamentally new narrative to say the least. We developed six operational principles to eliminate defects in value:

- Create management accountability systems to eliminate defects in value.
- Organize care around patients' needs anchored in primary care.
- Reduce mindless variation by augmenting mindful variation.
- Use data and technology to continuously innovate.
- Hardwire the connections upstream in the patient journey.
- Engage all staff in improving value.

Question: How was support generated for such a sweeping program?

It involved an "all-hands-on deck" campaign.

Senior management had to sell the framework to a lot of constituencies. It started with board members, leaders, and clinicians across the entire continuum of care. Employees were encouraged to think about defects in their own areas and the principles could be applied to eliminate them. To break down silos, senior management hosted a series of summits with leaders from dozens of departments to prioritize the largest defects—and create work teams to eliminate them.

Question: How were financial and non-financial incentives aligned?

We realized that it was necessary to align incentives among employees and clinicians, and to create a management system to guide our efforts. For example, we provided three free primary care visits for employees and added a financial incentive for our primary care physicians to complete 60 percent of their wellness visits for patients in the employee and Medicare populations. We instituted $0 co-payments for newer diabetic drugs while also providing physicians with a financial incentive that was tied to the percentage of their patients with diabetes with a hemoglobin A1C of <9.

As a practical matter, we focused on two groups of patients: those we employ and those we insure. We improved in improving the accuracy of patient attribution and implemented a team to continuously improve attribution.

We also provided real-time feedback on performance monitoring of efforts to eliminate defects in value. PCPs receive monthly dashboards outlining their performance on numerous performance measures. These include the percentage of patients without an annual wellness visit and the percentages and names of patients with uncontrolled physiological values, such as elevated blood pressure, high blood sugar, and high cholesterol.

UH hospital providers receive weekly reports on the percentage of patients going home after discharge, the percentage with a PCP follow-up within seven days, and the percentage using in-network skilled-nursing facility and home health services.

The hospital system began to include the percentage of patients being managed with evidence-based regimens for common conditions such as diabetes. Likewise, physicians get reports on discharging patients to home rather than to skilled nursing facilities and on reducing ninety day hospital readmissions.

So far, 6 percent of patients had a follow-up with their PCP after discharge. This increased to 72 percent in 2019 and to 85 percent in 2020. We are working on increasing the number of ambulatory visits for patients with chronic disease to be seen once a month for three months.

Question: What are cost savings to date?

Before this effort, employee plan costs increased by 6 percent in 2017-2018. From 2018-2019, costs increased by 1 percent. Costs were reduced by 13 percent in 2019 ($491 per member per month). For Medicare enrollees in the Shared Savings Program, costs decreased by 6 percent compared to the national average increase of 6 percent.

Question: What is the source of these cost reductions?

Hospital discharges decreased by 15 percent, skilled nursing facilities admissions decreased by 31 percent, length of stay decreased by 28 percent, post-acute spending decreased by 32 percent, and ED visits decreased by 13 percent.

The percentage of patients discharged to home increased from 66 percent in 2018 to 80 percent the following year, and to 85 percent in 2020.

Among our 52,000 Medicare Advantage patients, hospital admissions decreased by 30 percent.

Keep in mind that a number of defects in value remain and need to be worked on, especially in behavioral health, palliative care, and increasing the number of ambulatory touch points. These are being implemented as well.

I think our zero defects in care can eliminate 30 percent of healthcare spending that's being wasted, and we can improve value significantly.

Question: What are the most important learnings from this project?

I think the biggest lesson learned is that we need to lead with purpose based on key principles—rather than technology or data. There needs to be a galvanizing framework for organizing the work, like keeping people healthy at home rather than healing in a hospital. That was a powerful narrative for us.

Relationships and trust must grow among leaders across the continuum, so leaders need to meet regularly, learn, and improve together. Co-creating goals is important and provides horizontal connections for peer-to-peer learning and vertical connections for accountability.

Having a data infrastructure is essential to identify defects, segment populations, and produce dashboards to emphasize the focus on value. Hospital systems need to integrate claims and EMR data and grow their attributed patients in an ACO of another contracted arrangement.

Every employee needs to feel that they have two jobs: the job they were hired to do and the job of improving value.

It's difficult to ask medical practices to implement interventions for different payers. This requires additional outreach and collaboration between ACOs and patients.

Significant benefits can be achieved by aligning benefit design, incentives for patients, incentives for physicians, and care management teams.

Question: What did the overall framework consist of?

We used a framework that included defects in value, key principles, and a management system to realize results. We also paid attention to the "softer" side of change by inspiring and empowering people to eliminate defects in value. Both the technical and the adaptive components of leading change are important.

It's also important to celebrate what has been accomplished by pausing for retreats, taking stock, and then refocusing energy on eliminating defects in value.

Question: Any final thoughts on how eliminating defects can contribute to social determinists of care?

Every year we spend $1.3 trillion on suboptimal behaviors. We know we can save at least 9 percent of costs a year, and a lot more if we eliminate defects in value for *all* types of care. That would free up significant funds to pay to support social health investment in upstream community health programs.

A comprehensive zero defects strategy produces a triple bottom line: reduced cost and waste, improved value to patients and payers, and sustainable funding for Social Determinants of Health and eliminating health disparities.

Acknowledgement:

This interview was based in part on the published work of Peter J. Pronovost, MD, PhD; John W. Urwin, MD; Eric Beck, DO; Justin Coran, PhD; Abirammy Sundaramoorthy, MD; Mark E. Schario, MS, RN; James M. Muisyo, MSc; Jonathon Sague, MSN, RN; Susan Shea, MAA; Patrick Runnels, MD; Todd Zeiger, MD; Andrew Wilhelm, PhD; Sandeep Palakodeti, MD; and Amol S. Navathe, MD, PhD.

Chapter 4.

CommonSpirit Health Case Study

Introduction

CommonSpirit Health was created by the merger of Catholic Health Initiatives (CHI) and Dignity Health in 2019. The combined organization represents more than 2,200 care sites across twenty-four states and contributes more than $4 billion a year in charity, community benefits, and government program services.

One of the biggest challenges facing the new organization was the recognition that social determinants influence health, yet addressing these influences resides outside of the prevailing healthcare delivery model. That raised a fundamental question: What is the role of a health system like CommonSpirit in influencing non-clinical factors that drive health? It is widely acknowledged that non-clinical factors influence about 80 percent of a person's health.

Prior to the formation of CommonSpirit, CHI received a Robert Wood Johnson Foundation planning grant to answer that question. CHI developed recommended priorities, goals, and objectives. The work resulted in a comprehensive framework for thinking in seven domains across a multi-year horizon: the Total Health Roadmap (THRM). This work was continued through the merger, and the size and scale of CommonSpirit now provides broad opportunities for testing models and approaches in diverse community ecosystems. This work also entails overcoming significant obstacles and disincentives in the current healthcare system, including reimbursement practices of government programs and commercial payers.

Phase 1 of implementation was developed in Spring 2017 and focused on five THRM domains: social determinants, essential partnerships, CHI's community role, board competencies, and leadership competencies and composition. The strategic aims of the model align with the recommendations of the National Academies: increase community capacity to shape outcomes, engage in multi-sector collaboration, and make health equity a shared vision and value.[1] Aligned effort across the three priority areas were deemed necessary to make an impact on total health status. As anchor healthcare organizations, CHI recognized the need to work with others to move upstream and address the drivers of health in communities, advocating for total health and health equity. This requires leaders and board members who understand the complex drivers of health and to recognize accountabilities for collaborative work that will improve the health of patients and communities.

This phase was funded through a $2.5 million grant by the Robert Wood Johnson Foundation matched in full by the CHI Mission and Ministry Fund.

Primary care was the starting point since it is where individuals and families develop long-term relationships with providers. Work in Phase 1 focused on the integration of universal screening and referral for social needs and introduction of the Community Health Worker (CHW) role to assist primary care providers with addressing social needs and managing referrals. The ability to form collaborative partnerships depends on the knowledge CHWs and other caregivers and brings to the attention of clinical leaders and executives the influence of social needs on overall health.

Implementation Planning Process

CommonSpirit developed a lexicon of key terms to guide strategic planning: social determinants, social risk factors, social needs, and health equity.

- **Social Determinants of Health** (SDoH) are the conditions in the environments where people are born, live, learn, work, play, worship, and age that affect a wide range of health, functioning, and quality-of-life outcomes and risks. SDoH have a major impact on people's health, well-being, and quality of life.
- **Social risk factors** are constructs that reflect the influence of social processes and social relationships on health-related outcomes and are often considered in five domains: socioeconomic position; race, ethnicity, and cultural context; gender; social relationships; and residential and community context.[2]

- **Social needs** (also referred to as health-related social needs) are the manifestation of social risk factors and the impact of negative Social Determinants of Health—e.g., the patient is hungry, the patient is homeless, the patient cannot afford their medication. Social needs compromise an individual's ability to achieve better health and well-being (definition developed by CommonSpirit Community Health).
- **Health equity** means that everyone has a fair and just opportunity to be as healthy as possible. This requires removing obstacles to health such as poverty, discrimination, and their consequences, including powerlessness and lack of access to good jobs with fair pay, quality education and housing, safe environments, and healthcare.[3]

CommonSpirit's implementation planning process had three core intentions: *impact* relating to mission objectives, *influence* in terms of system outcomes, and *leverage* to advance strategic learning and sustainability.

The guiding principles for implementation strategy focused on five important values: person-centered care, empathy, partnership, humility, and equity.

- **Person-Centered:** We recognize that health is more than just the absence of disease and that a person's life is not defined by a diagnosis.

- **Empathy:** We practice empathy—seeking first to understand and then to assist.
- **Partnership:** We partner with patients—we do not make assumptions regarding current circumstances, nor do we pretend to know what is best without first understanding their priorities. We partner with community agencies by seeking to understand the barriers our partners face in developing and maintaining their capacities to serve.
- **Humility:** We practice cultural humility, as we realize that we will never be competent in understanding another's culture if we have not lived it ourselves. We practice cultural humility in our interactions with community partners as well—recognizing that the funding environment and cultural framework of healthcare is distinctly different than that of our social service, public health, and faith-based community partners.
- **Equity:** Equity is not the same as equality—to ensure opportunities for individuals to achieve good health, those with poorer health and fewer resources may need more time and effort to overcome their circumstances. As we learn more about the circumstances that have led to poorer health for our neighbors, we advocate and take action to change these circumstances.

CommonSpirit's underlying theory of change included three strategies. Each strategy is linked to concepts regarding influence, impact, or leverage. This chain of thinking is illustrated below.

Theory of Change

<table>
<tr><td rowspan="3">STRATEGY 1: We will transform our role as a healthcare provider by integrating universal screening for social needs in primary care

Aligns with the THRM Social Determinants domain</td><td>SO THAT we help providers address social needs</td><td>Characterized as influence – a change in system(s) and norm(s)</td></tr>
<tr><td>SO THAT patients achieve better health</td><td>Characterized as impact, as individual health will improve</td></tr>
<tr><td>AND THAT we contribute to local understanding of actual needs and effective referral and support pathways</td><td>Characterized as influence, as what we learn from our patients will inform changes in system(s) and norm(s)</td></tr>
</table>

STRATEGY 2: We will strengthen our role as a community organization by participating in local/ regional cross-sector partnerships Aligns with the THRM **Essential Partnerships and Community Role** domains	**SO THAT** we help to develop consensus and collaborative solutions aimed at closing gaps in the community's capacity to meet social needs	Characterized as **leverage**, as we anticipate a shift in resource allocation and funding strategies to close gaps
	AND THAT we share information to lay the foundation for future, more effective communication and collaboration	Characterized as **influence**, improved collaboration will change system(s) and norm(s)
	SO THAT we contribute to the national evidence base for the benefits of addressing social needs and tackling the Social Determinants of Health	Characterized as **influence**, as our contribution to the national evidence base will help change system(s) and norm(s)
	SO THAT we improve the understanding of leadership (at all levels) of the importance of this work	Characterized as **influence**, as improving leadership understanding and commitment will change system(s) and norm(s)
	AND THAT we develop an effective, collaborative approach for addressing social needs	Characterized as **impact**, as individuals will have access to better care

<table>
<tr><td rowspan="2">STRATEGY 3: We will strengthen leadership commitment by integrating the Total Health framework into leadership accountabilities

Aligns with the THRM Board and Leadership Competencies and Composition domains</td><td>SO THAT governing boards and leadership are accountable for sustaining a comprehensive approach to promoting health equity in the communities we serve</td><td>Characterized as influence, as improving leadership understanding and commitment will change system(s) and norm(s)</td></tr>
<tr><td>AND THAT addressing social needs becomes an integral and sustained component of quality healthcare</td><td>Characterized as impact, as individuals will have access to better care</td></tr>
</table>

The organization's strategic learning process with pioneer markets established the framework to increase the capacity to shape outcomes and engage in multisector collaboration. The intent was to make health equity a shared vision and value.

To integrate social needs screening in primary care means forming working relationships with public health agencies, social services, and community-based organizations to support individuals and families with social needs. Community collaboration was necessary to fill in the gaps in local resources and improve community health improvement plans, data sharing and information exchanges.

The planning process was slowed due to the COVID-19 pandemic and limited data was available to assess patient clinical outcomes and the potential impact of coordination provided by CHWs on clinical outcomes. However, the pandemic did highlight the impact of social determinants and inequities in community health. Further funding was secured for Phase 2 implementation (July 2020—present) to support the spread and scale of social needs screening, referral, and integration of CHWs.

Business Case

Making a case for business investment involves setting priorities for what is most important to an organization in terms of improving community health as well as determining what constitutes value for patients, staff, and stakeholders. It goes to the heart of an organization's mission, how investments are allocated, and recognizing organizational accountabilities for better clinical outcomes and cost reduction.

The THRM implementation team examined different ways to evaluate what constitutes value. There are at least six possible lenses and key questions for each approach, and these lenses were developed through participation in the Collaborative to Advance Social Health Integration, an initiative of Health Leads.

Lens 1: Impact on Clinical Outcomes and Quality

- Is there a difference in the clinical outcomes of patients after they receive social health support?
- Which clinical outcomes are impacted?

Lens 2: Patient Experience

- Has implementation improved patient experience and confidence in ability to manage their health?

Lens 3: Staff Experience

- Has implementation improved staff experience?
- What are the foundations of provider buy-in?

Lens 4: Productivity and Efficiency

- Is productivity and efficiency of the care team improved?
- How does technology development facilitate efficiencies in collaboration with community partners?
- How does technology improve efficiency?

Lens 5: Impact on Stakeholders

- What benefits have our providers, our care delivery systems, and our community partners gained?

Lens 6: Cost Reduction and Cost Avoidance

- How has total cost of care been reduced for the patient panel and/or for patients with complex needs and high utilization?
- Has utilization of high-cost care been reduced?
- Should other "costs" be considered, such as quality of life?

Pioneer Markets and Clinics

Three health systems (pioneer markets) in Colorado, Iowa, and Kentucky were selected to learn about key drivers and challenges related to implementing social determinants. Each local organization developed timelines and pathways for integration of screening, referral, and case management, as well as collaborative efforts with community partners. CHW job roles and training were also developed locally.

Centura Health (now CommonSpirit Mountain Region) serves Colorado, Utah, and Kansas through twenty hospitals and one-hundred-plus physician practices and clinics. The organization is developing a comprehensive social needs screening framework across care sites in conjunction with their electronic medical record system (Epic). The regional state Medicaid expansion program funds health coaching and social worker support for Medicaid patients, but not the costs of integration with value-based contracts. In Phase 1, three CHWs were employed. The state's Hospital Transformation Program emerged during Phase 1, which has advanced Centura's work on screening and referral for social needs and the development of a statewide social needs information exchange.

Centuras Heath's Strategy Map for addressing the impact of social determinants is illustrated below.

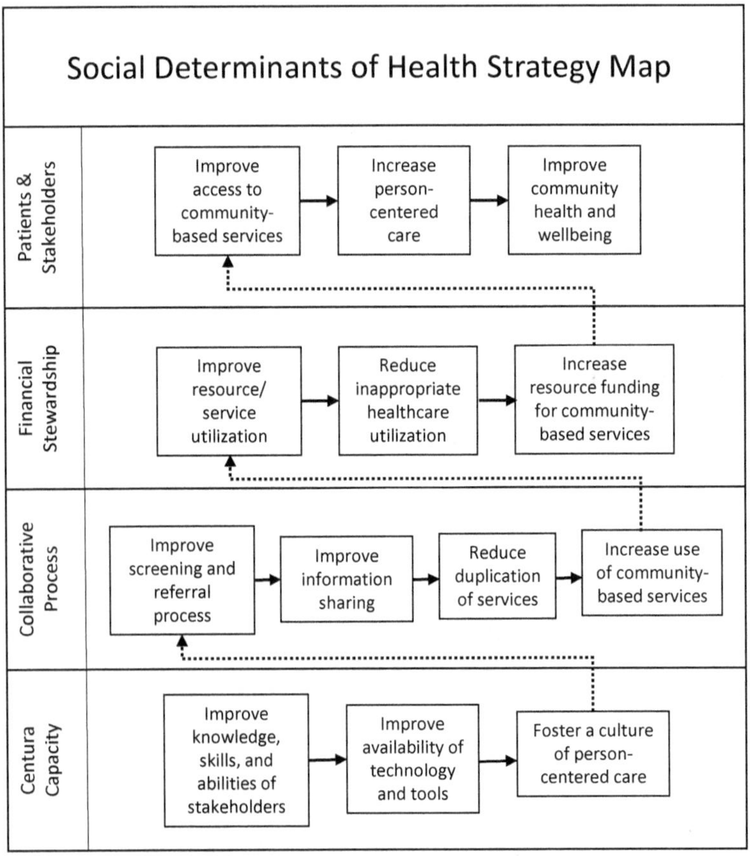

MercyOne, Iowa is comprised of 420 clinics, medical centers, and hospitals. The organization expanded the integration of CHWs in clinics and building new capabilities in the data platform that integrates screening and case management data with other population health functions. MercyOne's work is based in their population health services organization and serves as a model for replication in other CommonSpirit communities that have well-developed population health infrastructure and can leverage value-based contacts.

CHI Saint Joseph Health, Kentucky represents 135 locations in twenty counties, including hospitals, physician groups, and clinics. Screening and referral data indicated a need to close care gaps, smooth referral pathways, and increase awareness about how to manage social needs. The latter included gaining more information on creative workarounds developed by CHWs through their relationships with patients, families, and community partners. CHI Saint Joseph Health is working with the Commonwealth's legislature to inform development of new pathways of support for CHWs via Medicaid. In addition, these pioneer communities have provided essential insights on implementation in rural communities.

Strategic Learning Process

External evaluators reviewed quantitative data and conducted surveys, interviews, and focus groups to identify themes and lessons learned. Data and technology needs were identified, as well as barriers individuals and families encounter in managing their healthcare needs. Patient and family stories were particularly insightful as well as workarounds by CHWs through their relationships with patients, families, and community partners.

Phase 1 implementation, which overlaps with Phase 2, developed consensus on an operational framework and the development of best practices.

Screening Value

Another hallmark of CommonSpirit's Total Health Roadmap is universal screening. In fact, the necessity of universal screening is reinforced by THRM's initial analyses of patients who screen positive for social needs. The data indicates a broad distribution between Medicare, Medicaid, and private insurers. There is a risk of missed opportunities if only a subset of patients is offered access to support for social needs. Providers were relieved that universal screening was "payer agnostic" and did not require more work on their part during visits. The primary responsibility for data collection and referral resides with medical assistants and CHWs.

Screening for social needs in a clinical setting represents a new pathway to assess community health needs and to inform community health improvement plans. The screening tool posed questions drawn, in part, from the Health Leads toolkit, CMS screening tool, and items from the PRAPARE tool. An internal staff consensus arrived at the following nine questions on core social needs screening used in all pioneer clinics.

Core Social Need Screening Questions

Screening Question	**Circle One**
In the last twelve months, were you worried that your food would run out before you got money to buy more?	Yes No
Are you worried or concerned that in the next two months, you may not have stable housing that you own, rent, or stay in as part of a household?	Yes No
In the past twelve months, has the electric, gas, oil or water company threatened to shut off services in your home?	Yes No
In the last twelve months, did you skip medications to save money?	Yes No
In the past twelve months, has lack of transportation kept you from the doctor, work, or from meeting other needs?	Yes No
Are you worried about your physical or emotional safety where you currently live?	Yes No
Do you ever need help reading medical materials?	Yes No
Would you like help with any of these needs?	Yes No
Are any of your needs urgent? *For example: I don't have food tonight, I don't have a place to sleep tonight.*	Yes No

Ninety-six percent of pioneer clinic staff and 93 percent of leadership surveyed felt screening and referring patients to resources is valuable. The top patient needs identified through screening were food security, housing, and financial strain.

Across the pioneer clinics, one in five patients screened indicated one or more social needs. In Phase 1, 71,503 screens were conducted. Twenty-one percent of patients in Colorado, Iowa and, Kentucky screened positive for the following: food 25 percent, housing 14 percent, transportation 15 percent, utilities 14 percent, financial 16 percent, reading 11 percent, and safety 5 percent.

When asked about the benefits of using data on social needs, clinic staff thought the most important benefits were:

- Improved patient experience and satisfaction: 93.3 percent
- Improved clinical outcomes: 91.7 percent
- Improved provider and staff satisfaction: 86.7 percent
- Reduction in cost of care: 83.3 percent

As a faith-based organization committed to social justice, national and local CommonSpirit leadership includes Mission and Community Health functions. Community Health Leaders across CommonSpirit constitute a key group to comment on the value of social needs screening and referral, alongside the development of more effective community partnerships and collaboration to address resource and access gaps. These leaders were asked how social needs screening and referral data could be used to inform program development. Six options were given, and the level of importance is ranked below by the 31 respondents.

- To improve understanding of the barriers patients face in meeting their social needs: 96.8 percent.
- To gain a better understanding of the potential value of community health programs in improving health outcomes: 96.8 percent.
- To identify care gaps in the community that can be addressed in partnership with other agencies or sectors: 96.8 percent.
- To identify opportunities for collaboration with our communities to address upstream factors that contribute to social needs: 100 percent.
- To add depth to health needs assessment processes and analyses: 83.8 percent.
- To compare and contrast local data with state or national trends: 77.4 percent.
- To support case statements for grant funding and/or local giving: 80.7 percent.

Screening Tools

The selection and use of a common screening tool was a key component of the THRM strategy.

At the outset, fully validated screening tools were still in development, thus CommonSpirit explored various tools in development and engaged pioneer market clinical leadership and other mission leaders (faith community nurses) to assess the domains and types of questions to be used. The intent of the screening process is to identify patients who have needs and offer access to assistance to meet these needs. In addition, screening data has and continues to assist clinical and community health leaders in understanding the scope of needs in patient panels, which informs how and where clinics work with community partners to facilitate access and close resource gaps. Each pioneer market was able to add questions to the core screener used across all the markets. For example, CHI Saint Joseph added several questions designed to address potential changes in Kentucky Medicaid at that time and whether patients needed help in finding a local career center or job training program or help in understanding changes in state benefits. Kentucky's CHWs observed significant needs and added the following questions:

- Do problems getting childcare make it difficult for you to work or study?
- Do you need diapers, clothing, car seats, or school supplies?
- Do you need help with stress, mental health, or substance abuse concerns?
- Do you need help finding resources for an eye exam and reading glasses?
- Do you need help finding resources for a hearing exam and/or hearing aids?
- Do you need help finding resources for dental care?

Like the experience of other health systems, a drop-off between screening and completion of referrals in pioneer clinics was observed. In MercyOne clinics, for example, 1,885 patients requested help, but only 1,160 of those patients connected with CHWs and were referred to community resources (53 percent). Another 727 of these patients followed through with referrals (78 percent) and 601 had full or partial needs met (84 percent). This "funnel effect" was evident at each clinic (urban and rural) and reflects common difficulties in longer term patient follow-up.

Implementation Assessment

Three of the most important barometers of implementation activity are system readiness, organization challenges, and provider panel concerns.

System Readiness

To gauge the readiness to implement social determinants and screening, a questionnaire was administered to clinicians and system leaders at both the market and national level. It was used to establish a baseline perspective and to assess the difference between clinicians and leadership responses. Such a template could be adopted by other organizations in the SDOH planning and implementation phase. The questionnaire asked: "In your opinion, which basic needs are the most important/problematic for the patients you serve?" These are ranked from 1 (lowest) to 7 (highest) in order of importance and shown in column 2.

Social Needs Ranking by Clinicians and Leaders

	Clinicians	System Leaders
Food insecurity	5.82	5.29
Utilities assistance	3.37	3.32
Housing/shelter	5.15	5.24
Financial strain	4.91	4.54
Transportation	4.11	3.76
Literacy (ability to read and understand medical instructions)	1.98	2.58
Safety/exposure to violence	2.74	3.27

Food insecurity, housing/shelter, and financial strain were perceived as important issues in relation to health outcomes and social needs.

Pioneer Clinic Staff, Leadership, and Community Health Leads were asked to rate the most important challenges to implementation according to eight dimensions shown below on a scale of 1 (highest) to 5 (lowest; percentages reflect the proportion of respondents scoring 1 or 2).

Implementation Challenges

Challenge	Pioneer Clinic Staff	CommonSpirit Mission, Clinical, and Administrative Leadership	Community Health Leads
Lack of resources to address patient needs (either in the organization or community)	77.6%	93.1%	51.6%
Lack of effective screening tools	55.2%	62.1%	61.3%
Lack of integration with provider organizations	62.5%	82.8%	--
Lack of knowledge of how to screen and/or respond to identified needs	60.3%	55.2%	32.3%
Absence of actionable data and appropriate metrics to measure performance	44.8%	72.4%	45.2%
Difficulty of demonstrating return on investment (ROI)	49.1%	79.3%	74.2%
Lack of coordination with community-based organizations	59.6%	65.5%	35.5%
Lack of resources (e.g., time or personnel) to effectively screen patients	74.1%	79.3%	64.5%

There were notable differences among clinic staff, leadership, and community health leads, sometimes as much as a 20 percent-point difference. Leadership's biggest concerns were fourfold: lack of resources to address patient needs, integration with provider organizations, lack of actionable data and metrics, and demonstration of a return on investment. Understanding these differences in perception is essential to the program team in terms of developing messaging and program summaries for leadership review.

Each group gave low priority to availability of effective screening tools, knowledge of how to screen/respond, and coordination with community agencies. Responses of Community Health Leads differed from clinics and leaders in three areas. Leads expressed less concern regarding lack of resources, lack of knowledge on how to screen and respond, and lack of coordination with communities. This is likely due to their knowledge and use of screening tools and referrals outside the clinical setting as a part of their ongoing work. In addition, the Community Health leads surveyed represented the whole of CommonSpirit Health communities, a much broader group representing multiple and diverse communities.

Another set of challenges related to awareness about community resources and level of comfort in referring patients. Responses to awareness about community resources and level of comfort are shown below on a scale of 1 (highest) to 5 (lowest; percentages reflect the proportion of respondents scoring 1 or 2). There was a notable increase in the level of comfort (in a follow-up survey) in referring patients to these community resources in 2020 compared to the baseline survey administered in 2017.

Referral Awareness and Comfort Level

Community Resource	Awareness of Resources		Comfort in Referring	
	Baseline	Follow-up	Baseline	Follow-up
Housing/ shelter	41.1%	55.9% ↑	70.2%	80.0% ↑
Safety/ violence	41.9%	46.7% ↑	70.2%	73.3% ↑
Food security	52.0%	65.0% ↑	72.6%	81.7% ↑
Utilities	40.3%	55.0% ↑	67.8%	80.0% ↑
Financial strain	35.5%	48.3% ↑	62.9%	76.7% ↑
Transportation	47.2%	68.3% ↑	73.4%	78.3% ↑
Literacy	28.5%	31.7% ↑	62.9%	65.0% ↑

There were several reasons given by these respondents as to why patients were unable to complete referrals or reported barriers in getting needs met at referral agencies. Some agencies simply do not have sufficient capacity (or funding) to meet a community's full extent of social needs. Clinic staff suggested seven common reasons they were unable to complete referrals:

- **Application requirements:** patient needs help with paperwork, no access to fax machine to submit forms, long wait times
- **Access:** limited hours of service, hard to reach by phone, requirements for in-person appointments
- **Life circumstances:** dependence on others, patient moved, other issues arose
- **Misunderstanding:** missed follow-up by patient or resource; lack of understanding required documentation or completed forms
- **Alternative solutions:** patient located other resources prior to connecting with resource (e.g., family member provided help)
- **Patient health:** declines in patient health, caregiving for others prevented contact with agency
- **Transportation:** lack of resources, vehicles in disrepair, available transportation allowed only to doctor appointments, restrictions for Medicaid transportation, using city bus not amenable, other transportation resources very expensive, lack of reliability of available resources.

Barriers to getting needs met at referral agency:

- **Company or agency does not help**
- **Eligibility requirements:** income too high to qualify, other eligibility requirements not met, lack of legal custody for grandchildren

- **Language challenges**
- **Lack of follow-up from organization:** no return call, referral to other offices that do not follow through
- **Insufficient assistance:** transportation resources limited, discounts for medications still not affordable
- **Wait list:** timelines too long to address patient needs in a timely manner

Community Health Workers have been frustrated that some referral agencies are poorly funded and have long wait lists. *"It's like I'm referring to a dead end."* Gatekeeping procedures are often complex or laborious. *"Their way of getting people into their programs is very time consuming."*

Access is compromised by irregular hours and having not enough food banks and soup kitchens. "We ask a lot of resource partners without giving them money or the true resources to adequately met our patient's needs. And then for the patient, it is just another piece of paper." Even when referrals fall short, this service is comforting to most patients. "It's just having somebody there who cares to go through with them and kind of help walk through it with them."

CHWs were able to learn from patients about prior poor experiences or frustration with accessing resources and then develop alternative ways for gaining the support they needed.

Provider Panel Concerns

Screening for social needs in the clinical setting represents a new pathway to assess community health needs and to inform health improvement plans. While clinicians and system leaders believe in screening for Social Determinants of Health, priorities must be set in consideration of workflow issues and provider fatigue.

There may be resistance to the idea of a new project (or a redistribution of work), such as universal screening, among clinic staff who already feel overburdened in terms of workload. There is confusion about what new responsibilities will be required and where additional burdens will fall.

Total Health Roadmap staff made six suggestions to respond to these clinic concerns.

1. Early and clear communications and conversations with key staff members are critical. Discussions should be adjusted to consider the audience and the pressures felt in primary care settings.
2. Listening to providers to understand their stresses and pain points is fundamental.
3. Engaging and supporting provider and clinical staff champions is essential. This includes taking their advice and guidance on how to reduce interruptions in clinical workflow.
4. Early training is essential for CHWs and other clinic staff to understand and to define their clinic scope of roles.

The clarification process should be ongoing and address where overlaps occur.

5. Staff turnover and the need for retraining on the screening process will be an ongoing concern, particularly for front desk administrative staff and medical assistants.
6. Implementation teams need to be cognizant that a system's prior experience with this work may only have been with very focused efforts (e.g., familiar faces in the emergency room, high-risk patients at the time of hospital discharge, patients with significant chronic comorbidities).
7. Integration of CHWs in primary care to serve the needs of the entire patient panel represents a significant change in approach, as does the CHW's role in closing the loop on referrals.

While clinicians and system leaders believe in screening for Social Determinants of Health, priorities must be set in consideration of workflow issues and provider fatigue. It is important for clinicians to realize that ancillary support is readily available to address social needs of patients. The value of CHWs in taking on support for social needs is essential in freeing up providers to focus on individual health issues. Social workers and health coaches/nurse care coordinators can work at "top of license" for patients with complex health and behavioral health needs through support from CHWs in meeting patient social needs.

Paying for Social Needs

Among the chief concerns about paying for social needs screening are the source of reimbursement, screener costs, and equity considerations.

Source

A foundational issue that affects all aspects of strategy and healthcare delivery is "Who pays?" THRM asked pioneer clinics (staff and leadership) the following question: "Which parties do you think should be responsible for the majority of investment costs for addressing patient health-related social needs?" (i.e., government agency payers, private payers, public health and social service agencies, provider organizations). The three respondent choices were: "Solely responsible," "Partially responsible," or "Not responsible."

Neither clinic staff nor leadership felt "solely responsible," while leadership more often answered "partially responsible" than clinic staff. Leadership (100 percent) said government agencies and Medicaid should be "partially responsible." Clinic staff agreed (81—85 percent).

There were also differences between pioneer clinic staff and leadership on the importance of indicators for return on investment (ROI). A further question asked, "In your opinion, what are the most important indicators for determining ROI for implementing screening and referrals for social needs within a healthcare system?" from 1 "Extremely Important" to 5 "Not important at all" along a five-point scale; percentages reflect the proportion of respondents scoring 1 or 2.

Return on Investment Indicators

Indicators for ROI	Pioneer Clinic Staff	Leadership
Improved health outcomes for patients (e.g., controlled blood sugar or blood pressure)	91.4%	93.1%
Lower no-show rates for scheduled appointment	70.7%	62.1%
Lower re-admission rates	82.8%	82.8%
Fewer visits to the emergency room	87.9%	55.2%
Reduction in costs of care	93.3%	72.4%
Number of patients identified with needs that are successfully referred	86.2%	79.3%
Provider satisfaction	75.9%	65.5%
Patient satisfaction	89.7%	79.3%

Clinic staff thought a reduction in the cost of care was most important, followed by improved health outcomes and patient satisfaction. Leadership considered improved patient outcomes as the top preference. This was followed by lower re-admission rates, number of patients identified with needs that are successfully referred, and patient satisfaction.

Clinic staff indicated the value of additional indicators, including patient satisfaction with their experience at the clinic practice, access to mental health supports, and overall cost avoidance and life expectancy gains from mitigating chronic disease effects. Leaders' suggestions included reducing or eliminating racial disparities, improving reputation and community perception, enhanced community partnerships and trust, reductions in total cost of care, and adherence to CommonSpirit's mission.

When asked about the benefits of using data on social needs, clinic staff thought the most important benefits were improved patient experience and satisfaction (93.3 percent) and improved clinical outcomes (91.7 percent).

One of the organization's tasks in Phase 2 is to identify themes and opportunities for developing a revenue base to support universal screening and referral for social needs in primary care. The six main themes are:

Task 1: Develop strategies for articulating the value of screening and the work of CHWs to inform future development of value-based contracts.

- Assess what value-based contracts are currently in place in pilot clinics, identify payers, and open conversations.
- Develop methods for linking the work of CHWs to successes in patient outcomes and improved quality measures (i.e., contribution analysis).
- Assess Key Performance Indicators (KPI) unique to Medicaid or other payers and develop methods for assessing the contribution of screening, referral, and CHW work to KPIs.
- Explore use of self-sufficiency matrices to characterize movement of patients from crisis to well managed in terms of social needs (i.e., stratification by social needs)

that align with stratification of patient subpopulations by cost and medical complexity.

Task 2: Leverage new developments in Medicaid and Medicare (CMS innovation programs) that recognize importance of addressing social needs.

- Current pilot clinics have large proportions of Medicaid and Medicare patients: explore opportunities to reduce losses in clinics due to Medicaid contracting by improving no-show rates and reductions in inappropriate ER use.
- Characterize payer mixes and revenue sources in each pilot clinic, and open conversations with state Medicaid and commercial managed care organizations about the work of CHWs and value of screening and referral.
- Compare outcomes achieved with those reported by the CMS Accountable Health Communities work. (Note: referral completion rates in CSH pioneer markets are higher than what has been reported in CMS' first evaluation report.)

Task 3: Develop opportunities to contribute to improved measures in Merit-Based Incentive Payment System and Comprehensive Primary Care Plus frameworks.

- Learn the frameworks of these programs and where they are operating in pioneer and other markets.
- Develop metrics and contribution analyses to characterize support provided via screening and referral.

Task 4: Open broader conversations with Clinically Integrated Networks (CINs) and Accountable Care Organizations (ACOs) in operation in pilot markets.

- Develop opportunities for better collaboration with CINs and ACOs.
- Compare and contrast implementation in pilot markets with a view to CIN/ACO development to inform next steps for program development and development of synergistic roles for enterprise population health and community health in value-based care.

Task 5: Demonstrate value of health coaches and social workers practicing at top of license.

- Characterize whether shifts in work of health coaches and social workers occurred with the addition of CHWs, develop measures of this shift, track improvements in patient engagement and improved outcomes for chronic disease management and access to behavioral healthcare. This is particularly relevant for clinics where health coaches, social workers, and behavioral health specialists are well integrated.

Task 6: Leverage existing codes to secure payment for screening and referral.

- Explore Z codes to capture diagnostic data and advance

more effective use of coding to capture payment in existing frameworks.

- Assess potential administrative burden of using Z-codes and social needs payment codes, as well as the training that would be required for effective use in reimbursement, including opportunities to develop functions in case management platforms to auto-populate EMR coding modules.

At the same time, CommonSpirit believes that tracking the impact of clinical and community work addressing social needs entails a longer time horizon to assess program impact. It is also important to establish a balance between clinical outcomes and community-level indicators that mark progress in providing whole person care. This represents a significant shift from how ROI is calculated, which generally separates clinical outcomes from community outcomes. Community activities focus on gaps indicated in aggregate community-level data. With universal screening and referral for social needs within its systems of care, CommonSpirit will be developing additional insights regarding resource gaps, disparities in access, and overall capacity of local communities to meet needs identified through screening.

Screener Costs

To understand true costs of integrating effective screening and referral for social needs, CommonSpirit conducted a "look back" of costs associated with its work in pioneer clinics.

The first step was to conduct simple calculations of costs per screen alongside costs per "case"—meaning patients who identified needs and thus were provided the option of engaging with a CHW for additional assessment and referral. Centura Health conducted 26,053 screens during Phase 1 that identified 5,089 cases. This translated to $62 per screen and $316 per case. MercyOne indicated a cost of $49 per screen and $250 per case. CHI Saint Joseph indicated a cost of $56 per screen and $230 per case.

The second step was to consider the essential cost elements considering the patient panels served (pool of potential patients in need). Costs for integrating CHWs and universal screening and referral are estimated to be between $63,500 and $103,000 annually per clinic employing one full-time CHW. For clinics with a patient panel of 5,000, the costs range from $12.70 to $20.60 per panel patient per year in later phases of the rollout.

A refined approach to calculating costs is summarized in the table below and includes the following principles:

- The CHW Coordinator position is essential. The annual salary range for this position in Phase 1 was between $60,000 and $80,000, and the benefit rate averaged 25 percent. In Phase 1, implementation and maintenance of activities required 15-25 percent of the CHW Coordinator time (a proportion which may be reduced with spread and scale), resulting in costs between $11,250 and $25,000 per clinic.
- The annual salary range for a full-time CHW varied between $35,000 and $50,000, and the benefit rate

averaged 25 percent. As such, the range of costs for integrating a full-time CHW is $43,750 to $62,500.

- Training and continuous learning costs range from $2,000 to $5,000; participation in national conferences and regional training is encouraged.
- Travel is also essential, primarily for regional travel to partner agencies and an allowance for travel to one national or regional conference per year. Estimated annual allocations ranging from $1,500 to $3,000.
- Annual technology costs range from $5,000 to $7,500 per clinic. These costs include computer/IT costs, cell phones, and annual user fees for case management platforms.

It is important to budget for ongoing CHW training to enhance the following skills: patient communication skills, patient privacy and confidentiality requirements, and appropriate documentation and data management. CHW cost may be reduced by developing floating positions to support multiple clinics, and Coordinator costs can be reduced with spread and scale, i.e., a Coordinator can manage CHWs across multiple clinics.

Equity

Equity is at the heart of CommonSpirit's mission. A core belief is that THRM activity should be viewed through a lens that reflects a more encompassing set of performance measures in addition to ROI.

Performance metrics should reflect improvements in overall systems of care delivery and contributions to improved health equity in communities. This would include the following attributes:

- Measures must be important and relevant to a large population and have a significant public health impact; relevant to key stakeholders and have a significant impact for patients.
- Measures must be scientifically acceptable; evidence exists for linking structures and processes to outcomes.
- Measures have strong operational definitions (e.g., reproducible and valid).
- Measures must be feasible with ability to capture in clinical care; acceptable burden or cost of capturing data.
- Measures must be usable and actionable; ability to act in response to gaps in care.
- Measures must be responsive and improve with better care.

Another important question is whether new revenue streams have been identified to pay for continued screening. Payer-based programs are characterized in terms of the number of patients within a particular panel who are covered by the payer. From the THRM perspective, this misses the mark. From a provider point of view, the conversation needs to be flipped to focus on a more critical question:

> *"How can we combine resources available through conventional payment and value-based contracts across*

a patient panel to ensure that every patient who comes to the clinic for care has access to the supports and resources needed to achieve optimal health?"

It would be advantageous to pursue dual strategies: (1) a "clinic up" communication approach that leverages information from universal screening to judge the scope and depth of needs in clinic panels, and (2) a "systems across" approach that maps the scope of needs for local geographies to better understand community-level risk factors.

THRM is considering the development of social needs indices by assessing payer, income, and education, and by linking patient addresses to neighborhoods with lower health opportunity scores. This would stop short of using aggregate measures such as the CDC Social Vulnerability Index to stratify clinic patients based on where they live. That would miss opportunities for reaching patients with needs when applying community-level data to make decisions about who may be screened or provided access to resource navigation support.

A longer-term objective of the THRM for screening and referral is to develop pathways for addressing social needs as well as efforts to leverage existing diagnosis codes to secure reimbursement. The strategy and approach is payer-agnostic. It is to avoid stratifying patient populations by perceived need (i.e., insured by Medicaid) or diagnosis (diabetes, hypertension, or other comorbidities). Continuing with a universal approach is a core principle and essential to promoting equitable access to services for those who identify with social needs.

Community Health Worker Roles and Value

One of the most important goals of THRM is to better understand how addressing social needs can improve the efficiency, efficacy, and quality of ambulatory care. Breaking down silos between population health, ambulatory care, and community heath can be facilitated by appreciating the pivotal role that CHWs play in community health functions. The value of CHWs to population health and clinical leadership is evident through their day-to-day participation in multidisciplinary teams. The lived experience of CHWs is critical to accurately identify and meet social needs of patients.

Clinician Recognition:

These following commentaries from clinicians note the importance of Community Health Workers.

> Patients approach me for help with physical, mental, or emotional problems. These problems are usually a result of inadequate or complete lack of resources needed for human beings to attain health and happiness. The Community Health Worker fills a void that I can't.

"Screenings are critical to success and the ability to meet our patient's needs. People don't voluntarily divulge this kind of information unless they are asked. Healthcare workers can talk until they're blue in the face, but unless the patient has their most basic needs met, all treatment falls on deaf ears. To have patient engagement that's required for a positive health outcome, basic human needs must be met. First identified, then compassionately addressed and assistance provided."

"We're allotted twenty minutes for a visit to address all the medical needs of the patient. When they have social needs, CHWs are able address them and follow up with the medical plan too. If the patient doesn't have insurance, they can assist with that. If the patient can't afford their medications, they can assist with that. If the patient doesn't have transportation, they can assist with that. It allows for total patient care."

"Our CHW is an essential part of our Pediatrics team. Before she started, there were so many patients and families in need of assistance we couldn't provide, and that affected the health and well-being of children. When parents are worried about food, heat, housing, and transportation, then children suffer. Our CHW identifies resources in the community I've

> never heard of. Parents see that we really care about the health and wellness of their families, and that encourages parents to bring children in for well visits. The families have social needs that CHWs assist them with like food, beds, electricity, even education assistance. All these improve quality of life for the children, which improves the ability to be educated and grow into productive healthy adults."
>
> "Having a Community Health Worker here has made a big difference in many patients' quality of life and I'd go so far as to say even the quantity of life for several patients."
>
> "We're the sole Primary Care practice in our community that accepts Medicare and Medicaid. Our reputation and community perception are critical to the hospital's success. People will go elsewhere when they feel our system doesn't care about them as a community. The gratitude that our CHW receives can't be measured by money, but her work exemplifies the mission of our founding Sisters of Mercy."

CHWs channel the voice of patients to elevate awareness of clinical and community health teams on the barriers and challenges patients face in meeting social needs that compromise their ability to achieve better health. Hiring empathetic CHWs with lived experience is essential for the success of primary care teams, building relationships with front-line personnel, and forging effective community partnerships.

In turn, CHW Coordinators are an essential resource to tie together CHW activities across the market. Coordinators are often social workers or nurses with care coordination experience who serve multiple clinics by bridging primary care delivery and community health functions. Coordinators assist in the integration of social care into clinic workflows and leverage screening and referral data into useful information. This is used to improve collaboration with community partners to close gaps in services. They also contribute to better use of these data in leveraging community benefit dollars and community investment funds to strengthen the fabric and capacity of local communities.

Personal Stories

The following comments reflect personal stories that are an important complement to quantitative data gathered from each of CommonSpirit's health systems in Colorado, Iowa, and Kentucky (names changed to protect patient confidentiality).

> **Sharon**
> Sharon is fifty-nine years old, low functioning, and can't read or write. With the help of hospice, she's taking care of her husband who has dementia. One of our physicians brought her to our attention. Sharon identified needs for food security and was immediately set up with food

banks in the area. She also had outstanding medical bills, and we have helped her process financial aid applications. She also needed assistance with managing funds so that she could afford her prescription co-pays. She also needed new dentures that fit and had problems eating. We helped her fill out an application for new dentures and she has just been approved through a local foundation for ongoing dental care.

Sharon also heats her trailer with chopped wood. We've helped her reach out to Habitat for Humanity to upgrade her heat source from chopped wood and to do a home inspection for improved insulation and door and window repairs. Sharon couldn't do any of the work herself with the applications and didn't know where to get help. This is an ongoing process, and we will continue to keep in touch.

Smith Family

A few weeks after we had integrated CHWs, we met with the Smiths, a family of six that was the victim of a house fire. The house was a total loss. They had come to the clinic to check for smoke inhalation.

Because of the situation, we were able to connect the Smiths with Community Co-Operative Care (CCC). Through CCC, they were provided with clothes (three sets per family member) and food. When they find a home, CCC will furnish their home for free with used furniture. We also asked the mother if she received WIC and explained what the program was for. Mrs. Smith was able to connect with the county health department to get set up. For housing, we immediately called the local housing authority and was faxed a list of homes that were available for rent. Mrs. Smith followed up the next week to sign up for HUD benefits and get on their waiting list. The Red Cross provided $300 for a security deposit.

We also connected the Smiths with the county school resource department. By the end of the day, they had clothing and school supplies for their two school-aged daughters. We kept in touch for another three weeks to be sure that the family was able to secure the resources they needed.

Judith

As a result of screening, Judith came to me needing help with expenses for raising her grandchildren. At the start of our conversation, Judith was concerned that I wouldn't be able to help unless I knew of a resource that could provide the gallon of milk and loaf of bread her growing grandchildren went through each day. I didn't have a specific resource but knew of a program that supports grandparents who are raising their grandchildren. I connected Judith to this resource. At follow-up, I learned she had received $200 for each child for back-to-school clothes.

This reminded me of how important it is to reach out and meet with our community resources; otherwise,

I wouldn't have known about the grandparent program. Also, I take heart in knowing that sometimes I can help families meet their needs in a roundabout way. With Judith, I didn't have a resource specifically for her food needs, but I was able to help her find assistance with other expenses, which left more money in her budget for groceries. I think universal screening is key to identifying patients who need assistance. Without screening, we might never have identified Judith's concerns and the stress she was facing in raising her grandchildren.

Valerie

Valerie screened positive on the personal safety question. Before I met with her, I checked in with her provider. Valerie's provider was very surprised that she had answered yes to the screening question. When I met with Valerie, she hadn't told many others about her previous domestic violence experiences but felt this time she needed emotional support. I was able to get Valerie scheduled for counseling with a behavioral health provider who is co-located in our clinic.

Without screening, Valerie might have continued to hold onto her emotions around prior experiences and might not have reached out for help. I think this is a good example of how the screening tool helps patients feel more comfortable in asking for assistance with their needs.

Helen

In our rural area we have a lot of moms, dads, and grandparents who can't read or write. I was in the clinic lobby one day and met Helen, who is taking care of her fourth-grade great-granddaughter. I asked if she would like to fill out the screening form. Helen said she would love to, but she does not read very well because she only has a second-grade education. I explained that I would love to assist her by asking the questions and filling in the information. That way, if she needs assistance, I can help her as well as her granddaughter.

Helen let me know that she really needed a hearing aid. Helen had been using her brother's as hers are broken, and she can't afford new ones. So, we called a local audiology group to find out more about their "Hear Now" program. Helen needed a referral from a physician, so I reached out to her oncologist to get a referral. Helen is also a cancer survivor, and her oncologist was more than happy to assist. Helen qualified, completed her hearing test, and was fitted for new hearing aids at no cost through collaboration of the audiology group with our state university's rural health outreach program. Helen was very thankful for the assistance and looks forward to being able to hear her granddaughter's voice more clearly.

Training

CHWs and CHW Coordinators rated the types of training that would be beneficial in relation to: principles of community health work (rated second highest), goal setting with patients, individual social support (rated third highest), patient self-management, trauma-informed care, collaborating with medical professional, community health concepts, system navigation, adverse childhood experiences, teaching methods and strategies, home visiting, communication, presentation and facilitation skills, patient self-sufficiency measures, motivational interviewing and stages of change, behavioral health, stress management and conflict resolution for CHWs (also rated third highest) problem solving, how health insurance works (rated highest), substance abuse, data collection, and documentation.

Offering full-time employment, benefits, and career ladder programs for CHWs is essential in retention and for building a healthcare workforce that represents lived experience and lived expertise. A high school diploma or GED is recommended along with relevant work experience. Training in patient engagement, such as motivational interviewing, should be part of the onboarding process as well as shadowing other members of the clinic care and administrative teams for CHW to develop an understanding of their roles and responsibilities.

Conclusion

Equity is at the heart of CommonSpirit's mission and values. One of the purposes in developing the Total Health Roadmap is to address how CommonSpirit can improve its accountabilities and strategies for patient outcomes influenced by social determinants. The implementation process is based on active listening, multisector collaboration, and the foundational value of human dignity and social justice. Accordingly, CommonSpirit's approach to calculating return on investment is shifting from a conventional view related to clinical outcomes and to include community outcomes based on outreach activities and closing care gap in health disparities. As an organization, CommonSpirit is adjusting the lens through which national and local care delivery systems view sustainability. Conventional costs savings calculations must be balanced by stronger indicators of community health status that will guide targeted investments to remove barriers to inequitable care.

Improvement in health equity continues to be the defining objective of CommonSpirit's mission to build long-term capacity in the communities it serves.

Key Takeaways

Advancing the role of Community Health Functions in Health Systems

- The lessons learned and frameworks refined by the pioneer markets represent new opportunities for health system Community Health functions to play a better-defined role in developing the cross-sector **collaborations** and community **capacity** required for success in integrating social care into healthcare.

- Community Health leaders can apply the screening and referral data collected in primary care to add depth to community health needs assessments and to refine community health improvement plans to redirect resources toward advancing health equity.
- A better understanding of the community agencies and organizations called upon to support social needs may also assist in identifying additional collaborators that should be at the table during assessment and planning processes.

Value of Community Health Workers

- CHWs channel the voice of our patients and elevate awareness of clinical and community health teams regarding the barriers and challenges patients face in meeting social needs that compromise their ability to achieve better health.
- CHWs are a valuable addition to the primary care team but also play an essential role in development of effective community partnerships.
- The CHW Coordinator plays an essential role in bridging primary care delivery and community health functions—by assisting in integration of social care into clinic workflows and by transforming screening and referral data into useful information to guide improved engagement and collaboration with cross-sector partners to close gaps in community capacity.

Value for System Population Health Functions

- Universal screening is necessary for equal access (payer-agnostic) to equitable care as defined by patient needs and wishes rather than by payers or primary diagnoses.
- Primary care is a valuable starting place for development of universal screening and the integration of new services and support in a trusted care relationship that may span the patient's life course.

Additional Considerations for Mission, Community Health, Population Health Leaders

- A broader approach and a longer-term view is required for tracking the impact of clinical and community work intended to address social needs and to move upstream to tackle the root causes of negative social determinants and health disparities.
- A balance between clinical outcomes and community-level indicators/measures must be developed to mark progress in delivering holistic care.
- Seeking this balanced combination of measures and accountabilities represents a significant shift from the conventional approach of measuring clinical outcomes and return on investment separately from broader community outcomes (e.g., improvements in access, quality of social services).
- Health systems need to adjust the lens through which care delivery systems view sustainability. Conventional

> ROI or cost savings calculations must move to include stronger measures that reflect improvements in systems of care delivery as well as contributions to improved health *equity* in communities.

Executive Comments

Elizabeth Miller, PhD, is Director of Implementation of CommonSpirit's Total Health Roadmap.

There are no shortcuts to measuring impact.

Based on our initial work in Phase 1 and our understanding of the literature, we've come to the following conclusion: Tracking the impact of clinical and community work intended to address social needs and move upstream to address the root causes requires a broader approach and a longer-term view.

The usual cost-benefit analyses and ROIs do not reflect the reality of addressing root causes in a systematic way. Tackling root causes is necessary and far more complicated. It takes decades, not just a year or two. There are no shortcuts.

We believe this requires establishing a balance between clinical outcomes and community-level indicators that mark progress in providing holistic care and improving the ability of communities to sustain good health for their citizens. The challenge is figuring out a balanced combination of practical measures and stakeholder accountabilities. This represents a significant shift from tracking clinical outcomes and return on investment separate from community improvement outcomes. Both must be tracked in parallel to identify influencers and synergies that contribute to overall impact.

Measuring and tracking community-level outcomes—as opposed to process measures and outputs—is a challenge that requires not only community input, but community direction on what is most meaningful to community members in terms of specific outcomes. These efforts go far beyond tracking the usual disease prevalence rates and the practice of acting on perceived gaps in care that are based on aggregate community-level data.

Two bodies of work are essential for forward progress:

1. Screening and referral for social needs in our clinics and hospitals to understand the impact of social determinants on individual health and the challenges and barriers our patients face in addressing their own needs.
2. Using what we learn from patients to improve how we partner with our communities and where we direct our resources as part of local economic and social ecosystems.

We need to adjust the lens of how our national and local care delivery systems view sustainability of new services and programs, moving us from the conventional return-on-investment or cost-savings calculations to a broader framework of better, stronger indicators. This means crafting measures that reflect improvements in our systems of care delivery *and* in our contributions to improved health equity in our communities.

The challenge is to develop and refine metrics that signal improvements in community health status, which reflect the lived experience of the patient and the collective voice of the community. This calls for co-creating new measures in partnership with the community. That's the essence of making decisions and investments of time, energy, and resources through an equity lens.

This challenge is at the heart of our continuing journey.

Endnotes

1. National Academies of Sciences, Engineering, and Medicine. 2017. Communities in action: Pathways to health equity. Washington, DC: The National Academies Press. Available at http://nationalacademies.org/hmd/Reports/2017/communities-in-action-pathways-to-health-equity.aspx.
2. Healthy People 2030, U.S. Department of Health and Human Services, Office of Disease Prevention and Health Promotion. Retrieved March 28, 2021 from https://health.gov/healthypeople/objectives-and-data/social-determinants-health
3. National Academies of Sciences, Engineering, and Medicine. 2016. *Accounting for Social Risk Factors in Medicare Payment: Identifying Social Risk Factors.* Washington, DC: The National Academies Press. https://doi.org/10.17226/21858

References

Paula Braveman, Elaine Arkin, Tracy Orleans, Dwayne Proctor, and Alonzo Plough. 2017. *What Is Health Equity? And What Difference Does a Definition Make?* Princeton, NJ: Robert Wood Johnson Foundation. Available at https://www.rwjf.org/en/library/research/2017/05/what-is-health-equity-.html.

National Academies of Sciences, Engineering, and Medicine. 2018. *Implementing Quality Measures for Accountability in Community-Based Care for People with Serious Illness: Proceedings of a Workshop*. Washington, DC: The National Academies Press. https://www.nap.edu/catalog/25202/implementing-quality-measures-for-accountability-in-community-based-care-for-people-withserious-illness

Chapter 5.

Presbyterian Health Case Study

Introduction

As the largest private employer (13,000) in New Mexico, not-for-profit Presbyterian Healthcare Services is committed to improving the health of everyone in the state and contributing to a healthy economy. That means focusing on health equity and the Social Determinants of Health. Leigh Caswell, Vice President for Community Health, says, "Presbyterian views things from an equity lens— who's receiving the benefit and who's experiencing the burden."

Presbyterian facilitated community discussions across the state to prioritize determinants of health and develop specific interventions to impact health outcomes. This was done with an emphasis on equity for all participants and each county.

In alignment with community priorities, Presbyterian was awarded an Accountable Health Communities (AHC) grant of $4.5 million over five years from the Centers for Medicare and Medicaid Innovation in May of 2017. Milestones for Track 3 Alignment grantees are extensive:

- Establish relationships between hospitals, health centers, and behavioral service providers to screen either 75,000 Medicaid and Medicare beneficiaries or 51 percent of all beneficiaries within a geographic region.
- Deliver screenings electronically through clinical staff or arranged through a third-party organization.
- Update and maintain a database of services every six months.
- Submit operating procedures detailing the exchange of data and interventions.
- Report data to CMS on screenings, accepted interventions, intervention results, and availability and utilization of local services.
- Build and maintain active relationships with community service providers.

Program Direction

Presbyterian Health is building a culture of health through a Health Change Model that rests on four beliefs: health as a shared value, cross sector collaborations, stronger integration of health services and systems, and healthier and more equitable communities. The intended outcomes are improvements in population health, well-being, and equity; enhance individual and community well-being, manage chronic disease, and reduce toxic stress. (See Appendix 1: Presbyterian Health Change Model.)

In 2016, the Center for Community Health (CCH) was established to centralize Presbyterian's efforts to impact community health status and engage stakeholders to collaborate on interventions throughout the state. CCH formulates data-supported programs and pursues social impact investments as well as local and state government agencies.

As an anchor institution, Presbyterian leverages grants from federal and state sources, and philanthropic organizations. Presbyterian often functions as a statewide convener to solicit input through forums and tribal councils, and to measure collective impact.

Presbyterian is currently screening all patients for a full array of health and social needs, using CMS-validated eight questions. Three screening domains are illustrated in Appendix 2. (See Screening Domains.)

The AHC has been implemented systemwide with the aid of Community Health Workers hired to assess patients' unmet social needs and link them to appropriate community services. Says Caswell, "We're focusing on food, housing, transportation, utility assistance, and personal safety. Our efforts are based on data for key social determinants across all sites."

To implement the strategy, Presbyterian relies on the Unite Us platform to support the referral process in building and managing community resource networks. This has enabled clinicians and support staff to meet patients' unmet social needs, reduce Medicare inpatient stay and unplanned readmissions, and decrease Medicaid emergency department visits. Presbyterian's objective is to develop a seamless clinical-community partnership. Caswell further describes the objective: "We're working to build a closed-loop referral process so that Community Health Workers and community resource providers will be connected throughout the care process, especially in our rural communities."

The most recent community health assessment indicated four priority categories for each county. The most important priorities for Central New Mexico (Bernalillo, Sandoval, Torrance, and Valencia) were the following:

1. Behavioral Health
2. Social Determinants of Health
3. Access to Care
4. Healthy Eating and Active Living

A collective impact approach for community health improvement is used. It focuses on capacity building and partnering with local health infrastructure to use resources and implement broad-based evidence and practice-based community health activities to address significant health needs in the region.

Presbyterian's prevention framework for each county draws upon three categories of activity to guide initiatives and strategy.

1. Traditional clinical prevention by increasing the use of evidence-based services
2. Innovative clinical prevention by providing services outside the clinical setting
3. Community-Wide Prevention by implementing interventions that reach whole populations

To guide community interventions on social needs, Presbyterian developed twelve principles:

1. Data will be used to identify interventions.
2. Interventions will be consistent with best known evidence or practices.
3. Purpose of each intervention will be easy to understand.
4. Interventions will be simple and enhance existing initiatives.
5. Interventions will be practical.
6. Interventions will be sustainable .
7. Interventions will be engaging to the intended population.
8. Interventions will be age-appropriate and culturally relevant.
9. Interventions will promote equity while not reinforcing inequity in health outcomes.
10. Plan will be integrated with existing Presbyterian plans.
11. Presbyterian will collaborate with community agencies to strengthen adopted strategies.
12. Interventions will be evaluated and monitored.

Community health improvement services must also support the following guidelines:

- Be carried out or supported for the purpose of improving community health or safety.
- Be subsidized by the organization.
- Not generate an inpatient or outpatient bill.

- Not be provided primarily for marketing services.
- Not be more beneficial to the organization than to the community (e.g., not designed primarily to increase referrals of patients with third-party coverage).
- Not be required for licensure or accreditation.
- Not be restricted to individuals affiliated with the organization (employees and physicians).
- Meet at least one community benefit objective, including improving access to health services, enhancing public health, advancing generalizable knowledge, and relieving government burden.
- Respond to demonstrated community needs.

Implementing Plan Priorities

For each high priority health need, Presbyterian aims to build community capacity by connecting community health assessment with measurable outcomes, and specific strategies for each of the four highest priorities. System-wide strategies are included in the Implementation Plan with detailed strategies for each county. An overview of each priority, goal, objective, and strategy is shown below. (See also Appendix 3: Community Health Implementation Strategy)

1. Improve Behavioral Care

Preventing unhealthy substance use, including tobacco, alcohol, prescription, and illicit drugs by youth and adults, receiving care or insurance benefits from Presbyterian, and/or Presbyterian's workforce. This is done by increasing resiliency, promoting primary prevention, providing education about behaviors, and treatment resources.

Improving well-being for youth, families, and individuals. This is done by reducing stigma associated with behavioral health conditions and stigma associated with receiving mental health and substance use treatment; by increasing opportunities to find and receive the appropriate level of intervention and care. This is done by increasing access to and completion of substance use and other behavioral health treatments.

The behavioral health goal has measurable outcomes and specific strategies over three years.

Goal: Decrease drug overdose deaths in Central New Mexico counties over the next three years by 5 percent. CHA Community Indicator (annual trend): Age Adjusted Drug Overdose Deaths per 100,000 population.

Objective: Increase number of providers prescribing or providing Medication Assisted Treatment over next three years. **Outcome Measure:** Percent change in number of providers (source: Prescription Monitoring Program).

Strategy (12): Increase substance use disorder treatment and fill gaps in care by training and certifying providers in Medication Assisted Treatment.

Process Measure 1: Number of PHS providers trained to provide MAT to date. **Process Measure 2:** Number of non-PHS providers trainings to provide MAT to date.

2. Address Social Determinants of Health

Increasing identification of health-related social needs and connecting individuals to community resources.
Increasing community resource gap identification and strategic investment by Presbyterian and others in the social service system to improve the health of patient, health insurance members, and communities.
Increasing the number of policies, partners, investments, and programs that address the root causes of unmet social needs.

The social determinants goals have measurable outcomes and specific strategies over three years.

Goal: Increase connection of low-income individuals to healthy food resources. **CHA Community Indicator:** Percept population considered low income with limited access to healthy food by county (USDA).
Objective: Triple the number of food insecure patients utilizing Community Health food programs by 2022.
Outcome Measure: Percent of patients who completed food programs (denominator is number patients referred).
Strategy (2): Increase clinical opportunities to identify social needs that impact opportunities for health and well-being.

Process Measure 1: Number of clinical locations conducting screenings. **Process Measure 2:** Prevalence of food insecurity among patients.

3. Increase Access to Care

Increase individuals' ability to better manage their health and navigate health and social care.
Add members of the care team and supportive infrastructure to increase and enhance connection to appropriate assistance including behavioral health, chronic disease management, and social supports.
Grow capacity to meet demand for healthcare services.

The access to care goal has measurable outcomes and specific strategies over three years.

Goal: Promote equity and the elimination of health and healthcare inequities. CHA Community Indicator: Number and percent of LGBTQ+ high school students who reported persistent feelings of sadness and hopelessness.
Objective: Increase number of providers who are confident and able to provide high quality patient care to lesbian, gay, bisexual, transgender, questioning, + patients.
Outcome Measure: Number of Presbyterian providers (by specialty) who qualify for GLMA attestation for LGBTQ.
Strategy (7b): Help lead and support Presbyterian to become a provider of choice for Lesbian, Gay, Bisexual, Transgender, and Queer or Questioning (LGBTQ+).

Process Measure 1: Human Rights Campaign Health Equity Index Score. **Process Measure 2:** Number of staff attending optional, relevant trainings.

4. Support and Promote Healthy Eating and Active Living

Improve the nutrition of residents by increasing availability of healthy foods, education, and enjoyment preparing and eating healthy food.
Increase the ability of local food producers to provide healthy food to individuals and institutions.
Increase physical activity and improve infrastructure to promote safe and accessible places to exercise.
Improve prevention and self-management of chronic disease among populations served.

The healthy eating and active living goal has measurable outcomes and specific strategies over three years.

Goal: Decrease risk factors for morbidity and mortality due to chronic disease. **CHA Community Indicators:** Number and percent of high school students who are obese. Percent of adults who are at a healthy weight.
Objective: Maintain or increase consumption of fruits and vegetables by youth and adults over the next three years (< state average).
Outcome Measure: Youth and adults reporting consumption of five or more fruits and vegetables every day.

Strategy (4): Support nutrition education, long-term behavior change, and enjoyment of healthy food through cooking classes, tastings, demos, recipe creation, and other educational opportunities and events.
Process Measure 1: Pre/post measure of fruit and vegetable consumption. **Process Measure 2:** Number of classes held at PHS demonstration kitchens.

Community Impact

The Accountable Care Communities program is an innovations project for CMS, which extends to evaluating community impact programs (including Presbyterian) at a national level. Evaluation is based on using claims data to measure the impact on quality and cost of care. Direct impact on health outcomes specifically related to community health interventions remains a long-term goal for Presbyterian.

Presbyterian currently tracks metrics such as completed screenings, referrals and follow-up, resources provided, and whether needs were met. More data will be mined as screening is expanded across the organization through the Accountable Health Communities work.

As an example of what data is gathered, the following information is collected at the end of each quarter for virtual cooking classes:

- Demographics
- Food Farmacy patient participation in classes

- Number of referred patients per month
- Number of individuals with or at-risk for diabetes and other chronic disease
- Increased knowledge of nutrition and healthy cooking, food safety and healthy nutrition, practices, including for chronic disease
- Increased skills in healthy cooking
- Increased confidence in home meal prep, shopping on a budget, and making healthy food decisions, including for chronic disease
- Improved attitude/motivation toward healthy foods, trying new foods, and managing chronic disease through diet
- Improved fruits and veggies consumption, food safety practices, nutrition practices

Each program that is specifically for people with diabetes or another chronic disease program (e.g., Diabetes ReCHARGE, Kitchen Creations, Diabetes Self-Management programs) has its own measurement approach. For Diabetes ReCHARGE, for example, measures of self-care include progress toward behavior goals. An end of program survey (self-reported), measures change in habits and confidence, and pre- and post-A1C levels.

Every year Presbyterian tracks the impact of outreach efforts in each county. In Central New Mexico counties, program impacts for Bernalillo, Sandoval, Torrance, and Valencia counties are noted in relation to initiatives.

Bernalillo County (population 677,858)

In partnership with the Bernalillo County Community Health Council, in 2014, Presbyterian received a four-year, $3.6 million Racial and Ethnic Approaches to Community Health (REACH) cooperative agreement from the CDC to focus on improving poor nutrition, physical inactivity, and lack of access to chronic disease prevention, risk reduction, and management in two New Mexico communities through policy, system, and environmental changes.

Presbyterian was again awarded this funding for approximately $800,000 per year for up to five years beginning in 2018. REACH is part of a U.S. Department of Health and Human Services initiative to reduce chronic diseases, promote healthier lifestyles, reduce health disparities, and control healthcare spending. One example of this work is the Healthy Here Mobile Farmer's Market, which visits food-insecure neighborhoods and offers reduced price, locally grown produce during the growing season.

Presbyterian provided $36.4 million in funding, including financial assistance, to twenty-five organizations. An additional $5.8 million was leveraged from external funds. Participating in days of service were 430 staff and twenty-eight community volunteers.

Healthy Eating and Active Living

Wellness Referral Center is a community-wide resource that Presbyterian refers patients to. It received 3,831 referrals from thirty-eight community clinics and connected patients to community support services. These included ten cooking classes, dance classes, and eight options for chronic disease management sessions. A total of 1,374 individuals used at least one of these services.

The mobile farmers' market sold 7,995 pounds of food, twenty-nine patients redeemed $9,734 worth of vouchers at farmers' markets, and 42,564 pounds of healthy food was distributed to food insecure families. Presbyterian hospitals provided 7,002 free healthy meals for kids while 547 adult patients took advantage of the Food Farmacy service on a weekly basis.

Community Health Resource Center (on the Presbyterian Kaseman Hospital campus) houses a demonstration teaching kitchen where free classes are given by registered dietitians. The space is also used for ongoing dance and exercise classes (juggling, yoga, Zumba), dementia workshops, community gardening sessions, mental health first aid training, and Community Health Worker certification classes.

The resource center partners with Meals on Wheels, Three Sisters Kitchen, and Encuento to support local agriculture through a $400,000 matching grant with USDA Connecting Harvest to Health.

Prevention of Unhealthy Substance Use

Presbyterian implemented a wide-ranging strategy to address substance use and addiction. It established a telehealth program that provides behavioral health triage and consult services in hospital emergency departments. Education and training programs were developed to combat stigma and increase access to addiction and pain medicine through mental health first aid training.

Sandoval County (population 142,704)

Presbyterian contributed $5.7 million in funding, including financial assistance, to organizations in eight communities and pueblos. An additional $62,000 went to support the county health council, primarily for the health literacy ambassador program for young people, and $12,500 went to other community organizations in the county.

Healthy Living

Three-thousand dollats was awarded for free meals to kids, and additional support was given to children and families for play equipment. The Rust Medical Center hosts community classes on bariatric nutrition, breastfeeding support, senior care information, yoga classes for cancer patients, and periodic blood drives. Presbyterian employees supply sixty-five weekend backpacks filled with healthy snacks to low-income elementary school children.

Two-thousand dollars went to support tribal council youth programs. Two thousand books were distributed to elementary schools for the 10x10 health literacy program for high-risk children, and an additional 300 books in Spanish were given out. The after-school program on adolescent diabetes prevention received 120 books while 250 books went to Boys and Girls Clubs. A health inequities program serves 1,200 children from many neighborhoods and tribal communities.

Torrance County (population 15,519)

The amount of $36.4 million in community benefits, including financial assistance, was given for outreach efforts in three communities, and $62,00 was awarded to fund county health council activities.

Active Living and Healthy Eating

At hospitals, 7,002 free healthy meals were distributed, and forty elementary school students engaged in healthy eating activities with Farm to Table.

Active living initiatives included re-striping a cross walk for safe routes to school and the completion of a hiking trail.

Prevention of Unhealthy Substance Use

Substance use prevention social marketing campaigns reeached 27,111 students and parents, and seventy-five residents were trained to administer Naloxone/Narcan for opioid overdoses. Five senior centers hosted training on proper disposal of medications, and five medication lockboxes were distributed in the community.

Valencia County (population 76,027)

Sixty-two thousand dollars was allocated to support health council activities impacting five neighborhoods. Eleven thousand dollars was given to support the development of a rural health plan. Ten Presbyterian employees participated in service days, and nineteen community partnerships were strengthened.

Active Living and Healthy Eating

Health fairs reached 850 community members, and fifty-seven patient referrals were made by the Wellness Referral Center.

Community Wellness Council sponsored a facilitator to help community members create a culture of hope for at-risk youth through training sessions. The council also sponsored a book and action lab on preventing adverse childhood experiences and family trauma. In addition, community task force meetings addressed mentoring and early childhood and behavioral health needs.

Community Context

Behavioral Health

Community members indicated that behavioral health, particularly medication-assisted treatment for opioid use disorder, was not readily available. Transportation to treatment facilities was a widespread barrier, especially in rural areas. Interpersonal violence and child abuse were also quite prevalent.

Community-wide collaboration is central to improving access to mental health and behavioral health. Support services and treatment focus on community-based campaigns, school-based health centers, and peer support services.

Behavioral health initiatives encourage tobacco cessation and healthy substance use, including prevention and treatment.

Social Determinants of Health

Social Determinants of Health are addressed by connecting individuals' health-related social needs to community resources. This requires identifying gaps in care and making investments to improve patient health and community health status. Likewise, it means addressing root causes of unmet social needs and demonstrating measurable outcomes (e.g., reducing overdose deaths, meeting unmet food needs).

Improvements in build environment included walkability assessments, bicycle path lighting and re-striping bicycle lanes, adopt-a-highway program, Silver Sneakers enrollment campaigns for seniors at health clubs, and community runs and walks to encourage physical activity.

Social determinants involve programs to address violence, poverty, education, economic development, built environment, equity, and the root causes of unmet social needs. For example, if a patient has difficulty paying utility costs, Presbyterian's Community Health Workers can see if they are eligible for utility assistance. Or, if they are experiencing violence, a Community Health Worker may connect the individual with a local women's shelter.

Health-related social needs such as housing, transportation, violence, and food access may involve aligning services with other community partners or government agencies.

Access to Care and Services

Access to care and specialty care was a persistent problem because of distance, lack of insurance, and unaffordable prescription drugs. Access likewise includes expansion of population health workforce, stigma reduction, education and training, equity of care initiatives, and health literacy.

Access to care was bolstered through programs at educational centers, working with behavioral health specialists, training programs in Mental Health First Aid, and better coordination with hospitals and urgent care clinics. Mental Health First Aid is a skills-based training course that teaches participants about mental health and substance-use issues.

Many communities in central New Mexico now have Roadrunner Food Banks that provide access to healthy foods. In addition, partnerships between farmers' markets and WIC increase access to mobile food pantries and mobile farmers' markets in food deserts. Double Up Food Bucks enable SNAP beneficiaries to buy twice as much produce at farmers' markets and grocery stores.

Healthy Eating and Active Living

New Mexico has the third highest rate for senior hunger in the country at 11.5 percent. Presbyterian partners with Meals on Wheels, Three Sisters Kitchen, and Encuento to connect seniors with healthy food options. This initiative, Connecting Harvest to Health/Connectando con la Salud, is funded through USDA and has trained 135 Spanish-speaking home health aides in cooking and nutrition for seniors. More than 63,000 pounds of local produce has been purchased through the program and included in free meal delivery for 1,620 low-income seniors.

Caswell finds that making healthy choices around food is complicated and that "we have to work on different strategies to match up with cultural preferences and a host of access issues based on income, health insurance coverage, transportation barriers and environmental conditions. In low-income communities there is a lot less opportunity to make healthy choices." With this reality in mind, Presbyterian offers healthy food prescriptions and mobile farmers' markets to meet people where they are, not just at the hospital.

In the 2019 season, the mobile farmers' market provided food to 1,697 residents of Albuquerque's international district and south valley neighborhoods. It offered healthy, affordable fruits and vegetables, as well as educational classes and handouts on how to prepare the food in cost-effective, delicious, and easy-to-prepare ways. As an example, Presbyterian offers classes for people with diabetes to learn about meal planning, balancing carbohydrates, and adding more beans, fruits, and vegetables to their diets.

However, one of the most persistent problems was the preponderance of food deserts and lack of access to healthy food, compounded by poverty. Food insecurity, food quality, and healthy eating were identified as some of the most significant health issues in rural areas as well as Albuquerque.

According to Caswell, implementing food initiatives requires flexibility and ingenuity. "Rural areas have significant distance issues, and too many people rely on limited food choices at local gas stations. The local grocery stores might be fifty miles away."

Children at several Presbyterian hospitals receive free meals in the hospital cafeterias. Food is reimbursed by USDA Child Nutrition Programs and local agencies.

These projects are designed to improve nutrition and encourage indoor and outdoor physical activity. Initiatives include free healthy eating meals for kids, nutrition education for all ages, community gardens, community-sponsored agriculture, increasing access to healthy food, creating more parks and playgrounds, safe sidewalks, and bike and walking paths.

Healthy Eating and Active Living

During class sessions, in 2021, there were 2,525 adults who participated in 124 cooking classes and 234 active living classes. Participants were provided with 378 meals kits. Participants reported the following:

- 94 percent apply nutrition information they learned in class when making food choices.
- 92 percent increased confidence in cooking healthy meals at home.
- 91 percent agree that attending classes is helpful and valuable.
- 89 percent have tried a new ingredient they learned from class.

- 81 percent increased their consumption of both fruits and vegetables.
- 79 percent report decreased levels of stress after attending an active living class.

Each class provides opportunities to learn basic cooking methods, knife-handling skills, storing procedures, food safety tips for cooking together as a family, and recipe modifications. Classes provide guidance and nutritional support for management of chronic conditions such as hypertension, diabetes, and weight management. Active living classes aim to decrease stress while providing support to improve strength, flexibility, and promote overall wellness.

Patients were referred to the classes by 243 providers and forty clinics. Many participants manage a chronic condition such as diabetes (42 percent), hypertension (23 percent), kidney disease (26 percent), food allergies (6 percent), and other conditions (10 percent).

Food Farmacy

The Food Farmacy, which is available at two Presbyterian locations, prescribes healthy food for patients with food insecurity needs. Food pharmacies help patients with health issues like diabetes and hypertension to lower their A1C level and blood pressure. Seventy-one percent of patients reported achieving their goal of lowering A1C. Fifty percent achieved their goal of lowering blood pressure. Sixty-four percent experienced an increase in well-being.

Summary

Presbyterian Healthcare Services relies on multi-sector partnerships to further health equity and make it an ongoing priority. Social health determinants of health are central to Presbyterian's commitment to improving the lives of its members, patients, and employees in New Mexico.

Key Takeaways

- Interventions must promote equity to be sustainable.
- Addressing the root causes of health and health inequities is necessary to impact health.
- Community health interventions must be clearly stated, easy to read, and understood by patients and members.
- Partnering with local health councils and other community partners is key to implementing action plans.
- Health councils are trusted conveners for underserved populations, nonprofit organizations, and government agencies.

Appendices

Appendix 1: Presbyterian Health Change Model

Presbyterian's strategy to improve community health is to implement four top priorities (i.e., behavioral health, Social Determinants of Health, access to care, and healthy eating and active living) by building a culture of health. This change model explicitly recognizes health as a shared value, pursues cross sector collaborations, further integrates health services and systems, and supports healthier and more equitable communities.

The change model focuses on improving outcomes in four areas: (1) population health and equity, (2) enhanced well-being for individuals, (3) managing chronic disease and reducing toxic stress, and (4) enhanced well-being in the community.

Within this framework, specific programs are organized within four clusters of activity.

1. Community Health Assessment, Planning, and Implementation.
    - Health assessments and implementation plans
    - Convening and aligning
    - Community capacity building

2. Community and Clinical Linkages
    - Social needs and behavioral health support
    - Food Farmacy and free healthy meals
    - Wellness referrals
    - Evidenced-based chronic disease self-management
    - Infrastructure to support care teams
3. Health Equity
    - LGBTQ strategy
    - Social Determinants of Health
    - Data analysis and system change initiatives
4. Community Benefit
    - Place-based investing
    - Safe streets, local food systems, violenceprevention, policy and/or institution strategy
    - Maintain non-profit status

Appendix 2: Screening Domains

Domain	Question	Citation
Living Situation	What is your living situation today?	National Association of Community Health Centers and Partners, National Association of Community Health Centers, Association of Asian Pacific Community Health Organizations, Association OPC, Institute for Alternative Futures. (2017). PRAPARE.http://www.nachc.org/research-and-data/prapare/
Food	Within the past twelve months, have you worried that your food would run out before you got money to buy more?	Hager, E. R., Quigg, A. M., Black, M. M., Coleman, S. M., Heeren, T., Rose-Jacobs, R., Cook, J. T., Ettinger de Cuba, S. E., Casey, P. H., Chilton, M., Cutts, D. B., Meyers A. F., Frank, D. A. (2010). Development and Validity of a 2-Item Screen to Identify Families at Risk for Food Insecurity. *Pediatrics*, 126(1), 26-32. doi:10.1542/peds.2009-3146.
	Within the past twelve months, has the food you bought not lasted and you didn't have money to get more?	

Transportation	In the past twelve months, has lack of transportation kept you from medical appointments, meetings, work, or from getting things needed for daily living?	National Association of Community Health Centers and Partners, National Association of Community Health Centers, Association of Asian Pacific Community Health Organizations, Association OPC, Institute for Alternative Futures. (2017). PRAPARE.http://www.nachc.org/research-and-data/prapare/

Appendix 3: Community Health Implementation Goals and Outcome Measures

The overall priority is to increase well-being among New Mexicans. Outcome measures include increasing life expectancy at birth and reducing fourteen-plus poor mental health days in the last thirty days. In terms of reducing the impact of chronic conditions, outcome measures include lowering the prevalence of diagnosed hypertension and diabetes.

Four major categories have goals and outcome measures that document program impact.

Behavioral Health

- Decrease drug overdose deaths in communities served by Presbyterian.
- Increase treatment for alcohol and other drug use dependence for patients and members.

Social Determinants of Health

- Reduce household food insecurity for patients and community members.
- Improve the health of patients by supporting their social and economic needs to reduce inequitable outcomes.

Access to Care

- Increase health equity.
- Promote equity and elimination of health and health inequities.
- Decrease known inequities in health outcomes for the LGBTQ population.
- Decrease known inequities in access to and outcomes for perinatal and behavioral health.

Healthy Eating and Active Living

- Increase consumption of fresh, locally grown fruits and vegetables among adults and youth.
- Increase diabetes prevention and management in adult patients.

Executive Comments

Leigh Caswell is Vice President, Presbyterian Community Health

"Addressing Social Determinants of Health is critical to making a real difference in a community's health."

As a not-for-profit healthcare organization that has served the community since 1908, we're deeply invested in improving the health of the community. We realize that improving health also means investing in and partnering with communities in ways that extend beyond the care provided in our hospitals and clinics.

Addressing Social Determinants of Health—the economic and social conditions of people's lives that impact their health—is complex. But it's also critical to making a real difference in community health.

This work focuses on building on partnerships that address violence, poverty, education, economic development, built environment, equity, and the root causes of unmet social needs. Collecting data on what patients need and offering them the right resources is important. Presbyterian now asks every patient about their social needs, whether they have adequate food and housing, and connects them with resources through the electronic health record.

Other core priorities, identified through the community assessment process, focus on behavioral health, access to care, and initiatives focused on healthy eating and active living.

For example, to help improve behavioral health, peer support specialists help patients address substance use disorder needs following an Emergency Department visit. To encourage healthy eating, we provide a Food Farmacy for patients in need, diabetes self-management classes, and partner on a program that helps home health aides learn to prepare healthy food for senior clients.

Experience tells us that truly addressing the social needs of our patients and members requires strong partnerships with the community and our clinicians. In community health, our role is to connect the dots on behalf of the communities we serve.

Chapter 6.

Houston Methodist Hospital Case Study and Executive Interviews

Introduction

Houston Methodist is a hospital system with more than 3,000 physicians. One thousand are employed and 2,000 are aligned in private practice. In 2017, the organization made its first venture into financial risk with the Medicare Shared Savings Program (MSSP). It was part of a broader strategy to prepare the organization for value-based care.

In one year, the MSSP program significantly improved patient quality of care, reduced hospital admissions and readmissions, decreased post-acute facility and home health utilization, and lowered total cost of care. Getting there involved building the infrastructure and physician engagement for an Accountable Care Organization (ACO) from the ground up.

Houston Methodist's Coordinated Care program (HMCC) is an ACO led by physicians who joined HMCC ACO and met the ACO's standards and requirements. This includes 284 Primary

Care physicians. Sixty-five percent are employed by Houston Methodist and 35 percent are private aligned PCPs in the Houston metropolitan area.

Medicare MSSP Network

Houston Methodist Coordinated Care (HMCC) ACO, which is the first MSSP Track 3 program in Houston, faced steep goals from the start. Leaders needed to introduce and coordinate value-based care within an eight-hospital system. The team was tasked with developing a range of critical functions and capacities:

- High-value primary care network of employed and independent providers
- Inpatient case management team
- Data analyst team
- Population health advisor team for physicians and practices
- Nursing care management team with specific patient care programs
- Post-acute care network and management strategy
- Key performance indicators for all HMCC ACO teams
- IT infrastructure to track quality at the point of care
- Social Determinants of Health Assessments with Resources

HMCC ACO also needed to develop a network of collaborations with community partners to succeed in value-based care.

The first step was to form Houston Methodist Coordinated Care ACO. Developing a robust data and analytics strategy, which included predictive analytics to identify impactful patients, was central to HMCC. To that end, HMCC's leadership team tapped into claims data that provided key insights into quality, cost, and utilization goals. The population health advisors team also shared quality, cost, and utilization data with PCPs and specialists.

At the same time, the nursing care management team used predictive analytics to enroll, educate, and empower patients identified to be at risk for worsening health. These programs include Complex Care for patients with multiple co-morbidities, Transitions in Care for patients who were discharged from a hospital, and an Advanced Illness Care program.

HMCC also improved patient access and care coordination in key areas: primary care, urgent care, the ED, post-acute care, and home healthcare. Primary care physicians focused on ACO quality metrics and documentation to reflect the complexity of care provided to each patient, as well as making sure patient referrals and hand-offs were tracked. The post-acute team engaged nineteen skilled nursing facilities in the greater Houston area an implemented a home health review strategy with PCPs.

The case management team worked closely with physicians, patients, and home health agencies to achieve multiple objectives: make accurate recommendations to reduce home health over-utilization, and assess Social Determinants of Health and provide patients with specific needed services for a long-term care plan.

The organization's social work and case management team developed a value-based discharge planning model for MSSP patients that takes into consideration Social Determinants of Health. The model included a long-term care plan consisting of nonclinical and clinical factors when discharging patients.

As a result of these actions, PCP post-discharge follow-up appointments increased, and fall risk screenings increased as did depression screenings. The organization has also identified urgent care centers for after hours and weekend care to keep patients out of the ED when appropriate. A high priority patient access line and patient magnet, "Call your Nurse First," establishes continuity between nurse teams and patients.

Ensuring physicians had connectivity to ACO quality goals was also essential. The team worked with 113 private practice Primary Care physicians to achieve a level of IT interconnectivity with seven different EHRs.

Today, physicians access patient medical records, and the care team can access dashboards to monitor quality efforts and metrics in real time embedded within the EHR. The team's focus on quality at the patient, physician, and practice level is directed by real-time data and the review of outcomes.

In the 2020, HMCC ACO achieved the following:

- Avoidable hospital admissions decreased by 16 percent.
- All cause thirty-day hospital readmission rate was 15 percent.
- Avoidable ED Visits decreased by 21 percent.
- Even during a pandemic, PCP visits only decreased 3 percent due to virtual visit implementation.

- ACO Quality metric performance increased during the pandemic with an increase in depression screening and follow-up, increase in colon cancer screening with at home kits, and an increase in breast cancer screening.
- HMCC ACO ranked ninth nationally in quality performance from 513 Medicare ACOS with a quality score = 99.
- HMCC ACO ranked ninth nationally in Medicare savings per patient from 513 Medicare ACOS nationally with a 6.5 percent savings rate.
- HMCC ACO ranked fifteenth nationally in total Medicare savings received = $19.4 million.

With this success, the ACO is growing its primary care network. The number of primary care physicians has increased from 134 to 284, and Medicare beneficiaries have climbed from 16,299 to 38,000 in the fifth year.

Multi-Disciplinary Team Collaboration

HMCC conducts weekly team discussions on patient outcomes and care coordination to improve care.

During the COVID-19 pandemic, it became apparent that HMCC patients could end up being admitted to any hospital in greater Houston and that coordination among facilities was a necessity. Medicare patients can arrive by ambulance to any hospital when there is a medical emergency whether it is Hermann Memorial, Harris Health, HCA Houston, CHI-St. Luke's, or Houston Methodist.

The convergence of these trends reinforced HMCC's mission to treat the "whole person" regardless of their home address or condition. It likewise led to developing wrap around services that matched each patient's clinical needs, behavioral needs, and health-related social needs. The latter often give rise to a hospital admission or emergency department visit that could have been prevented through earlier detection and aggressive community outreach efforts.

Whole person care meant focusing on behavioral health needs, transportation needs, and food insecurity in addition to more customary hospital treatment like congestive heart failure and complications of diabetes. It requires coordinating care and patient follow up among hospitals.

Hospitals in Houston, including safety net facilities, recognize their interdependency in meeting the needs of a diverse population. No hospital in Houston has the breadth of services or financial capacity to meet the needs of hundreds of thousands of patients in their surrounding neighborhoods without the support and care coordination of each hospital and FQHC.

Population Health Paradigm

Houston Methodist Coordinated Care is a health system-based Accountable Care Organization and participates in CMS's Medicare Shared Savings model as part of its population health strategy. Social Determinants of Health services embedded in the EHR are utilized by HMCC outpatient nursing outreach as well as inpatient case managers/social workers for CMS Medicare enrollees.

Collaboration Teams

HMCC Nursing Care Management programs, available to Medicare Shared Savings patients, include transition care, complex care, and advanced illness strategies.

1. Transition Care Program Strategy: Reduction in Readmissions

Thirty-day program for high-risk patients recently discharged from acute and post-acute stays; focus is on follow-up appointments, avoiding inappropriate readmissions and ensuring smooth transition to home setting.

2. Complex Care Program Strategy: Prevent Avoidable Admissions

Ninety-day program for high risk, impactable patients with multiple comorbidities in the community; focus is on chronic disease management, health navigation, and individualized goal setting.

3. Advance Illness Care Program Strategy: Honor Patients' Wishes

Patients identified through predictive analytics as nearing last 12-18 months of life; focus is on palliative care management and end of life planning.

Post-hospitalization patient care plan focuses on an integrated delivery model with five elements that rely on coordination.

- Strategy focuses on appropriate patient resources for proper discharge planning coordination.
- Establish better patient care coordination between HMCC ACO inpatient and outpatient teams.

- Continuity of patient care with HMCC ACO inpatient team across the Houston Methodist system transforms care.
- Builds patient relationships.
- Initial HMCC ACO inpatient team assessment focuses on clinical and non-clinical Social Determinants of Health to provide appropriate patient resources.

The integrated care model also combines traditionally separate nursing functions into one HMCC ACO case manager role.

Utilization Review Nurse

- Determine medical necessity.
- Identify avoidable admissions in the Emergency Room.

Social Worker helps patient and families:

- Understand and cope with illness.
- Work through emotions of a diagnosis.
- Provide counseling for patient resources.

Case Manager

- Advocates for community resources.
- Advocates for consultation services during patient hospitalization.
- Is liaison between patient and medical team during hospitalization.

Case Examples

The following examples illustrate the importance and impact of an integrated care delivery model in relation to care coordination, skilled nursing facility outside the hospital, transition care nursing program, and inpatient admission following program completion.

Case 1: Care Coordination

> Ms. Jane Doe is a seventy-something-year-old female who was identified through predictive analytics as high risk for complex care and readmission. She has a medical history of COPD, asthma, congestive heart failure, atrial fibrillation, diabetics, chronic pain, bipolar depression, and anemia. Patient was offered the ninety-day Complex Care Program. A thorough assessment was completed, and patient-identified priorities were established.
>
> Through the depression screening, the nurse care manager found out patient had been experiencing thoughts of self-harm. The nurse proceeded with a further assessment of the individual's mental health and provided emotional support. Suicide contract was completed, and patient was referred to a psychiatric clinic and appointment was scheduled. She was provided with twenty-four-hour Suicide Hotline. Her primary care physician was notified of the new change. Due to COVID pandemic, patient participated in virtual

visits with the psychiatric provider and medications were adjusted appropriately.

Another concern for Ms. Doe was her declining memory. She was referred again to her Primary Care Physician PCP for an evaluation. Furthermore, the nurse care manager referred her to Baker Ripley Dementia Connection, a community partner that specializes in providing case management and resources for patients and family members managing dementia. Lena, another community partner that addresses social isolation, was also offered, though patient declined.

Patient had been experiencing worsening anemia, and nurse encouraged patient to follow up with her PCP. A referral was made to a gastroenterologist who recommended a colonoscopy. Patient was hesitant to complete the procedure, but with the nurse's encouragement, patient followed through and concerns from the test were addressed. The patient was grateful to have completed procedure due to family history of colon cancer.

Despite this individual's complex health concerns, patient has not had any inappropriate hospitalizations since program engagement.

Case 2: Skilled Nursing Facility Outside Hospital

Ms. CS was a seventy-something-year-old female who lived alone and had a history of chronic obstructive pulmonary disease, congestive heart failure, chronic back pain, liver cirrhosis, anxiety, and depression.

Because of her complex health condition and high anxiety, she was a high risk for readmission and for Emergency Department utilization. Her son lived out of state, so patient relied on an elderly neighbor. Upon discharge, Home Plate (a partnership between Houston Methodist Coordinated Care and Meals on Wheels) was set up for food security and a referral was made to counseling for anxiety and depression. Consent was obtained, and the nursing team began to coordinate with her son via telephone. It was revealed during these phone calls that the son had been attempting to relocate Ms. CS closer to him for support.

However, patient did not want to be a burden and declined. The nurse care manager assisted in facilitating communication between the two. The outpatient nurses "tag-teamed" with HMCC's inpatient team to ensure smooth transitions from home to hospital and vice versa. More than once, after patient had been discharged from the Houston Methodist Hospital System, the care team would receive notifications via Greater Houston Health Connect or Patient Ping that she had checked herself into another hospital system. The members of the HMCC team coordinated with case workers from these outside hospitals.

Eventually, for patient's health and safety, HMCC assisted Ms. CS in moving to a nearby assisted living facility. Frequent calls were made to this facility to educate the owner and her caregiver regarding her specific needs.

At this time, the number of her hospital admissions decreased significantly. Unfortunately, patient suffered another respiratory decline and was admitted and transferred to a skilled nursing facility (SNF) for physical therapy.

Meanwhile, the son had found a nearby assisted living facility and hoped to move his mother closer to him. HMCC team collaborated with the members of the SNF team and the son to get her prepared for the move.

Primary care physician, specialists, and pharmacy were established in her new home; appointments were scheduled, and prescriptions transferred. Oxygen equipment and other supplies were set up to make sure everything was available as soon as she landed.

On the day of travel, a member of the HMCC team travelled to the SNF to coordinate final paperwork and picked up prescriptions for her pain medications while another member of the team personally arranged transportation for her to the airport.

Case 3: Transition Care Nursing Program

As noted in the table below, patients who were engaged with a nurse care manager in Transition Care Program had a lower readmission rate compared to those high-risk patients who did not participate in a nursing program. Most patients not in a program either declined participation or were unable to be reached.

For the Transition Care Program, the readmission rate for those in a program showed a 78 percent rate reduction from 18 percent readmission rate for those not in a program down to 4 percent readmission rate for those who worked with one of our nurses.

Nursing Care Management Programs	Readmission Rate Patients Enrolled in Program	Readmission Rate Patients NOT Enrolled in Program	Decrease in Readmission Rate
Transition Care (n = 1,019)	4%	18%	78% Reduction

Case 4: Inpatient Admission Following Program Completion

The below table shows the inpatient admission rate from January 2020 to December 2020 of patients engaged in a program or within the thirty-day window following program completion versus those not in a program. Excluded from inpatient admission includes scheduled procedures/cancer therapies, patient leaving against medical advice, or transferred from another acute facility. "Not in a program" refers to patients who declined participation or were unable to be reached.

Patients who were in the Complex Care Program reduced their admission rate by roughly 19 percent (from 16 percent admission rate of the high-risk patients who did not participate to 13 percent admission rate for the patients who worked with a nurse in the Complex Care Program).

In the Advanced Illness Care Program, inpatients admission rates were reduced by 47 percent from a 19 percent admission rate for high-risk patients who declined participation to a 10 percent admission rate for patients who participated in the Advanced Illness Care program.

Nursing Care Management Programs	Admission Rate Patients Enrolled in Program	Admission Rate Patients NOT Enrolled in Program	Decrease in Admission Rate
Complex Care (n = 676)	13%	16%	19% Reduction
Advance Illness Care (n = 167)	10%	19%	47% Reduction

The executive leadership team attributes the resilience of patient navigation to passion. How else to explain their day-in day-out commitment to going the extra mile to identify, screen, and coordinate care for so many individuals and families with enormous unmet social and medical needs? The pressure and demands on staff are relentless as demonstrated by the exhausting response to COVID-19 throughout the organization.

Needs Assessment

Houston Methodist conducts a comprehensive needs assessment every three years that informs decisions on strategy, resource allocation, program design, and community investment. The main findings of the 2019 Needs Assessment Analysis noted the following:

79%	Lack of insurance
67%	Unable to pay/Too expensive
44%	Fear (not ready to face health problem)
41%	Can't take time away from work to see doctor
20%	Health services too far
18%	Language barriers/Do not speak the language
18%	Don't know how to find a doctor
18%	Unreliable/Insufficient transportation
5%	Cultural or religious beliefs
4%	Other
8%	There are no barriers

These findings indicate significant access barriers to care. In Harris County, 21 percent of the population is uninsured and 24.3 percent cannot afford to see a doctor. The impact of these barriers is poorer health outcomes due to the following reasons:

- Higher rates of preventable ED utilization
- Higher rates of preventable hospitalizations
- Duplication of services

- Lack of preventable services
- Gaps in community care
- Lower quality of care

Perceived barriers to care are greater for those receiving treatment for mental health problems, those with disabilities, and individuals with worse physical and mental function.

Lack of access to care also has a significant financial impact. Individuals lacking social support have 10 percent higher costs. Lack of a primary care physician results in 12 percent higher costs. Individuals with physical limitations have 9 percent higher costs. Substance abuse results in 89 percent higher costs. Financial distress results in 25 percent higher costs. Mental health diagnoses result in 38 percent higher costs.

Current models of care delivery fall short in addressing healthcare access. Unmanaged behavioral health for Medicaid beneficiaries, for example, spend 48 percent more when one or more behavioral conditions are present. Twenty-five percent utilize emergency departments because other sites are not open.

Social Determinants

Houston Methodist also screens patients during clinic visits to better understand what services are needed beyond the hospitals' wall that impact patient health. Roughly 80 percent of a patient's health is attributed to nonclinical factors often referred to as social determinants of care.

Major nonclinical social needs revolve around food insecurity (37 percent), housing and living security (35 percent), transportation

(13 percent), prescription affordability (9 percent), and health education (5 percent).

A more in-depth assessment was based on the following screening questions in the Social Determinants of Health Assessment:

Question 1. Alcohol Use

- How often do you have a drink containing alcohol?
- How many drinks containing alcohol do you have on a typical day when you are drinking?
- How often do you have six or more drinks on one occasion?

Question 2. Depression

- Over the past two weeks, how often have you been bothered by any of the following problems?
    - Little interest or pleasure in doing things?
    - Feeling down, depressed, or hopeless?

Question 3. Financial Resource Strain

- How hard is it for you to pay for the very basics like food, housing, medical care, and heating?

Question 4. Food Insecurity

- Within the past twelve months, did you worry that your food would run out before you got the money to buy more?
- Within the past twelve months, has the food you bought not lasted and you didn't have money to get more?

Question 5. Intimate Partner Violence

- Within the last year, have you been humiliated or emotionally abused in other ways by your partner or ex-partner?
- Within the last year, have you been afraid of your partner or ex-partner?
- Within the last year, have you been raped or forced to have any kind of sexual activity by your partner or ex-partner?
- Within the last year, have you been kicked, hit, slapped, or otherwise physically hurt by your partner or ex-partner?

Question 6. Physical Activity

- On average, how many days per week do you engage in moderate to strenuous exercise (like walking fast, running, jogging, dancing, swimming, biking, or other activities that cause a light or heavy sweat)?
- On average, how many minutes do you engage in exercise at this level?

Question 7. Social Connections

- In a typical week, how many times do you talk on the phone with family, friends, or neighbors?
- How often do you get together with friends or relatives?
- How often do you attend church or religious services?

- Do you belong to any clubs or organizations such as church groups, unions, fraternal or athletic groups, or school groups?
- How often do you attend meetings of the clubs or organizations you belong to?
- Are you married, widowed, divorced, separated, never married, or living with a partner?

Question 8. Stress

- Do you feel stress—tense, restless nervous, or anxious, or unable to sleep at night because your mind is troubled all the time—these days?

Question 9. Tobacco Use

- Frequency of Smoking/Smokeless Tobacco Use

Question 10. Transportation Needs

- Has the lack of transportation kept you from medical appointments or from getting medications?
- Has the lack of transportation kept you from meetings, work, or from getting things needed for daily living?

Question 11. Housing Stability

- In the last twelve months, was there a time when you were not able to pay the mortgage or rent on time?

- In the last twelve months, how many places have you lived?
- In the last twelve months, was there a time when you did not have a steady place to sleep or slept in a shelter (including now)?

Houston Methodist Coordinated Care program highlighted a number of Social Determinants of Health, which account for 80 percent of health outcomes as shown below:

Social Determinants of Health	Number Screened
Heavy alcohol use 3% (172)	6,153
Housing insecurity 2% (18)	947
Tobacco Use 6% (1,477)	26,749
Financial Insecurity 1% (16)	1,426
Depression 4% (842)	22,539
Stress 22% (223)	1,034
Food insecurity 3% (43)	1688
Transportation insecurity 3% (51)	1,732
Physical Inactivity 80% (858)	1,070
Social Isolation 35% (395)	1,131
Intimate partner violence 1% (7)	880

* Housing needs are rarely encountered for an insured population of Medicare beneficiaries.

To establish better patient coordination between HMCC ACO inpatient and outpatient teams, the initial inpatient assessment team focuses on clinical and nonclinical issues to provide appropriate patient resources.

These realities motivated Houston Methodist to develop a comprehensive program to address access issues, gaps in care due to fragmented medical care delivery, health behaviors, and life circumstances. If a need is identified during the assessment, the nurse looks further into the situation and coordinates next steps in collaboration with the primary care physician. A referral is then submitted to community partners and resources if the patient consents.

The HMCC model also includes two significant components: (1) a high-value network of physicians, and (2) an emphasis on collaboration that supports innovative partnerships benefiting patients.

High Value Network includes five place-based activities.

1. HMCC case management collaborates with Houston Methodist ED physicians and case managers to identify avoidable admissions.
2. HMCC social workers, case managers, and hospitalists collaborate for value-based care discharge planning and standardized post-acute placement using Medicare criteria for appropriate utilization of patient resources.
3. HMCC nursing outreach includes self-care education for home-bound patients (e.g., transitions in care,

advanced illness care, complex care), home healthcare coordination, and transitional care nurse visits.

4. HMCC's skilled nursing facility network is updated quarterly (including quality criteria) and nursing case manager follows up with patients in post-acute facilities.
5. HMCC includes same day clinics, virtual visits, and collaborates with Next Level Urgent Care, CVS Minute Clinics, and Dispatch Health to improve access for patients in need.

Collaborative Partnerships include seven vendors aligned with HMCC goals.

Baker Ripley offers disease-specific services such as dementia case management to ACO patients at no cost, including caregiver support and one-on-one caregiver consultations.

CVS Health care coordination provides ACO medication management program and ACO quality metrics outreach. CVS sends a letter and calls high-risk HMCC patients to offer personalized prescription schedule, home delivery, prescription synchronization, multi-dose packaging, and digital tools. Reminders for breast cancer and colon screening are on the medication bags of patients due for screening. CVS pharmacists also counsel patients on screening and giving them influenza vaccination.

Dispatch Health care coordination involves a house call to test and treat the same conditions, and at the same cost as an urgent care visit.

Greater Houston Health Information Exchange tracks MSSP patient discharges outside of Houston Methodist's system. It facilitates clinical integration by connecting disparate EHRs from hospitals, health systems, community clinics, physician office practices, and service providers across Southwest Texas.

Home Plate (Meals on Wheels) provides meals for MSSP patients with food insecurity. In 2020, this program provided 6,923 meals for patients in need.

Patient Ping is a post-acute strategy that identifies MSSP patients in real time when admitted to post-acute facilities in Greater Houston. The hospital's post-acute partners use the Ping platform, which provides increased visibility into SNF performance and improves care coordination with SNFs, long-term care, and hospice sites.

Lena Health Companion is an extension of the primary care provider and care team that offers health guidance, answers questions, and helps navigate heath resources for socially isolated patients. Lena Health also communicates patient concerns to the care team. There is no cost to HMCC patients.

Lena provides additional support and health guidance to patients while at home. Patients who benefit most live alone, are lonely, recently widowed, have been recently discharged from the hospital. Dual eligible also benefit from a Health Companion to navigate social resources as such as food pantries and income support.

Each of these programs contribute to the success of the HMCC model, which resulted in improved quality of care as shown below.

MSSP Building Blocks

The success of Houston Methodist's MSSP strategy is directly tied to the organization's ability to bring together core functions that support quality and cost savings. These, in turn, form the underlying foundation of the Care Coordination model.

MSSP's four core capabilities drive program performance and are related to quality, integrated platform, care management, and network performance.

1. Quality Metrics are a critical part of ACO performance.

- Comprehensive clinical rules engine that uses disparate datasets to find gaps in care for Medicare Shared Savings program quality metrics.
- Technology-enabled workflow that engages all care team members in closing gaps in care.
- Quality initiatives and programs compliant with Medicare Shared Savings Program and National Committee for Quality Assurance (NCQA) requirements.

2. Integrated IT is essential to data analytics that drive performance and business case.

- Ability to integrate and normalize claims, EMR and CMS data.

- Stratification engine identifies only "impactable" patients and matches them to the appropriate clinical program.
- Predictive Analytics necessary for Population Health Management.

3. Care Management drives medical expense savings.

Single patient profile that enables coordinated care across the care continuum.

- Integrated workflows with Primary Care Physician Practices.
- Jointly developed patient care plans that factor in socioeconomic, behavioral, and mental health.

4. Network Performance drives medical expense savings.

- Access to expanded set of data paired with analytics to identify key areas of network waste (unnecessary ED, home health, DME, SNFs).
- Physician education and alignment around the impact of value-based care initiatives (Quality and Utilization Metrics).
- Methodologies to encourage coordination and collaboration between all care providers, inclusive of specialists.

These building blocks are essential to improve quality of

care in the MSSP ACO program, as shown below:

ACO Quality Metric	2017	2018	2019	Improvement
Fall Risk Assessment	53.12%	90.82%	95.84%	42.72%
Influenza Immunization	68.75%	77.93%	87.15%	18.40%
Depression Screening	38.84%	83.96%	85.86%	47.02%
Colorectal Cancer Screening	43.63%	57.03%	74.01%	30.38%
Breast Cancer Screening	63.48%	69.32%	76.40%	12.92%
Diabetes HbA1c Control	83.07%	89.61%	90.00%	6.93%
Hypertension Control	58.79%	68.31%	70.00%	11.21%

Summary

Houston Methodist Coordinated Care is modeled on the institution's highest priorities of patient safety, quality, and service to diverse communities in greater Houston.

HMCC developed a comprehensive data and analytic strategy to support value-based care and nonclinical factors such as social determinants of care. This approach was necessary to provide "whole person care" and taking on downside risk for Medicare beneficiaries through its Accountable Care Organization.

Collaboration with its primary care physicians and numerous community partners was essential to achieving whole person and managing complex chronic conditions required by the Medicare Shared Services Program.

Key Takeaways

- A system-wide commitment to whole person care should define how, when, and where care is delivered.
- Access to patient medical records and real time-data

(24x7) is necessary for effective coordinated care.

- Multi-disciplinary collaboration (physicians, care teams) is necessary to improve care and outcomes.
- Wrap-around services (clinical, behavioral, social health needs) are necessary to prevent avoidable admissions and ED visits.
- Nursing outreach must include self-care education for patients.

Executive Comments

Julia Andrieni, MD, is President and CEO of Houston Methodist Coordinated Care.

Social Determinants of Health are just as important as clinical issues in improving population health.

The pandemic highlighted the importance of coordinated care to reduce disparities and close gaps in care. Wherever the patient was, we needed to loop them into a continuum of care.

We needed a new approach and that required developing infrastructure to track each patient across the whole system—IP, OP, ambulatory, skilled nursing, and especially home care.

Much of the infrastructure established during the pandemic for virtual care visits continues today. AI tools identify patient's health risks, nursing outreach, and collaboration with community partners.

What became clear is that if we weren't addressing

nonclinical factors like social determinants, then we couldn't impact chronic conditions or quality scores. How a patient presents at the hospital is just the tip of the iceberg.

Houston Methodist needed to know a lot more about each patient and that meant working hand-in-hand with other partners that provide services that we don't, like food and transportation.

If patients don't have access to healthy food and transportation or have a low health literacy level, how can we expect them to follow dietary guidelines, take medications as prescribed, and attend follow-up appointments to improve their diabetes?

Necessity also spurred Houston Methodist to address Social Determinants of Health to prevent admissions, as well as decreasing readmissions and ER use. That's essential when assuming downside risk for our 40,000 Medicare fee-for-service patients (Medicare Shared Savings ACO) and value-based care.

What matters most to patients is quality of care at the appropriate cost. Value-based care emphasizes whole person care and that means connecting patients with community resources, a multi-disciplinary team, and individualized service—clinical and nonclinical—to improve health.

We see patients and caregivers as fully engaged and empowered members of the healthcare team in this journey. We can't do it alone. Collaboration is key.

Patient Letter to Julia Andrieni, MD, CEO of Houston Methodist Coordinated Care

"A true hero isn't measured by the size of his strength,
but by the strength of his heart."
—Hercules

You may not be aware of this, but there is a superhero among us, and he works for you. I'm writing this letter to let you know of all the good that has come into our world because of Norman Lancit, otherwise known to us as Super Norm.

Last summer when my father was admitted to Houston Methodist and remained a patient there for over a month, Norman entered our lives. I remember feeling overwhelmed by the revolving door of all the hospital nurses, doctors, and staff who kept entering and exiting my father's room throughout the day.

Then, one day, this tall guy walked in with a big smile and a comforting presence. In all my confusion of meeting so many hospital staff, I remember not really understanding who he was or what he did, but I did remember one thing he said over and over as he gave us his business card: "I'm here to make sure your dad is taken care of and you can call me any time, twenty-four hours a day, about anything." I remember laughing in my head and thinking, *Yeah, right*. He proceeded to tell me that he cares for us like his own family and that he's the guy to call about anything.

Well, he was right. I ended up calling Norman about a number of things during out extended stay at the hospital, and he was always there for us, and he treated us like we were his family. I was never really sure how he managed it all. How did he get there so fast? How did he know that we would need that? How is he always able to answer my calls and texts? And to be honest, I still don't know how he continues to do it.

Therefore, we decided to start calling him by the name he truly earned: Super Norm. He was there any time we needed him and pulled off some miraculous feats for us at the hospital. I finally asked him outright, "Are you above the doctors? Do they have to do what you tell them?" Of course, I'm sure Norman wasn't comfortable with questions like that because he's a team player and is about as humble as you can get. But you need to know this: He's a superhero to us. Not a superhero in the way most people think of them. He's a superhero because of how much he genuinely cares about people. For Norman, it's all about people and the connections and relationships formed. He exudes compassion. You can tell this before he even says a word. It just radiates from him like a warm blanket.

It has been a year since my dad was in the hospital, and since then Norman has continued to be there. Throughout the year, we've kept in contact, because let's face it, he's our friend. We recently got together again for dinner and we're so happy to stay connected.

Executive Interview: Norman Lancit, Director of Transition in Care at Houston Methodist

The HMCC ACO program combines the functions of utilization review nurses, social workers, and case managers.

Compassion is central to providing whole person care.

Question: What is the approach of your department?

To start with, the ACO is totally different. We decided to create our own case management department instead of utilizing the existing Case Management Departments in the organization. Unlike most ACOs, our approach didn't target length of stay, but rather a holistic approach to coordination of care. We decided to emphasize the total needs of patients—not just solving the issue of "right now." The objective was to develop a care plan that would sustain healthy living and longevity of health.

This approach underscored the importance of whole person care. Our goal is to empower patients and educate them about their illness. This includes preventive medicine to help them build a road map to healthy living. We needed a more comprehensive strategy that went far beyond regular case management.

Question: Why were you selected for this role?

I've been in Case Management for more than twenty years, and still have the same passion as when I was a front-line Case Manager working in Detroit. It's important that patients know they have someone who will advocate for them, get to know them by building rapport to truly understand their journey, and focus on how to help them live a healthy life.

My training and experience had been working with the voiceless, those forgotten communities that have no resources and sometimes no family to support them. I wanted to make an impact and that meant going beyond a specific job title.

Question: What was the most important personal characteristic for this role?

More than anything else, what was needed is a big dose of compassion. That's why I think I was called for this work.

I learned so much from working in disadvantaged communities where most patients felt it was always about their insurance and not about compassion. Often their perception was that no one cared about the true reason why they were admitted, or couldn't afford medicines, or why they are taking specific medication.

Question: How does preventive health factor into this role?

Preventative care is especially important in disadvantaged communities. In the African American community, for example, many believe going to the doctor for an annual visit is a bad thing to do. And talking about their insecurities or health issues are taboo.

The only way you will ever help someone is by getting to know them personally. How else can you develop a plan of care when you aren't trusted?

I've been incorporating Social Determinants of Health since I started in 1998. Nothing has changed in terms of unmet social heath needs. But now I train my staff to get to know each patient, develop a life-long plan of healthy living, and find resources in the community to meet their needs. While every situation is different, earning the trust of patients and building rapport is always the key.

Question: How did you develop this patient sensibility?

I grew up in a family without health insurance. I remember tagging along with my mom from doctor to doctor, looking for help at free clinics. I'll never forget the embarrassment my mother felt not having insurance and not being able to see a medical professional because of it.

We were invisible, not worthy of being seen due to no medical insurance. This is an experience I'll never forget because it motivated me to serve those who need help regardless of social status, income level, or resources. I was determined to change the narrative.

Question: What do you look for in recruiting and training staff members?

I look for compassion. Passion for the job, staff that want to make an impact and be trendsetters. New staff orientation involves 3-4 months of intense training for new hires, and I try to shadow all staff one-on-one.

New staff are trained on three roles: case management, social work, and utilization review. We have fourteen clinical case managers, registered nurses, and social workers who make up the team with three senior care coordinators as support staff.

Question: Your job description is extensive. How is performance evaluated?

To be honest, I go beyond the job description because of my passion for patient care. The job description for my title, and my staff doesn't adequately describe what we do because I have transformed the role of case manager.

Our staff needs to know the *why* in order to do this work well. That's critical. As Dr. Andrieni says, once you figure out the why, then you can start a solid discharge plan for all patients. Knowing patients' journey and building trust is key and so important.

Question: What does this job mean to you?

I love this work. I love making an impact on people's lives, regardless of their life circumstances. My aunt always told me if you meet someone and don't leave an impression, then you haven't done your job. You missed an opportunity for them to say: "Wow! I'll remember this person for the rest of my life."

That's the narrative of this work. Helping the vulnerable and empowering them for a healthy living.

Chapter 7.

Cleveland Clinic Executive Interview

Elizabeth Bradley, MD, is Medical Director for the Center for Functional Medicine.
Michelle Beidelschies, PhD, is Research and Education Director for the Center for Functional Medicine.

"Addressing root causes is at the heart of Functional Medicine."

Question: How does functional medicine differ from traditional medical care?

The short answer is that functional medicine looks at the body as a whole and focuses on the root causes of disease rather than an isolated set of symptoms.

Question: When did Cleveland Clinic begin to focus on functional medicine?

In 2014, Cleveland Clinic was the first academic medical center to open a Center for Functional Medicine. The Center was tasked to demonstrate the value for the functional medicine model of care and to provide a solution for the management of various chronic diseases that burden the healthcare system. Additionally, we were interested in studying innovative care delivery models, such as shared medical appointments, or group settings.

The Center's approach focuses on a "food as medicine" approach that incorporates nutrition as well as lifestyle-based interventions such as exercise and movement, sleep, stress resilience, and relationships to prevent and mitigate chronic disease. All new patients see a provider as well as a registered dietitian and health coach as part of their initial visit. Patients also have the option to meet with a behavioral health therapist as well.

Question: Is the Center located on the main Cleveland Clinic campus?

The Cleveland Clinic Center for Functional Medicine is located on the main campus of Cleveland Clinic, as well as in a satellite location at a Cleveland Clinic family medical center. The Center also provides care as part of community initiatives in in-person and virtual care settings, including the Langston Hughes Community Health and Education Center, which resides in a resource-challenged Cleveland neighborhood.

Question: One of the recent studies focused on the effectiveness of the functional medicine-based approach to shared medical appointments. What was the objective of the study?

Our research approach evolved to align with our innovative care strategies, which eventually grew into offering shared medical appointments. We went from providing clinical care in an individual, outpatient setting at Cleveland Clinic main campus and family health centers, to expanding functional medicine services through shared medical appointments. So, it was only natural that our research followed suit to demonstrate the value of our approach. The shared medical appointment setting has enabled us to expand our research outcomes and gather more evidence on the model because they are smaller, and perhaps, more engaged groups.

In our landmark 2019 *JAMA Network Open* manuscript, we demonstrated that the functional medicine model of care delivered as part of individual, one-on-one appointments has significant and sustainable improvements on health-related quality of life. Then, we sought to compare health-related quality of life, biometric outcomes, and costs associated with functional medicine-based care delivered in a shared medical appointment setting and compare to care delivered through individual, one-on-one appointments.

We designed a ten-week program called Functioning For Life® (FFL). FFL integrated the multi-disciplinary team of caregivers (provider, dietitian, and health coach) into a group setting with no more than ten patients at a time. The goal of the program was to provide patients with the tools and education needed to be stewards of their own health, and to propagate this in their homes and communities. The FFL program included five condition-specific cohorts: weight management, autoimmune, digestive disorders, women's health, and diabetes.

Question: Can you say more about the research design?

The methodology compared changes in biometrics and health-related quality of life (HRQoL) patient-reported outcomes for two groups of patients: patients enrolled in Functioning for Life program (226) and patients with individual appointments (2,229) at Cleveland Clinic. In order to reduce bias due to confounding variables in the treatment group versus the control group, propensity score matching (statistical technique) was used.

Question: What were the main findings?

The general conclusion is that shared medical appointments SMAs are an efficient and effective way to deliver functional medicine care. But keep in mind that the context of care is especially important. In this study, functional medicine was delivered with a collaborative team for some of the most commonly diagnosed chronic conditions.

SMAs provide more opportunity for interaction with team members and for patient education than traditional care (individual appointments). SMAs reduces one of the most time-consuming elements of individual functional medicine visits. Namely, repeating the same baseline elements of dietary, lifestyle, and behavior change for each patient, one at a time versus a group setting. This allows more people access to care for common chronic conditions. The result is better care for patients and reduced provider workload.

Question: What specific metrics stood out in the study?

These metrics really stood out:

- Both groups had higher Patient-Reported Outcome Measurement Information System (PROMIS) scores (1.34 higher for individual visits, 3.12 for SMAs).
- Both groups also experienced improved biometrics (lower blood pressures and weight loss).
- SMA patients had a significantly greater improvement in PROMIS Global Physical Health (GPH) T-scores than patients receiving individual appointments (by 1.78 points).
- SMA patients were also more likely to experience improvements of five or more points (seen as a clinically important difference; 38 percent vs. 26 percent, NNT=8), but the differences were not significant (p=0.07). NNT stands for the "Number Needed to Treat," which measures the impact of a medicine or therapy by estimating the number of patients who need to be treated in order to prevent one negative outcome.
- SMA patients had a significantly greater improvement in their weight than patients receiving individual

appointments (-3.8 vs. -2.4 kg; mean difference of 1.4).

- Both groups showed equal improvement in their systolic and diastolic blood pressures.
- SMA patients received more caregiver time per patient than those in individual appointments (14.0 hours versus 3.5 hours).
- SMAs cost less to deliver and generated greater revenue.

By improving outcomes and reducing costs, this approach validates the functional medicine approach and is a compelling argument for expanding access to functional medicine for patients.

Question: What is unique about shared medical appointments?

If there is a "secret sauce," it would be the interpersonal dynamics among the patients and staff. During the ten-week period, group cohesiveness develops, and peer support offers reassurance about patients' concerns. This is a unique feature of group appointments.

Patients also have more time to get information about their specific health issues and more time with their physician or healthcare staff. There is plenty of time for additional questions about how to manage each patient's condition. Patients needing follow-up care for chronic conditions are routinely coordinated within the Cleveland Clinic.

Question: What was the role of patient education in the study?

Each cohort used a multidisciplinary team to provide condition-specific education related to nutrition, lifestyle, and behavioral health recommendations. We recognized that these factors play a significant role in determining health and that we needed to treat a patient's condition with a battery of resources if we wanted to achieve better outcomes.

During the ten-week regimen, four sessions were led by medical providers (MD, DO, NP, PA) and a health coach. Six sessions were led by a registered dietitian. A multi-disciplinary model was required to address the clinical and social health needs of patients.

Each session included education on lifestyle and behavior change. Each patient also received a limited medical evaluation with the medical provider.

The purpose of the education component was to empower patients to make positive decisions regarding food and become advocates for healthy lifestyles at home and in their community.

Question: Why are these findings particularly relevant for value-based care models and reimbursement?

"Pay for value" and "integrated care" models require a different approach to how care is delivered. Functional medicine and shared medical appointments change how we think about conventional healthcare delivery. The approach also leverages community settings rather than a hospital or outpatient clinic as the focus of care.

It also empowers patients, and that's a critical differentiator. One of the building blocks of social determinants and health equity is improving quality of life and closing care gaps. And that means incorporating a strong emphasis on making lifestyle changes such as diet and nutrition.

Question: What chronic conditions are addressed in the Functioning for Life program?

Six disease-specific programs have been developed and patients can select the ten-week series that addresses their condition.

- **Immune/Autoimmune Disorder Track:** conditions such as lupus and psoriasis.
- **Diabetes Track:** conditions such as diabetes, metabolic syndrome and pre-diabetes. Diabetic patients who are currently on insulin are eligible as well.
- **Women's Health Disorder Track:** conditions such as menopause, PCOS (polycystic ovary syndrome), and PMS.
- **Digestive Disorders Track:** conditions such as IBD, IBS, GERD/Reflux, and gastrointestinal issues.
- **Weight Management Track.**
- **Pain Management track:** conditions such as chronic migraine, osteoarthritis, fibromyalgia, and minor back pain.

Each weekly program is one hour long, except for sessions 1, 3, 5, and 9, which may last up to two hours.

Question: How applicable is the SMA model to community settings?

A nutrition and lifestyle-focused shared medical appointment is quite applicable in other resource-challenged community settings. Colleagues recently applied this model at the Langston Hughes Community Health and Education Center in the Fairfax neighborhood in Cleveland. The neighborhood population also had a number of health disparities compounded by Social Determinants of Health. For example, higher rates of heart disease, cancer, diabetes, and kidney disease than the surrounding community.

The program improved self-reported wellness and biometric outcomes in the resource-challenged neighborhood. Patients reported positive changes in energy level, gut function, and overall daily function as a result of the SMA program. A number of patients were able to sustain healthy behaviors for at least three months after the program ended.

This study demonstrates that such a healthcare delivery option (SMA) is a viable option in underserved communities where there is a disproportionate burden of chronic disease.

Reference

Nazleen Bharmal, Michelle Beidelschies, Marilyn Alejandro-Rodriguez, Kayla Alejandro, Ning Guo, Tawny Jones, and Elizabeth Bradley. "A nutrition and lifestyle-focused shared medical appointment in a resource-challenged community setting: a mixed-methods study." BMC Public Health (2022) 22:447.

Chapter 8.

Vanderbilt University Medical Center Case Study

Introduction

Vanderbilt University Medical Center is in Nashville, Tennessee. Health literacy is an important element of patient care and population health management strategies at the medical center.

Health literacy is defined as the degree to which individuals have the capacity to obtain, process, and understand basic health information and services needs to make appropriate health decisions.[1]

As important as health literacy is to navigate the healthcare system and manage chronic conditions, 90 million adults in the US have low health literacy.[2] It is associated with lower rates of preventive care, poorer disease control and greater mortality. Patients with low health literacy generally have poorer outcomes, greater utilization, and higher costs than others.[3,4]

In short, addressing health literacy is a national health priority. Vanderbilt University Medical Center recognized that understanding and addressing health literacy is a key factor in providing patient care and a good step toward assessing Social Determinants of Health throughout the organization. As a result, Vanderbilt researchers and clinical leaders partnered to implement health literacy assessments in clinical practice and conduct a series of studies to document the impact of health literacy on patient outcomes.

An Innovative Program for Health Literacy Screening

The medical center's challenge was how to operationalize health literacy assessment in day-to-day practice with 20,000 employees across the institution, including 5,000 nurses doing intake assessments, in a way that did not interfere with clinical workflow. Vanderbilt initiated a multi-year research program on health literacy screening beginning in 2010.

With the support of the institution's Chief Nursing Officer and other leaders, the group successfully incorporated a Brief Health Literacy Screen (BHLS) into the intake process for most primary care and hospitalized patients.[5] The items are administered in-person by nurses and recorded in the patient's electronic health record.

The screen incorporates a brief tool with three standardized questions for inpatient and outpatient settings:

- How confident are you filling out medical forms by yourself? (extremely, quite a bit, somewhat, a little bit, not at all)

- How often do you have someone help you read hospital materials? (all of the time, most of the time, some of the time, a little of the time, none of the time)
- How often do you have problems learning about your medical condition because of difficulty understanding written information? (all of the time, most of the time, some of the time, a little of the time, none of the time)

The three items each provide a score of 1 to 5, which are compiled to create an overall health literacy score of 3 to 15. Higher values indicating a higher level of health literacy. This information augments other assessments long performed by staff, including years of education, language preference, and preferred means of learning (e.g., verbal, written, video). Spanish is the second most frequently used language in the medical center, followed by Arabic. Medicaid covers 16 percent of patients and 5 percent identify as Latino.

Implementation of Health Literacy Screening

Nursing staff support was critical in implementing, evaluating, and sustaining the initiative. During the phases of obtaining buy-in, implementation, and monitoring, several key implementation outcomes were assessed:

Acceptability: Nursing and administrative leaders found the BHLS to be acceptable for use in clinical practice because it is short and follows a conversational and non-judgmental tone. These aspects are critical and differentiate the BHLS from other assessments of health literacy which are formatted more like tests, such as the Rapid Estimate of Adult Literacy in Medicine (REALM), Test of Functional Health Literacy in Adults (TOFHLA), and Newest Vital Sign.

Adoption: The intention to use the BHLS was demonstrated by leadership's commitment to incorporate the tool into the electronic health record and disseminate educational materials about assessing health literacy in practice to the large and diverse nursing staff.

Appropriateness: Frontline nurses and patients responded well to the new questions. Nurses have felt they are an appropriate reflection of patients' learning needs, which is the section of the intake in which the items are embedded. Patients have felt comfortable answering the questions, without feeling ashamed about difficulties they might have. Nurses precede the questions with the statement, "A lot of patients have trouble understanding the medical information they get at the doctor's office or hospital," which normalizes that patients can express their challenges.

Feasibility: These questions provide a valid and reliable assessment of health literacy in about one minute. This speed is critical for feasibility in busy clinical environments. During the first year, the screening completion rate among 51,063 hospital patients was 91.8 percent, while the uptake rate for 15,434 clinic patients was 66.6 percent.[5, p. 68]

Fidelity: To verify whether nurses in a busy clinical environment obtained similar scores from patients as non-time-pressured research staff, research assistants re-administered the BHLS to several hundred patients. Scores matched for the majority (60 percent) of patients, indicating a high level of fidelity overall. About 25 percent of the time, though, nurse-obtained scores were higher than those obtained by research staff on the same patients. Nurses' tendency to overestimate health literacy scores was greatest among male patients and those with lower educational attainment, which is something that future clinical implementations should keep in mind as a possibility.[6]

Sustainability: Administration of the BHLS has not been sustained in the outpatient clinics, largely due to streamlining of patient intake during implementation of a new electronic health record. However, it has been sustained for more than twelve years in the hospital setting. Completion rates remain high, at approximately 80 percent. To date, more than 450,000 health literacy screens have been completed.

Looking back, the main factors that contributed to BHLS success were leadership support, and project integration into medical center work flows as well as patient intake and documentation procedures. Key hospital leaders came on board during months of collaboration in planning and implementation. Project leaders capitalized on established nurse education activities to get word out about the program, as well as to obtain face-to-face feedback. Electronic health record data extractions were valuable for monitoring at the hospital and clinic levels.

Clinical Impact

The large screening effort has demonstrated that approximately 20 percent of hospital inpatients and 10 percent of primary care patients in the medical center have low health literacy. Routine assessment and documentation of health literacy has also enabled a unique program of population-based research on the association of low health literacy with clinical outcomes across a variety of medical and surgical conditions. These studies are driven by hypotheses that patients with lower health literacy may have undiagnosed medical conditions, worse self-management of known conditions (e.g., less engagement and adherence to recommended care), and poorer disease control, which could lead to poor health outcomes. In the surgical setting, low health literacy could contribute to slower recovery or higher complication rates after procedures.

The first of these investigations examined blood pressure among patients presenting to the Emergency Department over an eighteen-month period. Among 46,263 patients in this cross-sectional study, 22 percent had low health literacy. After controlling for other variables, patients with low health literacy were more likely to have elevated blood pressure readings (40.0 percent vs. 35.5 percent for those with adequate health literacy), extremely elevated blood pressure, and previously undiagnosed hypertension.[7]

Another study evaluated 1,379 patients discharged home following a hospitalization for heart failure and examined the independent association of health literacy with mortality during an average follow-up of twenty-one months. After controlling for age, gender, race, insurance, education, comorbidities, and hospital length of stay, patients with low health literacy had a 30 percent higher rate of death during the follow-up period.[8]

Several studies have examined post-operative outcomes. In one investigation that focused on 1,239 patients who had undergone major abdominal surgery over a three-year period, lower health literacy levels were independently associated with a longer hospital length of stay, but not with higher rates of thirty-day Emergency Department visits or ninety-day readmissions, which may have been averted by standardized follow-up protocols after hospital discharge.[9] In another study of patients who underwent radical cystectomy for bladder cancer, patients with lower health literacy had greater odds of developing minor complications, but not major complications.[10]

Most recently, staff evaluated the effects of health literacy and Social Determinants of Health, as measured by the area deprivation index, on telehealth visits. Telehealth visits have exploded during the pandemic, but concerns have been raised about equity in access. Video telehealth visits are superior to audio only, yet video requires additional steps to connect, and may be more difficult for some patient groups. In this study, 17,455 completed telehealth visits were evaluated, 1,375 (8 percent) of which were audio only. Patients who completed visits by audio only had significantly lower health literacy scores, and they also lived in communities with higher area deprivation index, indicating a higher burden of social risk factors.[11]

Patient Support Programs

Since it began in 2010, the health literacy screening initiative has raised awareness among staff and leaders about the prevalence of low health literacy, as well as the need for additional patient education resources. For example, the medical center has invested in supporting and growing a Department of Patient Education, which provides staff training on communication strategies such as the teach-back technique, provides direct input on patient-facing programs, and reviews and edits patient education materials across the clinical enterprise. The medical center has licensed a database of easy-to-understand written and video patient education materials, and regularly adds institutional materials to this library.

Targeted initiatives provide patient support in higher-risk situations, such as hospital discharge. A staffed Discharge Care Center provides routine follow-up of patients after discharge to home, through text message and phone (per patient preference). Structured communication protocols assess whether patients received their medications, durable medical equipment, and other anticipated services; whether follow-up appointments were properly arranged; if patients have any questions or concerns; and follow patients for the development of new or worsening symptoms. Programs such as this can mitigate risks associated with low health literacy or other social risk factors.

Broader Assessment of Social Drivers of Health

Vanderbilt University Medical Center's successful efforts to screen and address health literacy provides a roadmap for broader work related to social drivers of health (SDOH). In specific areas, such as the General Pediatric clinic, routine screening for food insecurity is performed, with referral to additional resources or social work evaluation depending on the level of need. Additional projects are currently underway in the Emergency Department, adult primary care, and urology practices, as the medical center scales up efforts.

As preparation for broader health system implementation, a multi-disciplinary mixed-methods study focused on universal screening of SDOH. The survey included 193 physicians, advanced practice providers, nurses, social workers, case managers, pharmacists, and administrators about attitudes and behaviors related to SDOH screening, and barriers and facilitators of screening. Qualitative interviews with sixteen leaders and front-line staff supplemented survey results. Participants believed routine SDOH screening is important, but only about 40-50 percent routinely screened patients regularly. Barriers included lacking resources to address identified needs (51 percent), time to ask (45 percent), support staff to ask (33 percent), and training in responding to identified needs (28 percent). Not surprisingly, social workers reported fewer barriers and greater familiarity with resources. If healthcare professionals are to be engaged in screening and addressing SDOH, addressing these barriers to implementation will be important for programs to successfully deploy, scale-up, and sustain.[12]

Conclusion

Since up to a third of adults in the US have limited health literacy,[2] it is important to understand how this applies to individual medical needs as well as community-wide medical and social needs. The research shows compelling associations of low health literacy with engagement in care and self-management, as well as worse outcomes for medical and surgical conditions. The prevailing guidance has been for "universal precautions," which assumes that most or all adults have some difficulty understanding and acting on health information, and that, therefore, all communication should be clear and follow best practice, such as teach-back. Realistically, it is difficult to direct additional time and effort to all patients. By screening health literacy levels, it is possible to follow an approach of basic universal precautions, with additional assistance and support for patients with demonstrated need.[13] Health literacy is a key factor in efforts to address social drivers of health.

Key Takeaways

- Successful screening depends on nursing and administrative leadership.
- Health literacy screening tools should be brief and acceptable to patients and staff.
- Screening should be incorporated into clinical workflows.
- Low health literacy impacts outcomes of medical and surgical care.
- Health literacy screening is a critical component of SDOH initiatives.

Important Facts

- 90 million in US have low health literacy, including more than a third of adults
- Low health literacy is associated with medical and surgical outcomes, including worse disease control, healthcare utilization, complications, mortality, and costs

Endnotes

1. Institute of Medicine. *Health Literacy: A Prescription to End Confusion.* Washington, DC: National Academies Press, 2004.

2. Mark Kutner, Elizabeth Greenberg, Ying Jin, and Christine Paulsen. *The Health Literacy of America's Adults: Results from the 2003 National Assessment of Adult Literacy (NCES 2006-483)*. Washington, DC: US Department of Education, National Center for Education Statistics, 2006.

3. Darren DeWalt, Nancy Berkman, Stacey Sheridan, Kathleen Lohr, Michael Pignone. "Literacy and health outcomes: a systematic review of the literature." *Journal of General Internal Medicine*. 2004;19(12): 1128-1139.

4. Nancy Berkman, Stacey Sheridan, Katrina Donahue, David Halpern, Karen Crotty. "Low health literacy and

health outcomes: an updated systematic review." *Annals of Internal Medicine*. 2011;155(2):97-107.

5. Courtney Cawthon, Lorraine Mion, David Willens, Christianne Roumie, Sunil Kripalani. "Implementing routine health literacy assessment in hospital and primary care patients." *Joint Commission Journal on Quality and Patient Safety*. 2014;40(2):68-76.
6. Kathryn Goggins, Kenneth Wallston, Lorraine Mion, Courtney Cawthon, and Sunil Kripalani. "What patient characteristics influence nurses' assessment of health literacy?" *Journal of Health Communication*. 2016; 21(sup2):105-108.
7. Candace McNaughton, Sunil Kripalani, Courtney Cawthon, Lorraine Mion, Kenneth Wallston, and Christianne Roumie. "Association of Health Literacy With Elevated Blood Pressure: A Cohort Study of Hospitalized Patients." *Medical Care* 2014;52(4):346-353.
8. Candace McNaughton, Courtney Cawthon, Sunil Kripalani, Dandan Liu, Alan Storrow, and Christianne Roumie. "Health Literacy and Mortality: A Cohort Study of Patients Hospitalized for Acute Heart Failure." *Journal of the American Heart Association*. 2015;4(5):e001799.
9. Jesse Wright, Gretchen Edwards, Kathryn Goggins, Vikram Tiwari, Amelia Maiga, Kelvin Moses, Sunil

Kripalani, and Kamran Idrees. "Association of health literacy with postoperative outcomes in patients undergoing major abdominal surgery." *JAMA Surgery*. 2018;153(2):137-142.

10. Kristen Scarpato, Stephen Kappa, Kathryn Goggins, Sam Chang, Joseph Smith Jr, Peter Clark, David Penson, Matthew Resnick, Daniel Barocas, Kamran Idrees, Sunil Kripalani, and Kelvin Moses. "The impact of health literacy on surgical outcomes following radical cystectomy." *Journal of Health Communication*. 2016;21(sup2):99-104.
11. Sarah Brown, Michelle Griffith, Sunil Kripalani, and Sara Horst. "Association of health literacy and area deprivation with initiation and completion of telehealth visits in adult medicine clinics across a large health system." *JAMA Network Open*. 2022;5(7):e2223571.
12. Sophia Kostelanetz, Mariah Pettapiece-Phillips, Jacy Weems, Tamarra Spalding, Christianne Roumie, Consuelo Wilkins, and Sunil Kripalani. "Health care professionals' perspectives on universal screening of social determinants of health: a mixed-methods study." *Population Health Management*. 2022;25(3):367-374.
13. Kristie Hadden and Sunil Kripalani. "Health literacy 2.0: Integrating patient health literacy screening with universal precautions." *Health Literacy Research and Practice*. 2019;3(4):e280-e285.

Chapter 9.

Essentia Health Case Study

Introduction

Essentia Health is an integrated healthcare system headquartered in Duluth, Minnesota. It includes fourteen hospitals, seventy clinics, six long-term care sites, and six assisted and independent living facilities. As of June 30, 2021, 907 physicians were employed along with 1,218 advanced practitioners, 3,746 nurses, and 8,172 other staff for a total of 14,043 colleagues. Clinic encounters number 1,608,866 each year with an average daily hospital census of 527 patients.

As a non-profit integrated healthcare system, Essentia Health believes that the highest quality care requires a regard for both the soul and science of healing and a focus on continuous improvement. The organization is committed to having a meaningful presence in the communities it serves in Minnesota, North Dakota, and Wisconsin.

Essentia Health has invested in numerous community health programs to carry out its mission of making a healthy difference in people's lives.

1. Addressing Social Needs and Influencing SDOH

Essentia Health received a Quality Award from the National Association of Accountable Care Organizations for its efforts on Social Determinants of Health and inequities. The award reflects Essentia Health's emphasis on service integration (social health needs), using technology to improve performance, enhancing quality while addressing disparities, and scaling interventions with community partnerships. "Addressing the Social Determinants of Health is a high priority at Essentia Health. Access to food, transportation, housing, and other basic needs impacts one's overall health, and creating tools to match patients' needs with the right community partner is foundational work," says Debbie Welle-Powell, Essentia Health's chief population health officer.

Food Insecurity

In the Central Hillside neighborhood, where Essentia Health's downtown Duluth campus is located, the food insecurity rate is 45 percent. Research shows that poor nutrition is a major risk factor for many chronic diseases and that food insecure populations are two times more likely to have a stroke, 1.7 times more likely to have diabetes, and 1.4 times more likely to have heart disease. Second Harvest Heartland, a local food bank, found that 67 percent of their clients had to make a choice between food, medical care or medicine at least once in the previous year.

To address this issue, Essentia Health piloted a screening program for social needs (including food insecurity, transportation, and financial strain) in three clinics. A Community Health Worker followed up and partnered with patients and their families to identify needs and create a plan to address them. Understanding that the COVID-19 pandemic placed a great deal of financial strain on communities, Essentia Health recognized that the need to help patients get connected to community resources is a top priority.

Impacting Social Determinants of Health

While working with a patient to address an immediate social need can be impactful for that individual, addressing the complexity of Social Determinants of Health one patient at a time is unlikely to make the lasting, systemic change needed for substantial improvements in the root causes of health disparities. In addition to the direct service provided for patients through this program, Essentia Health is also collecting valuable data that can support system change at the community level.

Essentia Health is working to develop community partnerships to further care transformation. By working across multiple levels of impact—individual, organizational, and community—Essentia Health is analyzing the broader context around poverty and inequity in the community. The focus is on identifying root causes and resource gaps, along with improving communication and coordination among services and resource providers.

Technology innovation was likewise identified as a necessary strategy to improve performance, particularly for unmet social needs. To generate a baseline of needed information, a social needs questionnaire in MyChart (Essentia's patient electronic health record portal) was developed and automatically assigned to all patients prior to their visit. It is also included in the rooming process for patients who are not active on MyChart. The questionnaire has been sent with 1 million encounters and completed 420,330 times (a 46 percent response rate).

Individual Level Impact

More than 20,000 patients have identified at least one social need. When a patient identifies they have a social need, an additional question asks if the patient would like to be contacted by a Community Health Worker to connect them to resources and services.

In addition to creating a new standard of work in primary care and pediatric settings, an additional level of outreach was conducted in May-June 2020 with a population of patients at high risk for severe COVID-19 illness. The goal was to create a model to identify those at high risk for a severe COVID-19 illness and connect them with timely healthcare resources so they could manage their chronic health needs. The outreach assisted them in meeting social needs so they could stay safely at home.

Through this project, the social needs questionnaire was sent to an additional 40,000 patients and offered to assist them with food, transportation, or financial needs. Risk factors that were considered in designing the target population criteria included:

eighty-plus years of age and comorbidities such as asthma, COPD, cancer, and inflammatory diseases.

As a result of these efforts, more than 4,000 referrals have been placed for Essentia Health patients to various community programs. Through the data captured since the beginning of the pilot, 13.5 percent of patients who complete the questionnaire report at least one social need. This is not evenly distributed across race and ethnicity. For example, 22 percent of American Indian/Alaskan Native patients and 17 percent of Black or African American patients reported food insecurity compared to 7 percent of white patients. Black and American Indian/Alaskan Native patients were also more likely to report financial strain and transportation barriers than white patients.

Overall, 9 percent of patients who report a social need are connected to a new community resource through the program. This has resulted in more than 2,000 unique patients being connected for a variety of social determinants, including food insecurity (1,246 patients), financial assistance (383 patients), transportation (220 patients), mental health (208 patients), housing (123 patients), and other topics, including alcohol use, intimate partner violence, legal aid, and stress management.

Between 2018 and 2019, Essentia Health saw significant improvement in the Care Coordination/Patient Safety domain for Medicare Shared Savings Populations (MSSP) with marked improvement in readmission, unplanned admissions, and ambulatory-sensitive conditions. There was also a marked improvement in depression remission and continued high quality scores in controlling diabetes and high blood pressure among this population.

Essentia Health's Accountable Care Organization (ACO) quality score, as determined by the Centers for Medicare & Medicaid Services (CMS), was 95 percent in 2019.

Organizational Impact

Essentia Health was able to scale a three-clinic pilot to the entire system of about seventy clinics in one year. One of the primary limiting factors was the capacity of community-based organizations that participate in the intervention. That led to the effort to find community partners who could quickly serve patients with a variety of needs across rural Minnesota, Wisconsin, and North Dakota service areas.

Four organizations were identified that could process and refer patients through the electronic health record (EHR). Additionally, relationships were developed to place referrals to eighty more organizations (not through the EHR), including senior services, county services, mental health providers, and housing resources.

During the second year, a partnership with Find Help was secured to build a more sustainable social care network called "Resourceful." The Find Help platform provides a way to streamline the referral process, as well as track and measure the success of connecting patients to local programs. Essentia Health, Generations Health Care Initiatives, Wilderness Health, and other partners collaborated to launch Resourceful. The vision was to create a social care platform to facilitate stronger coordination between helping professionals, patients, and the greater community.

Professionals can use the platform to search for social service programs and connect patients by sending a direct referral on behalf of a patient. By building relationships with key community partners through outreach and engagement, Essentia Health is creating a network of community-based organizations ready to serve community members and update referral statuses, forming a closed-loop network.

"We have been having conversations with community-based organizations for over a year about this project," says Emily Kuenstler, Community Health Director at Essentia Health. "There is a lot of excitement for the launching of Resourceful around the region. It is seen as a way for organizations to work more effectively together in meeting the needs of our community."

In the first eight months of launching Resourceful, more than 3,806 programs in Essentia's service area were added to an interactive community resource directory. The directory is accessible to healthcare providers through the EHR. It is also accessible to any community partner and the public. Of the 3,806 programs added, 490 programs "claimed" their listing, meaning that someone who works for the organization has reviewed the information for accuracy and decided on an appropriate next step to get in contact with the program. Many of the claimed programs have enabled referrals. Using a common platform to share information is a critical way to improve communication and coordination between organizations.

Community Impact

Food insecurity was one of the greatest identified needs in the social needs screening. Beyond connecting patients to community food resources, Essentia Health is also working with partners to address hunger in the community. The success of the referrals to community programs relies on the capacity of the local food resources to provide accessible, affordable, and healthy food. Through the organization's community benefit programs, Essentia Health donated $1.5 million to community-based organizations in 2020, including $300,000 for food insecurity initiatives.

These contributions were spread throughout Essentia's service areas. Essentia donated $125,000 alone directly to local food shelves. This includes a $93,000 donation to Second Harvest Northern Lakes Food Bank, reaching more than 80,000 individuals in northern Minnesota. Additional food shelves such as Second Harvest North Central Food Bank, Falls Hunger Coalition, Aurora Area Food Shelf, Mesabi Range College's food bank, and CHUM also received funding support.

In addition to food shelf donations, Essentia Health supported meal programs, such as $60,000 toward Damiano Center's Community Kitchen, the largest emergency meal provider in northeastern Minnesota. Free meals are offered at thirteen regular mealtimes each week and provided to anyone who is hungry with no questions asked. Damiano Center was able to pivot to a "to-go" meal program in response to COVID-19 precautions. Essentia Health's donation will feed 12,000 hungry individuals.

Essentia donated $38,710 to food access programs in schools across the organization's service area. Two schools received funds to implement a school garden program to increase the knowledge and access to healthy foods. The amount of $32,610 was awarded to support the Duluth Farm to School program. Through K-12 school gardens, lesson integration, classroom/cafeteria tastings and procurement, Farm to School programming focuses on increased consumption of fresh fruits and vegetables in youth, a better understanding of where food comes from and how it is grown, and developing a taste for fruits and vegetables using experiential learning tied to multidisciplinary standards. More than 13,000 students across Duluth are positively impacted by this program.

Essentia Health contributed more than $100,000 to farmers' markets in cities across the service area including Moorhead, Detroit Lakes, Grand Rapids, Virginia, and Duluth. A $50,000 contribution was made to the American Indian Community Housing Association to support their emergency food distribution programming and farmers' market efforts.

Essentia Health employees also volunteered 564 hours to organizations supporting food insecurity in Minnesota. These volunteer hours equate to a dollar value of $16,096. According to the Independent Sector (independentsector.org), the value of volunteer time in Minnesota is currently $28.54 per hour. Several Essentia Health employees are currently serving on boards of local organizations supporting food insecurity, including Second Harvest Northern Lakes Food Bank, Damiano Center, CHUM (a faith-based organization), and Iron Range Partnership for Sustainability.

The multifaceted partnership of financial donations, volunteer work and, leadership through board service helps community food access partners continue to operate and provide food to Essentia Health patients and the broader community.

Evaluation Framework

Essentia Health developed an interactive dashboard to measure several key performance indicators and map social needs across service areas. Through the data collected and visualized in the interactive dashboard, the team can start deeper work to consider the broader context around poverty and inequity in communities. Essentia Health is analyzing social risk drivers and root causes, identifying resource gaps, and improving communication and coordination among services/resource providers.

Additionally, Essentia Institute for Rural Health has received funding for a three-year community-based participatory research study to evaluate the impact of the program on outcomes and total cost of care as well as key drivers for and barriers to positive outcomes. By applying an equity lens, the research is intended to contribute to the evidence base and further understanding return on investment.

Essentia Health, Essentia Institute of Rural Health, and Generations Health Care Initiatives worked together to create a Community Advisory Committee and subcontracted with two community-based organizations to hire fifteen community consultants, most of whom are Black, Indigenous, or People of Color (BIPOC) and/or individuals who have personally experienced having social needs. The community consultants are working with the research institute to conduct an evaluation of the process, implementation and outcomes of the program from the perspective of someone in need of services. The intent is to learn from community members' experiences using the resource and apply lessons for improvement. Essentia Health aims to create trusting relationships among those they seek to support and continuously improve the program based on their experience.

2. Community Health Needs Assessment

Every three years, each Essentia Health hospital conducts a Community Health Needs Assessment (CHNA) to systematically identify, analyze, and prioritize community health needs. The process is conducted in collaboration with many community partners such as healthcare systems, local public health departments and organizations, or individuals representing the broad interests in the community. These include members of the medically underserved, low-income, and populations at higher health risk. Once the priority needs are identified, Essentia Health works with partners to design and implement strategies to improve health.

The plan is designed to draw upon community strengths and resources by using a Result-Based Accountability (RBA) framework. RBA uses a data-driven decision-making process to help communities and organizations get beyond talking about problems to taking action to solve them. Community members and partners are actively involved in setting priorities as well as designing solutions. A Tool for Equity Accountability was created to ensure that health equity is prioritized and opportunities are created to collaboratively engage people from affected communities.

During Essentia Health's last Community Health Needs Assessment process in 2019, eighty-two focus groups were conducted across the service area, including nearly 2,000 community members.

Throughout the CHNA process, Essentia Health follows five guiding principles:

1. Collaborate toward solutions with multiple stakeholders (e.g., schools, worksites, medical centers, public health) to improve community health.
2. Build trust through collaboration with community members.
3. Prioritize sustainable evidence-based efforts around the greatest community good.
4. Create clear, specific, realistic, and action-oriented goals to improve health outcomes.
5. Prioritize strategies that advance health equity, address structural barriers, or reduce health disparities.

Across Essentia Health's twelve Community Health Needs Assessments, there are a total of eighty-two strategies (about seven per community) being implemented with communities. During the second year in the three-year cycle, 92 percent of the strategies were completed or in-progress. The strategies include a combination of policy, system, and environmental change along with health education strategies. This work is made possible by partnerships and collaboration with more than 800 community partner organizations.

Examples of the types of strategies include:

- **Policy change:** Restricting access to tobacco across communities, public places, and worksites, and advocating for transportation resources
- **System change:** Working with school districts to create school-based mental health services, increasing access to medication-assisted treatment programs to treat substance use disorders, and adding new bus routes
- **Environmental change:** Increasing access to healthy foods through farmers markets and grocery retail and expanding bike lanes/multi-purpose trails
- **Education:** Diabetes prevention workshops, vaping educational campaigns, and creating mental well-being resources

Essentia Health implements several strategies across the entire system service area, working with partners in each community. Most of the strategies are personalized to each local community.

System-Wide Strategies

- Essentia Health started offering Mental Health First Aid (MHFA) to both Essentia Health colleagues and community members in 2019. The workshops were switched to a virtual format in 2020. Just as CPR teaches people how to assist an individual having a heart attack, MHFA teaches people to assist someone experiencing a mental health or substance use crisis until professional care is obtained.

Since June 2019, 557 people have attended the eight-hour training program, including 142 Essentia Health colleagues. After the training, 99 percent of participants reported feeling confident that they could reach out to someone who may be experiencing a mental health crisis. And 100 percent of participants reported that they would recommend the training to others. Plans are underway to train every employee in several local fire and police departments.

- Essentia Health developed a video and toolkit for use by teachers and community groups to educate students and the public about the dangers of vaping. The ten-minute video utilizes a peer-to-peer education model by featuring only youth voices and has been viewed more than 8,000 times in the past year. To evaluate impact of the campaign, pre- and post-surveys were completed by 748 high school students. The surveys show a decrease in the percent of students who would be somewhat or very likely to try an e-cigarette after completing the program.

  The surveys show an increased understanding of the harmful health effects of vaping after completing the program. The video and toolkit have been used in eighth through twelfth grade classrooms across all Essentia

Health markets. The materials are publicly available on Essentia Health's website and have been shared with schools across the United States.

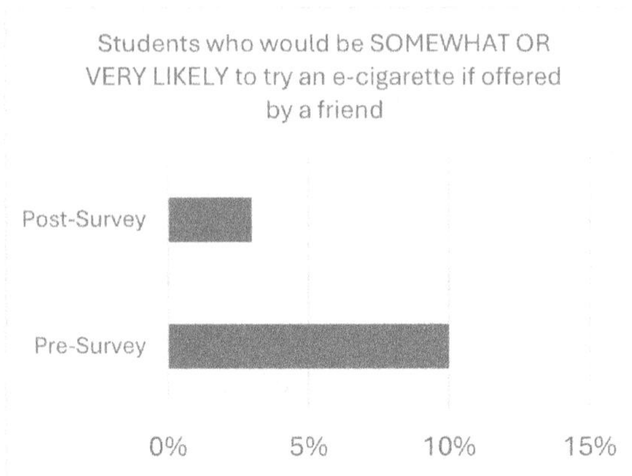

Representative Local Strategies

Crow Wing Energized, a grassroots movement backed by Essentia Health and Crow Wing County, supports the National Diabetes Prevention Program in the Brainerd Lakes area. "We're preventing problems before they happen," says Kara Schaefer, community health educator for Essentia Health, who also leads the program's classes. "It's a proven program that's split into two sections—core classes for sixteen consecutive weeks and then once a month for the remainder of the year. It goes beyond teaching healthy eating and exercise habits. You have a curriculum to encourage group talk and idea sharing." The program is free for participants. Since 2019, 1,464 participants have completed the year-long program.

Crow Wing Energizes also leads a worksite wellness coalition that holds challenges like *Rethink Your Drink,* which encourages organizations to adopt policies to remove sugar-sweetened beverages from vending machines and cafeterias and encourages individuals to drink water. In 2020, eight worksites participated in the challenge, including 562 individuals. The worksite wellness team also works with employers to encourage physical activity such as walking meetings, yoga, and creating trails or paths for employees to use during breaks.

Over the past eight years, Crow Wing County is starting to see an increase in the percentage of adults engaged in moderate or vigorous physical activity and an increase in the percentage of adults eating five or more servings of fruits and vegetables.

According to the 2021 County Health Rankings, Crow Wing County now ranks forty-first out of eighty-seven counties in the state for health outcomes. This represents significant improvement from 2018 when it was ranked sixty-first.

Becker County Energize is a collaborative across Becker County led by Essentia Health. A collaborative was launched to improve mental health of youth in the Frazee community. More than fifteen community-based organizations in this rural community came together to support the development of *CornerStone*—a new community and youth center designed by and for students to support well-being. The goal is to enhance community relationships, create a positive empowering space for youth, and become a thriving attraction in the community. A local church donated a building, and more than forty youth and one-hundred adults volunteered to support this vision.

CornerStone creates a safe space for youth to congregate without drugs and alcohol, with programming designed to support holistic wellness and advance life skills.

Cornerstone is in the progress of launching a Farm to Table Bistro and Coffee Shop as part of a student entrepreneurial program. This unique and dynamic opportunity provides a mechanism for youth to develop an array of entrepreneur and workforce skills. Additionally, it helps fill a need for healthy food options in the community.

Data from the Minnesota Student Survey is showing an improvement in Frazee student mental well-being. The percentage of students reporting "not at all" to feeling down, depressed, or hopeless increased in both eighth and ninth grade. Additionally, the percentage of students reporting that adults in the community care about them has improved from 2016 to 2019.

Olivia, a Frazee student, provided her testimonial: "A lot of kids in Frazee suffer from mental health issues because there are not a lot of things to do. CornerStone makes me feel more useful. I feel like I am a part of the community—I can help with things in the community, and I like that feeling."

Summary

Essential Health's mission is making a healthy difference in people's lives by improving the root causes of health disparities in the community. This calls for system-level change in terms of food insecurity, transportation, behavioral health, and financial stress.

Key Takeaways

- Collaboration with community partners must include addressing the priorities of at-risk populations such as medically underserved and low-income patients.
- Community members and partners must be collaborative in setting priorities and designing solutions based on health equity, removing structural barriers to care, and reducing disparities.
- Matching patients with the right service partners in the community is a prerequisite for better outcomes and patient satisfaction.
- Clinical care alone cannot fully address health inequities. Addressing individual social needs is only part of the solution. Hospitals must engage in systemic community level approaches to make lasting impact.
- Community health priorities must be set by local communities—each rural community is different with unique needs and assets.

Executive Comments

Debbie Welle-Powell is Chief Population Health Officer, Essentia Health

Social needs must be part of care plans.

As an integrated health system in the Midwest, Essentia has been on a journey to provide comprehensive high-quality care to the communities we serve. In fact, we often describe our work as a moral obligation, a calling to stay and work through the challenges of rural healthcare together.

If you look at Minnesota's county-level data on health outcomes and healthy behaviors, we have a higher than average number of smokers, obesity levels, and alcohol and substance use in our service areas.

Same for social and economic factors. We have higher unemployment rates, income inequality, children living in poverty, and lower graduation rates. Yet, our mission is to make a healthy difference in people's lives. To deliver on that promise, it requires a holistic approach to meeting the needs of our patients and communities. Unless we have healthier communities, it's very hard to reduce healthcare costs.

Our prescription for health is threefold: prevention and wellness, influencing policy, and strengthening community partnerships. This entails screening for social needs and making long-term investments in community.

We know that change isn't easy. We work hard to make the right thing to do the easy thing to do.

Healthcare systems like Essentia Health were challenged by the pandemic to deliver necessary care differently. Prior to COVID, we offered limited retail e-visits and some remote patient monitoring. When the pandemic hit, we took a quantum leap forward, redirected our change management capability, and fast-tracked adoption of digital technology.

With the technology platform in place (built), we moved quickly to direct-to-consumer services that kept our patients safely in their homes. This included screening for immediate social needs, especially food insecurity, which increased dramatically.

Integrating the social needs of our patients into their clinical care plans allowed us to take a more comprehensive and holistic view of improving the health of our patients.

Chapter 10.

Christensen Institute Executive Interview

Ann Somers Hogg, MSPH, is the Director of Health Care Research. She was formerly Assistant Vice President of Strategy and Transformation at Atrium Health.

The Clayton Christensen Institute for Disruptive Innovation is a nonprofit, nonpartisan think tank founded on the theories of late Harvard Business School professor Clayton M. Christensen. The Institute offers a unique framework for understanding many of society's most pressing problems by elevating the conversation surrounding these issues through rigorous research and public outreach.

Question: You have said that to thrive in the future, healthcare organizations need a transition plan to be financially viable and to continue serving their communities. What does this imply?

We've analyzed the healthcare landscape and found that healthcare organizations don't have the business models in place to sustainably address drivers of health (also known as Social Determinants of Health), which is a requirement for successful value-based care.

In the US, 90 percent of healthcare spending is for medical care, which only accounts for 10-20 percent of health outcomes. Yet, up to 80-90 percent of outcomes are attributable to drivers of health. So effectively, the US pays 600 percent more for medical care than it should. If we want to reduce disparities and improve health outcomes across the country, we must address DOH. And today's traditional, fee-for-service business models are not set up to succeed at addressing DOH because they're focused on sick care rather than addressing the root causes of disease. Addressing the root cause of illness is a fundamentally different value proposition than solving an illness once it arises. And to deliver a new value proposition, we need new business models.

Question: Why aren't such investments being made in what improves people's lives?

The healthcare system doesn't incentivize prevention. Instead, providers are incentivized to perform services that treat illness instead of keeping people healthy. This incentive structure perpetuates the business models that profit from fee for service.

Question: How is this changing?

The ACA was one effort to promote value-based care and address the drivers of health. It requires nonprofit hospitals to perform community health needs assessments every three years and to develop a strategy to address those needs. Additionally, CMS's Innovation Center launched multiple programs around DOH, and updated reimbursement models to incentivize upstream interventions.

However, these interventions are largely ad hoc and mostly tied to existing business models. They are a bolt-on to the current system rather than a redesign or transformation. And without a transformed business model, DOH success is less likely.

At the same time, our research revealed that innovators around the country are building *new* business models around four key components:

1. Addressing the needs of both consumers (i.e., patients) and customers (i.e., payers and employers)
2. Establishing payment models that incentivize serving those needs
3. Measuring what matters to those served
4. Connecting dots across the disconnected healthcare ecosystem and its community partners to achieve these goals (what we refer to as a "partnership ecosystem.")

Traditional healthcare business models fall short in meeting these customer-centric criteria because they threaten the existing profit model. As business models mature, they become too rigid to alter the resources, processes, and profit formula they have established in order to repeatedly deliver on their value proposition.

On the other hand, innovative health and care organizations are designing approaches that fill the gap between what consumers and customers want, and what traditional organizations offer. In 2021, the for-profit DOH industry had fifty-eight such startups, which represented $2.4 billion in funding, and a valuation of more than $18.5 billion. These companies offer a fundamentally different value proposition than traditional offerings.

Question: Can traditional healthcare organizations partner with others to impact DOH?

Absolutely. But today, most don't have the required interfaces with others to make a sizeable impact on drivers of health. They're organized around partner and vendor relationships to execute against their core business model's priorities of providing best-in-class, illness-based care. This leads to disconnected and incomplete DOH efforts.

In contrast, innovators have created partnership ecosystems comprised of multiplayer, interconnected webs to tackle DOH problems. Those that are most effective leverage an enabling technology platform to fuel interdependence across these partnerships.

Question: What works best?

Based on our research and interviews, we found the most effective models at addressing DOH are paid through value-based arrangements. These included global capitation or participating-in-payment models that have both upside and downside risk.

Question: What is the role of philanthropy in this model?

Philanthropy can be a bridge to a long-term funding model and a mechanism to leverage when learning which DOH efforts are most effective for a given population.

Question: You distinguish between drivers of health and Social Determinants of Health. Why is that?

At the Institute, we believe it's important to think about these terms through the eyes of the consumer.

In recent decades, the healthcare industry has used the term Social Determinants of Health (SDOH) to refer to the societal, population-level structures that influence health outcomes. But there are multiple competing definitions for SDOH, all suffering from a high level of complexity and the exclusion of the individual's perspective.

Drivers of health offers clearer language to describe the individual's ability, and the health ecosystem's necessity, to improve the causal drivers of health and life outcomes. These structures that drive health outcomes are *drivers*, not *determinants* set in stone.

The DOH phrase challenges the assumption that these factors are predetermined and highlights our individual and collective agency to drive change, thus enhancing health and life outcomes for all people. It likewise addresses the limiting nature of the word "social," as drivers of health encompass the social, environmental, and economic systems that influence how people live, work, play, pray, and age.

Question: You cited Humana as an example of prioritizing DOH. Can you say more?

Humana's Bold Goal program launched in 2015 and has become an industry model of innovation in assessing the impact of helping members address DOH. Its efforts seek to address the needs of the whole person, by focusing on what is truly important to individuals and families: living happier, more productive lives. Humana measures the success of these efforts with the CDC's Healthy Days tool.

It is a four-question, self-administered questionnaire where individuals assess the number of mentally and physically unhealthy days they've had over the last thirty days. In a recent report, Humana shared what happened when it applied this measure to Medicare Advantage members and communities during the COVID-19 pandemic in 2020. Some key findings that stood out were:

- A 2.4 percent reduction in physical unhealthy days for Medicare Advantage enrollees.

- 2.2 percent reduction in overall unhealthy days for Bold Goal communities.
- A decline in unhealthy days across health plan populations, ranging from -6.3 percent for low-income members to -2.7 percent for dual-eligibles.

Communities with fewer unhealthy days in 2020 versus 2015 included Baton Rouge, Knoxville, New Orleans, and San Antonio.

Humana is a notable leader in how it demonstrates the impact of its DOH efforts on the outcomes that matter to the people served. Additionally, the findings led to further refinements in targeted interventions to further improve individual and community quality of life measures. What's particularly important is that Humana measures DOH success through the eyes of consumers rather than trying to use traditional quality measures, which fall short in terms of impact and relevance. Healthy Days looks at multiple aspects of health that better reflect the intent of DOH interventions on community health.

Question: How does the Christensen Institute assess how a business model effectively addresses drivers of health?

New value propositions require new business models. As a result, our research showed that organizations seeking to impact DOH must alter their business models to effectively deliver on a value proposition that promotes prevention and health. This means all components of the business model—value proposition, resources, processes, profit formula, and priorities—must work together in a way that allows the organization to sustainably deliver on its promise to consumers and customers. Our research revealed that organizations effectively impacting DOH incorporated the following components into their business models:

- Their value propositions focused on enabling consumers and customers to achieve their goals, or desired progress.
- From a resource perspective, they realized they couldn't tackle DOH all on their own. As a result, they harnessed a partnership ecosystem, which was supported by an enabling technology platform.
- When it came to processes, they recognized the critical role of trust in their model, and they hard-coded processes to establish and maintain trust with those they served.
- Lastly, they measured what mattered to their consumers and customers and aligned their revenue streams to these outcomes.

Question: Healthcare organizations wanting to develop DOH capacity face a "make or buy" decision. What is the best strategy?

This question of "What is the best strategy?" was the focus of our report *Improve or transform: Choosing the right business model to deliver health.* The short answer is that business model change is not one-size-fits-all. The right strategy for a given leader depends on their company's context. By context, I mean various aspects of the organization's current situation, such as:

- Its mission, vision, and beliefs about the future
- The current business model structure and viability
- The leader's willingness to take on risk in an uncertain environment.

In *Improve or transform*, we provide a "how to" guide to walk leaders through the process of determining which strategy is the right fit for them. We share that one strategy—improve—will lead to more success in the short-run, while the other—transform—is more likely to yield longer-term success. So, each strategy has a different purpose; a different set of requirements; and different challenges, benefits, and risks.

In *Improve or transform,* the Christensen Institute analyzed leading organizations that employed various strategies. Atrium Health and Advocate Aurora Health represent two different strategic approaches. Since the publication of the report, these entities have been combined into one health system: Advocate Health. These case studies are copied from that report below.

Case Study: Atrium Health

Atrium Health is a large, integrated nonprofit health system located in the Southeast. It provides a continuum of care across the Carolinas, Georgia, and Alabama. The mission is to "improve health, elevate hope, and advance healing for all." Accordingly, it established social impact and health equity as a strategic priority. The effort was led by the senior vice president and chief community and social impact officer for the forty-hospital system.

The new strategy was already aligned with its mission and could deliver on its DOH and social impact efforts by making improvements to its existing business model. However, leaders recognized they needed additional capabilities that were not inherent to Atrium's core business model of healthcare operations and care delivery. Key additions included the following:

Value proposition

Address the most critical community health needs as highlighted in the Community Health Needs Assessment (CHNA).

Resources

Form a new social impact valuation team with expertise in grant writing and intervention evaluation.

Find help for an enabling technology platform to support connections to community-based organizations.

Hire Community Health Workers.

Processes

Use existing CHNA collection process to inform strategy and investments.

Expand process to screen patients for social needs.

Provide low-interest loans for housing partners to preserve naturally occurring affordable housing in the region. The social impact work enhanced and built upon the long-standing community benefit structure.

Add processes to ensure closed-loop referrals to outside entities. Community Health Workers are responsible for delivering this activity.

Profit formula/Priorities

Fund social impact work with balance sheet assets, grants, government funding, and philanthropy.

Align most measures of success for social impact to existing success measures, including new measures such as DOH screenings and closed-loop referrals.

A key to Atrium Health's success in implementing this approach was aligning its social impact goals to existing success measures. This meant priorities did not need to fundamentally change to incentivize carrying out the work. Instead of creating a new measurement system, and the need to change the resource allocation approach, it employed existing measures of success and made the targets for these measures higher. The higher targets incent leaders and staff to carry out the processes required to achieve them. The one exception is the measurement of DOH screenings and associated closed-loop referrals, which were not previously captured.

The start of the undertaking was an uphill battle that required communicating to on-the-ground and frontline leaders about the importance of investing in nontraditional resources and processes. A critical example was the requirement to address clinical and community-level data that would allow providers and care teams to better understand individuals' DOH and address them effectively. However, few staff were initially interested.

In addition to the organization's perseverance to overcome challenges, the keys to Atrium Health's ability to successfully execute this strategy were four-fold:

1. CEO and board support: Without support from the highest level of the organization, strategies that require changes to the business model would not succeed.

2. Partnership ecosystem: The network of entities working together to tackle DOH issues included community-based organizations addressing housing challenges, large corporations dedicated to improving health disparities, medical school partners such as Wake Forest University School of Medicine, and startups.

3. Dedicated resources for the work: A dedicated leadership team is critical for success. It enables the social impact strategy to be carried out without constantly asking the core business for additional resources.

4. Strong financial position: To support this work, Atrium Health leverages a diverse pool of funding that includes balance sheet assets, grants, government funding, and philanthropic donations that includes a $10 million gift from Bank of America.

While Atrium Health's improvement strategy is appropriate for its current situation, it has an ambitious goal to reduce the life expectancy gap in its most vulnerable communities. Given the sizeable difference between this goal and its core value proposition, the organization will need to transform its business model, instead of improving the existing one, to realize this objective over time. This is because an organization cannot deliver on a new value proposition from within an old business model. The resources, processes, profit formula, and measures of success are simply not set up for that to work.

Atrium Health is harnessing an improvement strategy to invest in the future with a focus on social impact and health equity to address the drivers of health to deliver on these goals. The effort supports the current strategy while preparing for a value-based environment. These capabilities support social impact as well as enhanced value to consumers and customers.

Case Study: Advocate Aurora Health

Advocate Aurora Health is a not-for-profit health system with locations across Illinois and Wisconsin. The organization is driven by its purpose to help people live well. In the mid-2010s, the organization noticed nationwide trends indicating its core business of healthcare services could face a continued structural decline in profitability. As a capital-intensive business, market declines in reimbursement could compromise Advocate Aurora's ability to continue delivering on its mission. Its core business was at risk of being disrupted.

To stave off possible disruption and declines in core business profitability, the executive team and board made a commitment to invest in innovating the core business and establishing a new growth strategy to promote long-term viability. Namely, becoming more involved in the consumer health and wellness space with a vehicle to enable that objective.

Because consumer health and wellness offerings are not a core component of Advocate Aurora's healthcare operations business model, a transformation strategy was required to create a new growth engine. Advocate Aurora's executive team and the board aligned on the importance of investing in a new growth engine. They secured a capital allocation to build Advocate Aurora Enterprises (AAE) with a two-fold strategy: to impact health at scale and to improve the financial health of Advocate Aurora. To achieve these goals, AAE set out to acquire companies focused on improving consumer health and wellness.

The key business model differences of AAE from that of Advocate Aurora's core entity can be summarized as follows:

Value propositions

- Diversify revenue streams and new growth opportunities for Advocate Aurora.
- Impact consumer health and wellness at scale, beyond current market footprint.

Resources

- Adopt an asset-light approach.
- Create a dedicated team that is separate from Advocate Aurora's core business resource.

Processes

- Invest in and/or acquire companies that help people live well at every stage of life.

Profit Formula

- Receive capital allocation from Advocate Aurora.
- Invest in and/or acquire companies with direct-to-consumer revenue sources.

Priorities

- Measure EBITDA (same as core).
- Track lives touched by companies invested in or acquired.
- Create and track a Health Impact Index.

The Health Impact Index was designed internally and based on the quality-of-life measures used by AAE units. Through surveys and additional tools, AAE determines if its portfolio companies are improving the health and wellness of consumers (e.g., Senior Helpers provides in-home personal care services to help people age in place).

By creating an index, AAE can continue to use the same measures as it adds portfolio investments with additional areas of consumer health focus. Establishing measures of success is essential to determine if a business is effectively meeting its consumers and customers' needs and goals.

This undertaking was not without its challenges. Critical challenges to overcome included balancing the realities of business model theory with the gravitational pull of the core business. Leaders had to manage employees' tendencies to carry out the processes they had been taught over many years that supported the core value proposition that may be counter to those of the new growth engine.

The leadership team realized that acquiring a new growth business was necessary (versus incubating one) if the organization wanted to scale quickly. AAE's transformation strategy embodied a Transformation—Buy approach focused on investment and acquisition.

Keys to success were outlined that would enable AAE to deliver on its goals:

1. **Aligning with the board of directors:** This includes alignment on the importance of investing in a new growth engine, while also investing in innovation for the core organization.
2. **Having the CEO's continued support:** Specifically, the CEO supports AAE to be completely unfettered from the core.
3. **Separating from the core:** AAE was created and is maintained as a wholly new organizational structure.

4. **Innovating the core and transforming for the long run:** As the healthcare market and future profitability evolves, there must be an emphasis on swift action to innovate and transform the core in the long run.
5. **Being patient:** The transformation process takes time. This recognition is critical to success.

To support these goals, Advocate Aurora's Transformation Oversight Committee included an eight-leader subset of the organization's executive team. The CEO, COO, CFO, CSO, and four key operational staff meet weekly to deal with the strategy and resource allocation issues that arise as a new growth engine runs counter to the core business model's resources, processes, and priorities. To date, the committee has adroitly exercised oversight in balancing competing interests as they arise.

As leaders seek to establish new growth businesses through a Transformation—Buy strategy, much can be learned from Advocate Aurora's approach. In short, patience, persistence, and perseverance are critical leadership characteristics to employ for this strategy.

Question: Any final thoughts?

There's a pathway out of today's predominant fee-for-service, sick care business model, and it starts with creating business models that support addressing drivers of health. Focusing on what matters to consumers and customers, establishing payment models to support addressing those needs, measuring whether consumers and customers achieve their goals, and connecting dots across the disconnected ecosystem are foundational steps on this journey.

Business model change isn't easy. But when it's required, it's worth the effort. In our research, leaders that pursued a transformation strategy acknowledged that while it required the organization to take on risk, trying to survive the course by keeping or improving their current business model posed greater risks.

Thank you.

Reference

Atrium Health and Advocate Aurora Heath-Advocate Aurora Enterprises case study material was based on "Improve or transform: Choosing the right business model to deliver health." Ann Somers Hogg, November 2022, Christensen Institute. https://www.christenseninstitute.org/publications/doh-improve-transform/

Chapter 11.

Montefiore Health System Case Study

Introduction

Montefiore Medical Center (MMC) is in the Bronx and serves many socioeconomically distressed patients. As such, Montefiore has developed many programs to help address Social Determinants of Health. These include funding community development, launching a housing-at-risk program, deploying community training and employment opportunities, operating a food pantry, offering free/steeply discounted healthcare, funding medico-legal partnerships, and providing donations and funding to local Community Based Organizations (CBOs).

In 2018, MMC developed a social needs screening tool to use across its primary care practices. The purpose of screening is to identify social needs and match them with community services to improve patient and population health. MMC is a large urban health system in Bronx, New York, with four hospitals, more than one hundred ambulatory care sites, and 22,500 employees. The Bronx is the nation's poorest urban county; 30.5 percent of residents live in poverty compared to 15.5 percent statewide. The Bronx consistently ranks last in the Robert Wood Johnson County Health Rankings of sixty-two New York State counties.

Montefiore Medical Group (MMG) includes twenty-one primary care locations across Bronx and Westchester counties. Nine sites are Federally Qualified Health Centers (FQHC) and six are teaching sites. In addition, Montefiore's Community Pediatrics Program (CPP) is made up of two FQHCs and a mobile clinic in the South Bronx and serves both children and adults. For a sense of scale, MMG sees 207,000 primary care patients each year and CPP treats 6,500 patients.

Internal Screening Tools

A multi-disciplinary committee of representatives from Montefiore care management, social work, community health, pediatrics, family medicine, clinic administration, and DSRIP was formed to recommend a system-wide tool for SDH screening. The committee's main requirements for the screening tool were for questions to be succinct, relevant to patient needs, actionable and, where possible, previously validated. The group was committed to achieving a streamlined workflow, even though the electronic health record system (Epic) did not have a built-in social health screening module at the time. The screening process was not meant to overburden staff and patients. Nor should it detract from the physician encounter as screening fatigue was an important institutional concern. In the absence of a single gold-standard screening tool, an inventory of screening tools was conducted by the multi-disciplinary working group (e.g., nurses, social workers, doctors, community population health representatives) to identify whether it was best to adopt a single tool that was already in use or, if modifications were necessary, to understand what domains and types of questions should be included.

Several departments across the system had previously developed "home-grown" screening tools. Montefiore's Care Management Organization (CMO) provides a host of services for patients in value-based contracts, including care coordination, patient education, provider relations, credentialing services, community health programs, data analysis, and reporting. At the time of the initial review, CMO was conducting a comprehensive assessment of psycho-social and other risk factors as part of their telephonic care management intake. This can take upwards of one hour to complete and covers more than twenty domains, with multiple assessments as part of each domain, including a review of benefits enrollment and eligibility, social supports and needs, healthcare utilization, and depression and anxiety screening.

As a more pragmatic and scalable approach, Montefiore Community Pediatrics Program (CPP) previously developed a fourteen-item SDH "stressor" tool as part of its paper-based Pediatric and Prenatal Parent Questionnaire. This Stressor tool had been previously compared against PHQ-4 scores and was tailored to include questions that were highly correlated with PHQ-4 patient reported outcome instrument for Social Determinants of Health scores. The CPP stressor tool approached the social determinants from a simple framework: "How much do the following issues cause you stress?", with a three-part response of "none," "some," or "a lot." Domains assessed a range of problems: housing, financial, legal, violence in the home or in the neighborhood, living with a partner/family member with mental illness, alcohol dependency, chronic medical conditions (separate questions), and not having enough food.

Medical residents had also shown an interest in screening patients for SDH. In 2013, the Social Pediatrics program standardized social history taking for their faculty and residents using a modified version of the IHELLP mnemonic device. IHELLP stands for **I**ncome, **H**ousing, **E**ducation, **L**egal, **L**iteracy, **P**sychosocial. It is used to take a social history during a patient encounter. The introduction of this mnemonic tool was associated with increased rates of screening for food and housing insecurity.

At the time of the assessment, only the "I-HELLP" social risk findings were documented and stored as free text, rather than structured fields, in Epic for a limited number of patients. The I-HELPP approach was not feasible for system-wide implementation because it collected social history data in an unstructured manner. The detailed CMO assessment was also not appropriate for quickly screening a high volume of patients since it took forty-five minutes to complete. The CPP tool was included in the list of potential tools to use since it included structured questions, and its reliability had been established.

External Screening Tools

When the assessment was initiated in 2016, relatively few external social needs screeners had been developed. The Center for Medicare and Medicaid Services (CMS) Accountable Health Communities (AHC) Health-Related Social Needs Screening (HRSN) tool was initially attractive but has drawbacks. It was not efficient (e.g., separate questions for each kind of interpersonal violence), not designed for low literacy levels due to the varying nature of answer responses (e.g., some multi-select, some Likert scales), inclusion of important topics was not directly related to social needs (e.g., physical activity and alcohol use), and the twenty-six questions would take too long to complete. In addition, many of the measures proposed by the HSRN tool were already assessed elsewhere within the Montefiore EHR (e.g., smoking, language, mental health/PHQ-2).

Similar issues were raised for the Protocol for Responding to and Assessing Patient, Risks, and Experiences (PRAPARE) tool, created by the National Association of Community Health Centers. The tool had numerous types of multiple-choice options and nested tables. The housing availability answer choice for "I do not have housing" was confusing to patients who might otherwise consider living with others as having housing.

Other screening tools used by other organizations serving the Bronx were also evaluated.

The Institute for Family Health had developed a five-item social needs screener that assessed housing, food security, healthcare access, violence, and community safety. Their tool was embedded in Epic and model workflows were developed. While the committee liked the simple yes/no answer format, the five questions included were felt to be too brief, domains assessed were too broad (e.g., "issues with housing"), and the question on community safety, while touching on an important issue, was one that the clinical team was ill-equipped to handle.

Additional instruments evaluated were the New York State Medicaid Health Home enrollment, including the Functional Assessment of Cancer Therapy—General Population (FACT-GP) and the Health Home Functional Questionnaire. Again, the questions were too non-specific. The homeless question required a "yes/no" response to "I am homeless." The five homeless questions ask for a yes/no response to "I am homeless" and, (1) I need assistance dressing myself, (2) I need assistance eating, (3) I need interpretation services, (4) I have people to help me if I need it, and (5) I go to my doctor/clinic to address my behavioral/ medical needs.

The Adverse Childhood Experiences (ACE) instrument, which was being used by some programs, was discussed, but the questions lacked an actionable timescale that would facilitate immediate action. For example, asking about what happened in your childhood may not be highly indicative of your situation today.

The 2016 Health Leads Social Needs Screening Toolkit, which included eight primary questions and two follow-up questions in "yes"/"no" format was appealing given its previous validation, relative brevity, and simple response options. Domains assessed included food insecurity, housing instability, utility needs, transportation, financial resource strain, and exposure to violence. The Health Leads toolkit also proposed alternative screening questions that increased the flexibility of the instrument. The toolkit met many of the group's requirements.

Initial Screening Tool Selection

The most promising tools were the CPP screener ("Stressor Screener") and the Health Leads Social Needs Screening Toolkit ("Social Needs Screener"). While there was interest in launching a standardized tool across the ambulatory setting, no consensus could be reached about which tool to use. The turf issue centered on using the fourteen-point screener with strong backing from an outstanding medical group in the system that was well funded by grants and very innovative. There was debate about which domains were most critical, which phrases and answer-sets were at the appropriate literacy level, and how many questions would be sufficient to identify need without overwhelming patients or staff. There was consensus around concrete social needs like food, housing, and transportation, but divergent views on social and emotional issues like losing a loved one or experiencing neighborhood violence. While interpersonal violence is a validated question, it remains very limited in terms of defining violence. In many neighborhoods in the Bronx, day-to-day violence can extend from the home to the neighborhood (e.g., gang violence), which is not addressed through this question. In addition, the evaluation work group did not think that

Montefiore could do much about neighborhood violence and, thus, there was no reason to screen for it.

The Stressor Screener was shortened from fourteen to eleven questions and the Social Needs Screener was shortened from eight to seven questions, with some minor modifications made to selected questions (e.g., adding clarifying text and examples). Both screening tools addressed similar issues such as housing problems, food insecurity, transportation, and financial barriers to accessing healthcare, lack of childcare, and interpersonal violence.

Patient and provider feedback was elicited via a small pre-pilot evaluation to see if a single tool was viewed more favorably, and to assess mode of data collection (e.g., via paper or a tablet). Both tools were developed as paper screens (English-only) and briefly used in two MMG clinics and presented to the MMG Patient Advisory Council to gauge patient and provider acceptability as well as informing workflow development. Overall, both tools had high provider support (i.e., no majority dissention) and patient acceptance.

Only a few respondents reported discomfort with questions. However, two questions did cause patient discomfort: "Why are you asking me these questions—do I look homeless?" and "Who is going to see this data, and why are you asking it?" Most patients surveyed by the Patient Advisory Council felt that SDH information was pertinent to their clinical visit and that MMG would be able to help them with these issues. Patients noted a preference toward completing the screener on paper rather than tablets due to concerns about privacy and the cleanliness of tablets.

Providers were also receptive to this initiative but were aware of patient screening fatigue given the number of forms that are completed during registration. In some medical practices, Community Health Workers helped patients fill out the questionnaire. Providers were also concerned about site staffing and resources to address SDH issues identified through screening; therefore, early-test sites were chosen based on the presence of social worker and/or CHW support.

Pilot and Workflow Refinement

After a one-month testing period, the SDH committee regrouped to share feedback and to seek consensus on a single screening tool. The initial testing showed no preference or benefit to using one tool over the other. One of the forms with fourteen items had been successfully piloted and was strongly preferred by one group, in part because it was supported by a volunteer staff. The other screening tool had ten items and was compatible with the Epic record system. The committee chose to formally expand both tools. Although MMC's intent had been to use a single screening tool across the primary care network, the group felt the main mission was screening and connecting patients to resources, not survey design and validation, and that scaling screening in the near-term was more important than perfecting a single tool. Including both forms also furthered consensus in the group.

The paper screening tools (translated in English and Spanish) were distributed to MMG and CPP practices. Both screens were built in Epic so that patient responses could be discretely captured in the medical record, tracked over time, and would facilitate reporting.

Given the lack of evidence-based guidelines on which patients should be screened and the frequency of screening, sites were given discretion to determine which populations would be screened and which of the two pilot tools to use. The two CPP sites chose to use the eleven-item stressor tool and to continue their focus on pre-natal and post-natal mothers. The twenty-one MMG sites predominantly used the seven-item tool, though four used the stressor screen. Each MMG site targeted different patient cohorts, some focusing on new patients, others on recently hospitalized patients or on screening patients of certain providers on selected days. Screening specific high-risk patients (e.g., those with uncontrolled diabetes or asthma) was not possible because front desk staff did not have access to clinical elements in patient charts.

Patients were given paper versions of the screens to complete in the waiting area or in the exam room, and answers were entered into Epic by clinic staff (e.g., LPNs). Screeners were available in multiple languages, so interpreters were not necessary. CHWs occasionally assisted. Physicians reviewed the results with patients and offered to connect patients to clinic-based social workers and/or CHWs who could assist if the patient screened positive for any social needs. A positive response to interpersonal violence was treated as urgent and required an immediate warm hand-off to social work.

Pilot Results

Both pilot screening tools were available for use from March 2017 through March 2018. Pilot feedback from clinic teams and summary screening results were reviewed monthly by the committee. A total of 18,964 patients were screened using either of the two pilot tools (17,380 completed the Social Needs screener and 1,584 completed the stressor screener). During the pilot, the stressor tool was used by five sites and 54 percent of patients indicated "some" or "a lot of stress" due to one or more of the questions; 13.9 percent indicated "a lot" to one or more of the questions. The Social Needs screener was used by eighteen sites and 21.2 percent of patients reported issues with one or more of the seven items. The stressor tool was expected to have a higher positivity rate because more social domains were included. The stressor tool was piloted in a vulnerable community in the South Bronx and included three response options rather than two. For both tools, most patients who screened positive reported only a single issue; allaying fears that implementing a system-wide SDH screening process would overwhelm clinics.

Because modifications to previously validated questions were used in many cases, the objective was to establish the criterion validity of the revised Social Needs screener. The sample size for the CPP screener was too small and had previously been compared to PHQ-4s. The relationship between the number of social needs (categorized as 0, 1, 2, and ≥3) was compared to data on smoking status, diagnosed diabetes, obesity, asthma among adults, and having ≥2 emergency department (ED) visits in the prior year for children and adults. There was a positive association between number of social needs and smoking (p-trend<0.001), diabetes (p-trend=0.017), asthma (p-trend=0.004) and frequent ED visits (p-trend<0.001), but not obesity (p-trend=0.68). For obesity, there was a positive association among women but not men, consistent with the literature. Given the established social gradient for each of these outcomes,[1] early results suggest that the initial SDH screener reasonably captures data on social risks experienced by patients.

It is important to distinguish social needs and social risk from what is meant by the broad category of Social Determinants of Health. Social Determinants of Health are circumstances that people are born into and include conditions of daily life like work and aging. Such conditions are shaped by economic policies, social norms, and political systems and may have both positive and negative impact on health. Social needs focus on self-identified needs at the level of an individual that are non-medical in nature, such as not having enough food or housing instability. Social risk factors refer to adverse social conditions specific to a community or neighborhood such as poverty, unemployment, and housing affordability/quality. These conditions may be prevalent in a community and are associated with poor health. People may live in communities with multiple social risks but may identify fewer immediate social needs specific to their household.

Final Tool Development

The group also discussed how to assess and document whether a patient wanted help with any reported SDH issues. A decision was made not to include the question "Do you want help with any of these problems?" on the screen so as not to discourage patients from getting the help they needed. The group wanted to ensure that providers took the time to discuss the SDH responses with patients and did not rush any conversations because they assumed that the patient was not interested in help from the patient response. Instead, the working group agreed that it would be sufficient for providers to ask patients this question verbally and document the response in Epic after reviewing the SDH responses. The decision to set a uniform standard as to which patients would be screened, and how often, was postponed gaining both site level buy-in and further experience and expertise on the matter.

The screening tool went through three iterations. Version 1 (May 2017-April 2018) modified Health Leads Survey tools, resulting in seven questions. Version 2 (April 2018-December 2019) increased the screener to ten questions and added household quality questions. Version 3 (December 2019-present) had several edits, including reducing the "look back" in the questions related to transportation, medication, and housing. By going from "In the past twelve months…" to "In the past three months…", the social workers felt the question would pick up more recent and acute issues as opposed to problems that had existed a year ago but were now resolved. The social workers also wanted to increase the acuity of the question that screened for interpersonal issues (finding it hard to get along with [...]) by adding "finding it so hard to get along with [...] that it is causing you stress." Lastly, a question was added to the bottom of the screening tool asking patients if they wanted help with any of the issues.

The final tool is shown as Figure 1 in the Appendix. The ten-question SDH screening tool which was already available in English and Spanish was translated into eight additional languages: Albanian, Arabic, Armenian, Bengali, French, Haitian Creole, Khmer, and Brazilian Portuguese. The tool was then integrated in Epic and rolled-out across primary care sites. The previous stressor screen was restricted in Epic to the CPP sites, which had existing research studies they wanted to complete with that version of the screener. Site medical directors and administrators were notified of the new tool's availability in advance of the change and paper copies of the screens were distributed to sites in advance of decommissioning IHELP and prior versions of the old screens.

Screening Findings

The goal of the screening is not to determine the population-level distribution of social needs, but rather the distribution among patients seeking outpatient care. This provides clinics with an assessment tool that could lead to additional outreach to address unmet social needs. There were some key differences in who was screened (n=24,794) and who was not screened (n=158,718) during the implementation period from April 2018 through December 2018. Differences were due primarily to the differential uptake of the screener by some departments (e.g., pediatrics and family medicine practices were most enthusiastic about screening families with children because it was a pressing issue; less so with internal medicine practices).

It was important to compare screened and unscreened patients coming to clinic visits. Screened patients tended to be younger (median age was 26.2 versus 35.9). There were no differences in screening for gender (59 percent female versus 60 percent) in the comparison group. Screened patients were more likely to be on Medicaid (50.9 percent versus 44.4 percent), and somewhat less likely to be on Medicare (15.8 percent versus 18.6 percent) and commercial insurance (33.3 percent versus 36.9 percent). No differences in preferred language of the patient were observed.

During the implementation period, 20 percent of patients screened positive for at least one social need. Forty-eight percent of these patients (9.7 percent) reported ≥2 needs. Housing quality (6.5 percent) and food insecurity (6.2 percent) were the two most prevalent needs. Housing quality refers to the presence of mold, bugs, pests, secondhand smoke, and leaky roofs—all of which can be remedied through integrated pest management and registering complaints to get leaks fixed. The prevalence of each individual social need is presented as Figure 2 in the Appendix. Positive screens for food insecurity by neighborhood are shown as Figure 3 in the Appendix.

One advantage of documenting the results of SDH screening in Epic is that data is loaded in the Montefiore Data Warehouse and can be used to support future analytics, linking clinical data and SDH screening data. Once the screening tool and workflow logistics were resolved, the focus turned to enhancing the referral process to community-based organizations.

Lessons Learned

The two-year experience in adapting and integrating social needs screening in twenty-one primary care practices resulted in a tool that balanced breadth of SDH domains and brevity of screening questions. The ability of MMC to intervene on any identified needs was considered important in the final decision of which questions to include. Important lessons were learned in launching social screening:

1. Clinical teams, including physicians and medical leadership, supported social needs screening, but had concerns about the additional workload.
2. Once it was clear social workers and Community Health Workers would be responsible for identifying resources and connecting patients to care, clinical teams were much more eager to implement the process at their sites.
3. Getting agreement on a single SDH tool is a challenging process and requires significant discussion and consensus-building. Setting firm criteria upfront for a screening tool can drive consensus.

4. Concerns of work-overload were tempered by sharing results of the test and pilot implementations, which consistently showed that three quarters of patients who screened positive reported only one or two issues.
5. Some patients were reticent to be referred for help if told they were going to see the "social worker." Reasons for these refusals were varied, but the majority stemmed from the misperception that these social workers were government social service case workers. This triggered concerns about how the SDH data would be used. As a result, the screening question was changed to "Would you like to speak with someone on our team who can help you?" Accordingly, the response rate and patients were referred to social work with a warm handoff, or a social worker or CHW would call back.

Community-Based Directory

To link patients with SDH issues to community-based services, Montefiore decided to procure a Community Based Organization (CBO) resource directory to facilitate closed loop referrals. This allowed providers to know if patients received services they were referred for. A working group of social workers and CHWs vetted several CBO referral management technologies and selected NowPow.

As of December 2018, Montefiore's 1,194 staff across thirteen departments had access to NowPow and 15 percent use it regularly. The rate of uptake was slowed because staff was pressed for time to learn how to use the directory. A wide net of staff were credentialed to use NowPow, including physicians, nurses, Community Health Workers, social workers, quality improvement managers, and clerical staff. Social workers, CHWs, and care managers are among the most active users.

To promote adoption, the project management team established forums with internal NowPow users and NowPow customer success team members to routinely review utilization data, troubleshoot implementation, and share feedback with NowPow. This informs future product enhancements and reconciles discrepancies in the service directory (e.g., hours of operation, food pantry closure).

As MMC was implementing NowPow, staff reached out to neighboring health systems across the region to coordinate efforts around SDH interventions and CBO engagement. MMC is now partnered with six large health systems and the New York City Department of Health & Mental Hygiene who are also using NowPow to connect patients to CBOs. This working group meets every 6-8 weeks to discuss and make decisions about NowPow product development and deployment. In the meantime, sub-working groups have been established to facilitate decisions and share information around four issues: compliance, analytics, service information improvement, and network development and CBO engagement.

Next Steps

MMC has embraced social needs screening as an on-going organizational priority and an essential component of high-quality healthcare. Now that the screening has gained traction in primary care networks, MMC is exploring multiple avenues to standardize, streamline, and scale the SDH portfolio of interventions.

SDH screening parameters need to be defined across MMC. While the American Academy of Pediatrics suggests screening pediatric patients for unmet social needs at every well child visit, no guideline exists for adults. At the time, MMG has organized a SDH working group to engage clinical champions and establish standardized screening populations and frequencies for adult and pediatric patients. Further discussions and evaluation will determine how to expand SDH screening to other clinical footprints, including inpatient and emergency department settings, and how to support a standard approach for the overall health system.

In preparation for Medicaid risk adjustment of healthcare premiums using ICD-10 codes, MMC is looking to incorporate ICD-10 SDH-related z-codes in the patient's problem list. However, coding the screener responses using ICD-10 is a challenge since there are often a multitude of hyper-specific z-codes per SDH domain. This complicates efforts to standardize codes and SDH domains across screening tools within and between organizations. As such, a paper tool was developed to help Revenue Cycle and social work teams match potential codes to questions that would help inform which codes were most relevant and what information needed to be documented in the EHR to support billing, presented as Table 2 in Appendix.

A major barrier to implementation is staff that primarily deals with the social needs (e.g., CHWs or social workers) do not have permission to add assessments as part of their role-based access in the EHR, a function limited to select providers (e.g., MD, psychologists). Revenue Cycle and social work teams are designing workflows to streamline the process of adding these z-codes to the problem list in preparation for future risk adjustment for SDHs and other value-based payment activities.

Identifying and addressing social needs at a patient level is important, but using analytical tools like GIS mapping allow visualization of areas that have an elevated burden of social risk by neighborhood, zip code, or census tract. Montefiore uses social needs screening data to create hot spot maps of different SDH issues. These findings are shared with city agencies to foster dialogue around CBO resourcing and funding. As part of these efforts, a private foundation has committed to augment the emergency food system supplied by a CBO servicing one of the hotspots for food insecurity, shown as Figure 3 in Appendix. As Montefiore screens more patients for unmet social needs, overlaying hot spotting data with maps of CBO resources could be a useful way to identify discrepancies between neighborhood need and resource availability.

Another area of opportunity is to support CBO partnerships and develop resourcing and contracting strategies that strengthen capacity as they receive an influx of referrals through referral management technologies, such as NowPow. These technologies can be implemented on the CBO side and, if the CBO desires, referrals can be directly transmitted between health systems and the CBO. However, CBOs need resources to adopt and implement referral tools like NowPow, and additional staffing to implement workflows that include processing and closing out referrals from health systems. MMC is meeting with CBOs and convening discussions to set shared expectations for making and acting on referrals (e.g., timeliness, defining "urgent" referrals) so that each party is aligned on operational procedures and enhancing patient experience.

Having access to SDH screening and referral outcomes data will also help health systems like Montefiore understand the cost burden of SDH, impact on patient health, and total expenditures of referring patients for services that address SDH issues. Additional analyses will be necessary to quantify financial and clinical implications.

MMC created Social Needs Screening Guidelines for Health Systems and is included as Table 1 in the Appendix. Suggested z-codes for SDOH screening questions is shown as Table 2 in the Appendix.

Conclusion

After years of acknowledging, but not acting on Social Determinants of Health, the healthcare delivery system is finally making sizeable and tangible investments to integrate social and clinical services. Though Montefiore has a legacy in addressing psycho-social needs within vulnerable populations, the organization still faces challenges when broadening social needs screening and intervention outside of the traditional care management cohort.

For health systems designing screening and outreach interventions in clinical settings, it is important to engage clinical, social, and community experts (via forums) to help devise SDH strategies and implementation procedures. As more health systems join in this effort, there is opportunity for more sophisticated collaboration with other stakeholders, including payers, on policy, program, and reimbursement development. The healthcare industry's momentum on addressing social needs holds great potential for innovative system redesign and improving population health outcomes.

Key Takeaways

- Block-level data is far more precise and actionable (i.e., solutions) than zip code information.
- Many home-grown screening tools are limited by collecting unstructured data, which is not adequately captured by electronic health records. Creating structured screening tools and embedding them in the EHR takes a significant amount of effort and time.
- Screening tools should be designed for low literacy populations and translated into the linguistic preferences of patients.
- Screening topics should be directly related to specific social needs to facilitate immediate action.
- Understanding clinic culture is a prerequisite to gaining support for screener implementation.
- Physician support for screening tools (and SDH) is increased when personnel (e.g., social workers and Community Health Workers) are available to minimize work-overload.

Executive Comments

Amanda Parsons, MD, MBA, is Deputy Chief Medical Officer for MetroPlus Health Plan in New York City. She was formerly Vice President of Community and Population Health at Montefiore Health System in New York.

Among the biggest lessons learned from the screening program was the impact of collecting the right kind of data that leads to solutions.

We collected an enormous amount of compelling data on patients' social needs and mapped it at the block level. That's a powerful tool because it's actionable. It draws attention, ignites solutions, and leads to funding and new investment. We saw this time and time again at the clinic in our health system. To address inequities, we have to move from speech to action, and using data in innovative ways can support those efforts. In our experience, timely and relevant data can be used to guide program development, target resources, and measure outcomes.

With block-level data, you can tell why patients aren't getting to the clinic from certain neighborhoods because the bus routes are too far away. You can intervene and work with the city to change bus routes. With block-by-block data, you can see how to target food bank distribution to families that need it the most. Same for blocks with rodent-infested apartments and moldy homes associated with high rates of family asthma. You can do something about the problem when you show this kind of data on code violations to government agencies who oversee building safety and quality. It gets results.

Kevin Fiori, MD, MPH, MSc is Director-Social Determinants of Health, Office of Community and Population Health, Montefiore Health System, New York City.

In a multi-hospital system, one of the biggest challenges is understanding the culture of each medical clinic as a prerequisite for social needs screening.

I think we spent a lot of time debating the merits of different social risk screeners and not enough time on thinking through what social needs categories we can deliver on at each of our clinics. Figuring out how to effectively address unmet social needs is the biggest lift for the health system right now. It will involve multiple approaches such as social service directories, like NowPow, and growing social sector partnerships.

What we did well was getting everyone to the table—front office staff, nurses, PAs, NPs, MDs—and understanding their roles and priorities for implementing screens. And it makes a big difference whether clinics have social workers and CHWs on board.

We tried to strike a balance between screener length and feasibility. Social need screens had to be simple, easy to use, and actionable. Understanding the culture of the clinics and gaining their support was critical. To date, we have screened more than 60,000 patients for unmet social needs, a testament to the planning and engagement work by the Office of Community & Population Health.

Appendices

Table 1. Next Steps: Social Needs Screening Guidelines for Health Systems

PROJECT CHARTER

Goal Statement: Develop universal social needs screening questions, workflows, and quality measures.
Timeline: 8/1/2020-7/31/2021

Problem Statement

- Social needs screening varies by population and frequency across MMG/MMC sites.
- Social need referral workflow implementation is inconsistent across MMG/MMC sites.
- No social need quality measure currently exists to incentivize providers to screen.

Patient/Client/Customer Value

- Compile complete data on social risk prevalence within patient population.
- Enhance access to clinical and community resources to

address patient social needs.

- Improve patient satisfaction with care.
- Increase appropriate task shifting from providers.
- Develop social risk profile for patients across the health system.
- Identify associations with major clinical outcomes (ASC, hospital readmissions, missed appointments).
- Become a national leader in social needs population-based assessment and engagement.

Objectives/Deliverables

- Complete implementation readiness needs assessment.
- Design timeline for universal screening roll out across network by November 30, 2020.
- Operationalize referral pathway for internal/external resources to address social needs by March 31, 2021.
- Complete training plan for MMC staff related to screening/referral by April 30, 2020.
- Finalize social need quality measure(s) by July 31, 2021.

Table 2. Suggested z-codes for Social Determinants of Health screening questions.

SDH Screening Question	Preferred ICD-10 z codes	Possible alternate codes
Are you worried that in the next two months, you may not have a safe or stable place to live? (eviction, being kicked out, homelessness)	**Z59.1** Inadequate housing **Z59.0** Homelessness	**Z59.8** Other problems related to housing and economic circumstances **Z59.9** Problems related to housing and economic circumstances, unspecified
Are you worried that the place you are living now is making you sick? (has mold, bugs/ rodents, water leaks, not enough heat)	**Mold** - **Z77.120** Contact with and (suspected) exposure to mold (toxic) **Bugs/rodents, water leaks, not enough heat** - **Z59.8** Other problems related to housing and economic circumstances - **Z59.9** Problem related to housing and economic circumstances, unspecified	**Z77.118** Contact with and (suspected) exposure to other environmental pollution **Z77.128** Contact with and (suspected) exposure to other hazards in the physical environment **Z77.9** Other contact with and (suspected) exposures hazardous to health

SDH Screening Question	Preferred ICD-10 z codes	Possible alternate codes
In the past twelve months, has the electric, gas, oil, or water company threatened to shut off services to your home?	**Z59.5** Extreme poverty **Z59.6** Low income	**Z59.7** Insufficient social insurance & welfare support **Z59.9** Problems related to housing and economic circumstances, unspecified **Z59.8** Other problems related to housing and economic circumstances **Z72.89** Other problems related to lifestyle **Z73.89** Other problems related to life management difficulty **Z73.9** Problem related to life management difficulty, unspecified

SDH Screening Question	**Preferred ICD-10 z codes**	**Possible alternate codes**
In the last twelve months, did you worry that your food could run out before you got money to buy more?	**Z59.4** Lack of adequate food & safe drinking water	**Z59.5** Extreme poverty; **Z59.6** Low income; **Z59.7** Insufficient social insurance & welfare support
In the last twelve months, has lack of transportation kept you from medical appointments or getting your medications?	**Z59.8** Other problems related to housing and economic circumstances **Z75.3** Unavailability and inaccessibility of healthcare facilities	**Z59.9** Problems related to housing and economic circumstances, unspecified
In the last twelve months, did you have to skip buying medications or going to doctor's appointments to save money?	**Z59.7** Insufficient social insurance & welfare support **Z91.128** Patient's intentional under-dosing of medication regimen for other reason **Z91.14** Patient's other noncompliance with medication regimen **Z91.19** Patient's noncompliance with other medical treatment and regimen	**Z59.5** Extreme **Z59.6** Low income

SDH Screening Question	Preferred ICD-10 z codes	Possible alternate codes
Do you need help getting childcare or care for an elderly or sick adult?	**Z74.2** Need for assistance at home and no other household member able to render care **Z63.79** Other stressful life events affecting family and household	**Z73.9** Problem related to life management difficulty, unspecified
Do you need legal help? (child/family services, immigration, housing discrimination, domestic issues, etc)?	**Z65.3** Problems related to other legal circumstances	**Z63.32** Other absence of family member **Z63.79** Other stressful life events affecting family and household
Are you finding it hard to get along with a partner, spouse, or family members?	**Z63.0** Problems in relationship with spouse or partner	**Z60.2** Problems related to living alone **Z63.5** Disruption of family by separation and divorce **Z60.4** Social exclusion and rejection
Does anyone in your life hurt you, threaten you, frighten you, or make you feel unsafe?	**Z91.410** Personal history of adult physical and sexual abuse **Z63.0** Problems in relationship with spouse or partner	**Z56.81** Sexual harassment on the job

Figure 1. Paper version of English SDH screen used by Montefiore Medical Center.

ENGLISH

PLEASE PLACE PATIENT LABEL HERE

Your care team is interested in your complete wellness. Please take a moment to answer the questions below prior to seeing your doctor. **This is an optional questionnaire.**

		YES / NO
	Are you worried that in the next 2 months, **you may not have a safe or stable place to live?** (eviction, being kicked out, homelessness)	Y N
	Are you worried that the **place you are living now is making you sick?** (has mold, bugs/rodents, water leaks, not enough heat)	Y N
	In the last 12 months, did you worry that **your food could run out** before you got money to buy more?	Y N
	In the last 3 months, has the **electric, gas, oil or water company threatened to shut off services to your home?**	Y N
	In the last 3 months, has **lack of transportation** kept you from medical appointments or getting your medications?	Y N
	In the last 3 months, did you have to **skip buying medications or going to doctor's appointments to save money?**	Y N
	Do you need **help getting child care or care for an elderly or sick adult?**	Y N
	Do you **need legal help?** (child/family services, immigration, housing discrimination, domestic issues, etc.)	Y N
	Are you **finding it so hard to get along with a partner, spouse, or family members that it is causing you stress?**	Y N
	Does anyone in your life **hurt you, threaten you, frighten you or make you feel unsafe?**	Y N

Do you want help? Y N

Phone Number: ______________________

Best time to Call: ______________________

Montefiore-Einstein Social Determinants of Health Screen
As of: March 1, 2020

Montefiore | EINSTEIN Albert Einstein College of Medicine

Figure 2. Overview of SDH screening data from Montefiore Medical Center based on the first completed screening only (n=24,794).

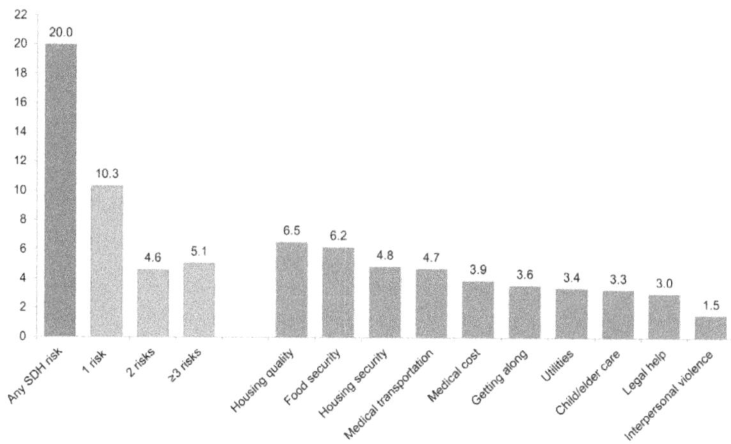

Figure 3. Number of positive food security screens by Neighborhood Tabulation Area in the Bronx. Labeled neighborhoods are those with ≥56 positive screens.

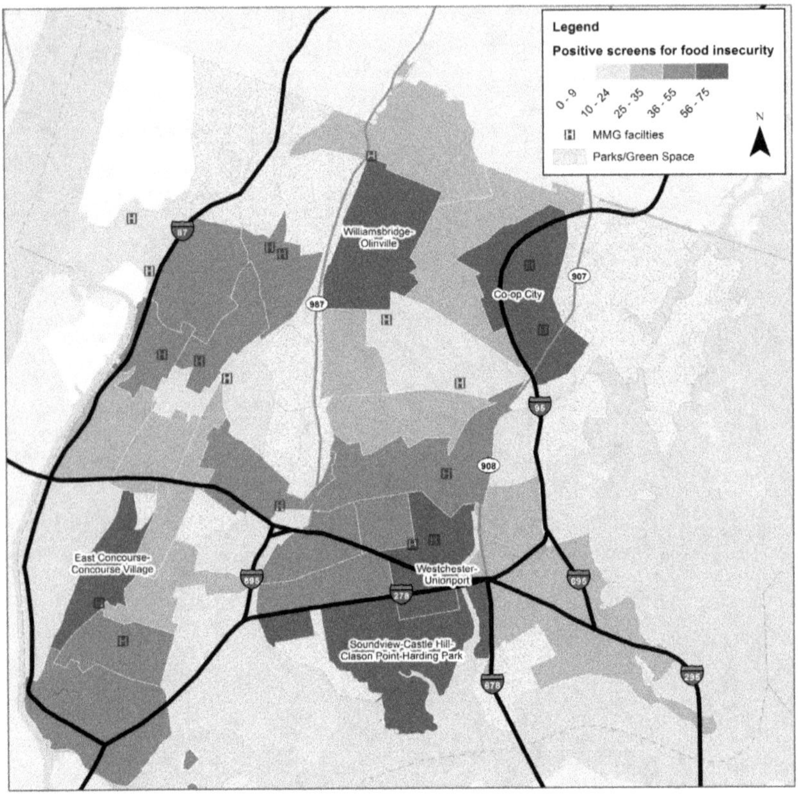

Endnote

1. "Social Risks Among Primary Care Patients in a Large Urban Health System," Caroline G Heller, Amanda S Parsons , Earle C Chambers, Kevin P Fiori, Colin D Rehm; *American Journal of Preventive Medicine*, 2020 Apr;58(4):514-525. doi: 10.1016/j.amepre.2019.11.011. PMID: 32199514; PMCID: PMC7362999.

Chapter 12.

University Health Case Study

Introduction

University Health (UH) is considered Kansas City's essential hospital, serving individuals and families struggling with social hardships and economic barriers to health. UH's social health strategy rests with making personal connections with an extremely diverse population. This includes immigrants, refugees, people facing housing insecurity, and communities of color. For this population, navigating social barriers poses special challenges.

One of the challenges facing UH providers and staff was communicating with patients and family members whose native language was most often Spanish, Somali, or Arabic. Few of these individuals spoke English and even fewer had familiarity about navigating healthcare systems such as UH. Additionally, many of these patients and family caregivers had no knowledge of how to access community services and public assistance programs.

The health system recognized that linguistic challenges were an obvious barrier to patient care. However, the deeper divide was cultural. To treat patients from diverse cultures, staff would need to be hired and trained not only as interpreters, but also as *cultural* health navigators. These navigators would need to work within the context of each patient's unique culture and become proficient in navigating the complexity of America's healthcare system.

Cultural Health Navigation

The Cultural Health Navigator (CHN) position is a hybrid of Medical Interpreter and Community Health Worker. Through the creation of these positions, UH sought to achieve multiple ends: bridging the language barrier faced by many of their patients, assisting with navigating the medical system, addressing social needs, connecting to primary and specialty care, and securing insurance and financial aid.

Five interpreters applied for the new positions, funded through a grant from the Reach Foundation. Three were fluent in Spanish, one in Arabic, and one was Somali speaking. All had immigrated from Sudan, Somalia, or South America.

The interpreters attended training conducted by members of the Social Determinants of Health (SDOH) Leadership team. The training included topics such as Trauma-Informed Care, Empathetic Interviewing, Social Determinants of Health screening, Electronic Medical Record (EMR) documentation, and working with upset individuals. All five interpreters additionally received Missouri's Community Health Worker certification.

Camaraderie between staff members of different cultures developed through personal stories and shared meals in their common meeting space. Everyone came to appreciate one another's rich culture, values, and beliefs. "Breaking bread" together afforded team members the opportunity to enjoy experiences, look out for one another, and become an extended family.

New patients also found their way to the Language Access Department and were warmly welcomed and helped with their needs. Social cohesion among staff and navigators became an essential ingredient of program success and served as an anecdote to burnout and job stress.

The creation of the Cultural Health Navigator positions symbolized the UH commitment of "meeting the patient where they are" by honoring their culture and building a bridge to adopted communities based on trust. It did not happen overnight but developed and matured alongside UH's efforts to incorporate Social Determinants of Health screening and assistance with the services provided to patients and families. CHNs became cultural ambassadors to immigrant and refugee communities, an essential bridge between the health system and underserved neighborhoods in Kansas City.

A "Safe Haven" Introduction

One of the first steps taken by the SDOH Leadership team was to set up a portable table every Friday just inside one of the main entrances to the hospital located in downtown Kansas City,

Missouri. The location was strategic because of heavy foot traffic. The table was placed close to the clinic elevators, pharmacy, a US Bank branch, and the cafeteria. Staffed by the Social Work department as well as by interpreters from the Language Access Department who were trained as Cultural Health Navigators (CHNs), the resource table served as an easy access area for patients and community members to seek assistance with their social needs or with navigating the healthcare system.

As word of the table spread, it soon became a "safe haven" meeting place for non-English speaking and homeless patients. Here they received assistance from compassionate staff who understood their culture as well as their struggles. As CHNs and Social Workers greeted and assisted patients in meeting their social needs, they began to build trusting relationships. Often patients would bring back family members, neighbors, or friends seeking help.

Social Determinants of Health Screening

The work of the CHNs sits within the context of a larger effort by the organization to incorporate screening and assistance with the Social Determinants of Health (SDOH) into the work of UH clinics.

The SDOH program was initiated by a small group of staff from different departments within the hospital. The staff had limited resources but worked together to reach a common goal. It was a "learning by doing" process that required UH staff, interpreters, and navigators to work as valued and respected team members, regardless of different backgrounds and cultures. The conference room in Quality Resources, where these meetings took place, became known "the cool kids' table." At the table, differing strengths, abilities, and points of view came together to balance one another, bridge departments, and work collectively to accommodate what was needed to provide the best services to patients.

The Patient Voice

The voice of the patient was a significant asset in the development of the SDOH process. As a prelude to initiating the SDOH program, 100 patients and family members were interviewed by the Manager of Patient Advocacy and Engagement to learn which Social Determinants of Health most affected them and their community. Four areas of greatest need arose from this dialogue: transportation, housing, food security, and financial constraints about the price of medications.

The voice of the patient continues to remain an integral part of the work as the SDOH initiative matures. Members of the Patient and Family Advisory Council (PFAC) are regularly updated regarding the progress of the work and are encouraged to offer suggestions and provide feedback to the SDOH Leadership team. Additionally, a member of the PFAC serves on the SDOH Leadership team.

The Screening Process

Since housing was already being addressed through the hospital's Behavioral Health department, the decision was made to screen patients in ambulatory clinics for food security, transportation, and the ability to afford medications. A simple three-question screening tool was developed, adopting the questions from the Health Leads screening tool:

1. In the past twelve months, have you missed a doctor's appointment or going to the pharmacy because of transportation?
2. In the past twelve months, did you ever eat less than you thought you should because there wasn't enough food?
3. In the past twelve months, did you ever skip medications to save money?

Patients who screen positive are offered a list of resources that may assist in meeting their need. If the need is immediate or could cause imminent harm, the medical assistant or nurse notifies the social worker or nurse care manager to assist with the need right away. A list of all patients screening positive is supplied to the clinic manager with the monthly data report, and the SDOH Leadership team asks the clinic to follow up with the patient within three weeks.

Each patient's social needs are recorded in the medical record system, allowing providers to read the information in conjunction with each appointment. The Social Work Department updates the lists of available social health services and community agencies every six months.

Cultural Health Navigators screen patients through a more conversational format than generally used by medical assistants in the clinic setting. CHNs contact a patient through a language interpreting referral. Once this contact is made, they establish a relationship with the patient, ask guided questions that lead to uncovering the need(s), then continue working with the patient until the need has been resolved. Additionally, CHNs screen for the patient's ability to access primary and specialty care as well as insurance. CHNs use a "teach a person to fish" philosophy, establishing the needs the patient chooses to prioritize and then teaching and modeling the behaviors that lead to resolution of the need. The objective is for patients to gain enough knowledge, skills, and confidence to continue on their own.

Patient-Centered Screening

The SDOH Lead Team at UH strongly supports efforts to screen patients and their families with non-clinical barriers to care. Initial SDOH efforts to implement screening targeted eight primary care clinics, as well as Diabetes and Endocrinology.

Efforts have since been expanded to include specialty clinics such as women's care and birthing care. The team has placed an emphasis on promoting equitable care and closing care gaps in maternal/fetal outcomes between whites and persons of color. That required more extensive screening than provided in primary care clinics. This enabled staff to take a deeper look into the unmet needs of patients being served.

A series of PDSA (Plan, Do, Study, Act) cycles were implemented in the OB/GYN clinic. Evaluation of the data occurred in two- to four-week cycles. Patients were provided with the American Academy of Family Practice (AAFP) Social Needs Screening Tool, a fifteen-item screener developed by AAFP. The form screens for the food, transportation, and finance issues already being screened by the hospital, but adds questions on housing, employment, education, childcare, and personal safety.

During initial screening cycles, three more questions were included to gather input on the survey itself.

1. "Were you okay with being asked the questions on the form? Why or why not?"
2. "Is there anything you suggest we add to the form?"
3. "Would you rather answer these questions yourself on paper, receive screening by text before the appointment, answer on a tablet, or have someone ask you the questions?"

Given the fact that the country was struggling with the COVID pandemic, the survey also asked: "Has COVID affected you in a negative way? If yes, how?"

SDOH staff and physicians wanted to learn more about specific issues created by the pandemic, and what further support was needed.

Taking the time to ask additional questions proved instrumental in refining the questionnaire to better capture patient concerns. Three insights stood out.

Insight 1:

When asked how they wanted to receive the screening tool, more than half of respondents (53 percent) wanted to receive the questions on paper. Twenty-five percent of those who answered said they would prefer receiving the questions in a text prior to their appointment. Only 13 percent wanted the nurse or MA to ask them questions at check–in. Interestingly, a mere 9 percent preferred answering the questions on a tablet upon arrival, which is a common method of screening in the digital age.

Evaluation of patient responses led to much discussion and soul-searching by the SDOH team.

While previous screening cycles in primary clinics led to efficiently adding questionnaire data to the electronic record, the team learned a valuable lesson in honoring the patient perspective. The team elected to honor the voice of the patients by using a paper screener while also moving forward with embedding patient data in the electronic record for documentation by intake personnel.

Insight 2.

Some team members were concerned with the sensitive nature of the interpersonal violence questions found on the AAFP form. The team surveyed patients to elicit their opinions. Ninety-three percent (239 of 257 answering the question) said they were comfortable with having the questions asked. Comments from patients indicated they felt the doctor needed to know this information. Several patients reflected that asking the question illustrated a sense of caring.

Insight 3.

During the COVID pandemic, the team felt it was important to gain an understanding from patients about their vaccine status. The survey asked patients if they received the vaccine and, if not, why they have chosen not to do so. Having this information readily available to the practitioner allows for an immediate opportunity for targeted conversation with the patient. This aids in resolving their concerns, addressing possible misinformation, or providing needed education.

Asking directed questions and making the effort to listen to the patient voice has been crucial to refining the screening processes in the OBGYN clinic. Data on patient perceptions has led to new staff awareness and action. A poignant lesson learned is the value of pausing to listen to the patient voice. This critical step has educated the organization and strengthened strategies to assist patients through a person-centered approach to care.

The SDOH team learned that slowing down to listen is an essential step in educating the organization on how to best to meet patient needs.

Social Health Services

In 2019, social work services were provided to 27,649 patients and amounted to 45,095 hours of interventions. Social work and spiritual care services are available seven days a week at each hospital location and operate in some community-based clinics during regular clinic hours.

Social workers have a master's degree in social work and are licensed as either a Licensed Master Social Worker (LMSW) or a Licensed Clinical Social Worker (LCSW). Services provided include:

- Psychosocial assessment
- Healthcare directives
- Discharge planning (home transitions or institutional placements)
- Financial Assistance (federal, state, and UH programs)
- Community information and referral (employment, financial, emergency assistance, housing, transportation, food insecurity, access to healthcare)
- Protective services (adult, child, institutional abuse/neglect, interpersonal violence, sexual assault)
- Counseling (crisis, adjustment to illness/hospitalization, grief, and loss)
- Mental health and substance use disorders (identification, support, connection to treatment)
- Identification of at-risk populations based on the nursing admission data base/adult screening and the LACE index score

LACE data is embedded in the electronic medical record system and a report is run every morning for inpatient social workers for all patients with scores of eleven or higher. Those patients are assessed by the social workers for psychosocial and discharge planning needs.

The department modified the tool to include mental health and substance use disorders in the calculation since those are frequent co-morbid conditions seen within the UH patient population.

Social Health Services supports a variety of additional programs aimed at meeting the immediate health risk needs of patients such as help with prescriptions, transportation, food, homelessness, and trauma-related behavioral assistance.

Prescription Assistance

More than 5,000 patients a year visit UH Medication Assistance Program pharmacies, with most filling multiple prescriptions on a regular basis. Direct 340B pricing is available to qualified UH patients. Eligibility is based on criteria established by UH Financial Counseling and criteria that is specific to each medication manufacturer. Criteria for UH patients include uninsured status, federal poverty level, and UH service area.

UH operates two Medication Assistance Program (MAP) pharmacies, one on each campus, which provide prescription services to qualified low income, uninsured patient populations. Medications dispensed from MAP pharmacy locations are made available from pharmaceutical manufacturer donation agreements and charitable organizations. UH also partners with

Walgreen's pharmacies, on-site and throughout the community, to provide discounted prescription pricing directly to qualified UH patients. This is made possible via 340B program contract pharmacy arrangements. UH invests over $1 million a year to provide Medication Assistance Program pharmacy services.

Transportation Assistance

Transportation on the city buses is free. Lyft rides are subsidized by UH. The Logistics Center provides transportation to patients living in designated catchment areas who do not have a Medicaid transportation benefit. Logistics Center contracts with Circulation Platform (Lyft) and Express Medical (Wheelchair Van) and services are paid for by UH.

Food Security

UH partners with the Jackson County Health Department and Harvesters to provide a pop-up food pantry on the second Tuesday of the month. About 128 families are served through this pantry each month. Any food left over at the end of the day is donated to a local homeless shelter.

Behavioral Health Assistance

UH ensures behavioral health services are available to low-income residents and persons who are homeless. UH provides requested assistance to individuals experiencing homelessness through the Housing First initiative at the

Center for Trauma Informed Innovation. The Center works with organizations, school districts, and businesses across the country to highlight how trauma affects behavior. The Housing First initiative is funded by FEMA (Federal Emergency Management Agency) and SAMSA (Substance Abuse and Mental Health Services Administration).

Cultural Health Navigator Profiles

University Health's sensitivity to the special needs of its immigrant and refugee populations is greatly enhanced by its five-person team of Cultural Health Navigators. Each brings unique skills, passion, and credibility as members of the community.

Susan Oweti

Susan Oweti immigrated from the South Sudan to Canada in 1997. She settled in Kansas City in 2001 where her husband, also from South Sudan, was living. She has been an interpreter for five years and is currently on her third year as a Cultural Health Navigator. Susan speaks English, Arabic, and Shilluk dialogue, spoken in Sudan and South Sudan.

> I've been a Cultural Health Navigator for two years and help patients with scheduling clinic appointments and connecting them with the right resources in the hospital. They are scared, don't speak English, and do not understand our culture here. They have no relatives here. As an immigrant, also from a war-ravaged country,

I understand their sorrow and pain and being homesick for their families.

My job is to assess their needs, make sure they get to the right clinic, get the right medications, explain how to take them, and hold their hand at each step along the way. I'm passionate about my work and my patients. I'm lucky to be here. I know life can be short. There is no promise of tomorrow. So, I give 100 percent every day. This could be my last day.

I'm proud to help non-English speaking patients. I like being the warm, welcoming part of University Health, someone who understands their day-to-day needs. Patients don't know anyone here. We have groups that meet in the community. We try to keep our culture and share our food. Simple things count.

Odily Rowland

Odily Rowland is from Honduras and settled in Kansas City in 1998. She began working as an interpreter in 2009 and has worked as a CHN for the past two years. Ms. Rowland speaks English and Spanish.

I have a unique position at University Health that covers the entire hospital—ER, all the clinics, all the medical specialties. It's been harder since COVID-19. We must wear a mask and that makes communication difficult. A lot of trauma happens at night.

> Our women suffer serious abuse, and it's hard to hold their pain. Some women arrive who are pregnant and vulnerable. They've been through so much. Last year, our patients' families couldn't be with them because of COVID. They couldn't touch or hug, so we must do that for them. It's a big responsibility and communication was more difficult because we all wore masks.
>
> The best part of my job is to make a difference every day in their lives, to bring some light into their dark. My patients know that I love them, that I care for them. I build trust every day. That's my job. It's an honor.
>
> My boss has done a special job choosing people who have so much love and compassion and humanity. It's my passion that keeps me going, passion for my community.

Lorena Zambrano

Lorena Zambrano immigrated to the United States from Colombia. She is fluent in both English and Spanish and worked as an interpreter since 2013 before moving into the Cultural Health Navigator role.

> Our patients have such a difficult time getting through the system—transportation, food, appointments, medications. I must jump right in and advocate for them, especially about how to pay for treatment and meds. They have so little money and finding work is very difficult because of immigration status.

When patients can find work, they want to pay something even when they have so little money. So instead of sending them to collections, I step in and help them with eligibility programs like Medicaid. And I advocate for them when the diagnosis is serious like diabetes, and they don't know what to do about it. I always go the extra mile and make sure my patients know what to do next.

The hardest part is when I'm trying to find help and hit walls. Not everyone has the passion and willingness to help others. That's what we do; we jump right in and offer that piece.

In my previous job as an interpreter for medical and legal issues, I could only do so much. When I was working in the juvenile system with moms, I was not allowed to explain to them what was going on. I was not allowed to go beyond my role. It was so frustrating. But as a CHN, I can explain to patients what's going on and what to do about it.

I know how it feels to be an immigrant trying to deal with an illness in a new country. I remember when my young son was very sick and not knowing what to do until someone was able to explain things to me in my native language. It made all the difference, and I was so grateful.

Zuhur Hiiray

Zuhur Hiiray is from Somalia and has been in Kansas City for seventeen years. She has been a medical interpreter for fifteen years at University Health and a CHN for two years. She volunteers in her community to accompany non-English speaking individuals to appointments to interpret on their behalf and speaks English and Somali.

> Many of our patients cannot read or write. A few weeks ago, a patient in his fifties called me at 9:30 p.m. He had severe diabetes, his toe was badly infected, and he was making plans to travel out of state soon to visit relatives. He didn't know what to do.
>
> I arranged transportation to the hospital and made an appointment for the next day with the podiatrist to examine his leg—before he made any more travel plans. He knew me and trusted me. He knew I would take care of things.
>
> His leg was very bad and needed three weeks of treatment at the hospital. What would have happened had he not trusted me? His leg would have been amputated.
>
> Trust is so important. My patients can call me at any time, day or night—especially for patients who work days. I'm there for them.
>
> Last year, a patient asked me to stay with her through a troubling biopsy. She was so scared and nervous. Her blood pressure was very high. I stayed with her and

offered emotional support. Her blood pressure went down. The doctor was pleased that I could stay and make the patient comfortable. Now the doctors are placing orders for Navigators.

Sometimes I just get a text with just a picture ID. I know that means they need me to make an appointment and follow through with them. I'm grateful to be a part of their life in that way—to advocate for them and teach them how to navigate the health system.

One time a patient was checking out and I was not with him. When I came back to the office, I saw that he didn't make a follow-up appointment. I called him. He thought the doctor's note on his paper was an appointment. Someone has to say, "I wonder if he made his appointment." CHNs know to always follow up.

It takes heart to make that connection, to go the extra mile. I'm grateful every day that I can touch one or two or three people's lives. It makes me happier.

Gabriella Gardner

Gabriella Gardner is the director of Language Access and Multicultural Health Navigators and has been at UH since 2010. Gabriella speaks English, Spanish, and French.

What makes me proud of our team is their love and compassion. We have a word in Spanish "*te le encargo*," which means I'm leaving this person in your care, and there's nothing you won't do to make that happen. This is so much more than the rigid role of interpreters that must abide by the ethics and standards of language interpreters.

When I first came here, I asked interpreters what they liked and didn't like. They all saw the need to do more, to have one-on-one conversations with patients. That's how they create wonderful trust and relationships, through natural conversation with patients and staff.

Team members tell me stories about how they had to step out of interpreter roles to best serve patients, to meet their needs. Each member is so intelligent and smart. They are the boots on the ground. They follow a patient through every clinic, do patient rounds. We are their voice. We hold their hands, we lift them. We are always patient and positive, constantly teaching.

Doctors and nurses and staff trust us. Now they place orders for Navigators.

We collect data on how well we're doing every month, meeting our goals, but numbers don't do justice to the humanity and love our team show patients every day. Whether the patient speaks Somali or Arabic or Spanish, we're all cousins, brothers, and sisters. Our patients know they're in good hands. They trust us because we're here for them.

Summary

CHNs are a hospital's most important asset in communicating the "patient voice" of immigrants and refugees who are not English-proficient or reticent to disclose personal information due to cultural norms or fear of immigration agencies.

Key Takeaways

- Immigrants, refugees, and communities of color face significant hardships and barriers to access medical care and social health needs.
- Cultural Health Navigators are the cornerstone to bridging cultural, social, and economic barriers that separate marginalized communities from mainstream medical care and social health services.
- CHNs have credibility with underserved neighborhoods and act as medical center ambassadors, which is a prerequisite for addressing health disparities and health inequity. Disparities data is contingent on CHN-administered screening and documenting personal information of such patients in electronic health records.
- To be effective, screening tools must honor the patient voice and cultural perspective.
- Patients do not necessarily prefer answering personal questions on a tablet despite widespread use of digital technology.

Executive Comments

Charlie Shields is President and CEO of University Health.

Cultural Health Navigators are an essential building block of our care team and Social Determinants of Health initiatives.

The Cultural Health Navigators are a great example of our motto "Brightest Minds, Biggest Hearts." The Navigator team empowers patients to take control of their health by presenting the comprehensive care we offer all patients, in a way that's understandable and culturally sensitive. The latter point is especially important in meeting people where they are. It's a prerequisite to guide them toward better health.

Hospital executives, program staff, and Patient Advisory Council members need unvarnished feedback on how patients experience our care and the barriers they encounter—especially immigrant patients. The lived experience of Cultural Health Navigators is a tremendous asset that enables us to embody "whole person care" and forge a trusted relationship with vulnerable communities in Kansas City.

This small and mighty group has helped save lives and close gaps in care. Whether it's communicating with a patient about their need for immediate care, or by helping remove financial barriers for a life-saving medication. The team carries the experience of vulnerability, and uses it, along with their knowledge of how the medical center works, to offer the best care possible. Our patients are so grateful.

We're indebted to the Cultural Health Navigation team for their passionate commitment to our patients and our community.

Health Plans and Self-Funded Employer Plan

Chapter 13.

Blue Cross Blue Shield of Massachusetts Case Study

Introduction

Blue Cross Blue Shield serves three million members in Massachusetts. It provides a wide range of services to its health plan members and is committed to serving marginalized populations through corporate citizenship programs and an overarching commitment to address racial inequities.

As a community convener, Blue Cross is in a unique position to facilitate and fund strategic partnerships across the Commonwealth. This entails supporting multi-year collaboratives with organizations on promising ideas and training programs (one- to five-year funding) in specific communities. This includes heath advocacy with stakeholders around the objectives of food, environmental, and racial justice.

The new corporate citizenship mission is focused on helping all Massachusetts residents lead healthy lives and create more equitable and just communities across the state. This means eliminating physical and societal barriers that lead to health inequities. To make these efforts sustainable, the strategy is based on three drivers: food justice, environmental justice, and racial justice.

- ***Food Justice*** promotes access to healthy and culturally relevant food, while building a sustainable food system. It is being advanced through the new South Shore Food Bank, a collaboration between the Weymouth Food Pantry and The Greater Boston Food Bank. It will improve access to nutritious food for eighteen communities in the South Shore. The food bank, supported with a $70,000 grant, will serve as a distribution center for clients south of Boston and will enable these organizations to pick up fresh nutritious food on a regular basis, and put it in the hands of community members who need it.
- ***Environmental Justice*** means overcoming the disproportionate impact of pollution and environmental degradation on under-resourced communities.

  It is being advanced by nonprofits to ensure equitable access to green spaces and improve environmental conditions in communities that bear the effects of the region's industrial and transportation hubs. Chelsea and East Boston are home to 100 percent of Logan Airport's jet fuel and 80 percent of New England's heating fuel, road salt for 350 cities, airport parking lots, and freight forwarding companies.

  Environmental stewardship is also being supported by providing East Boston students with hands-on experiential learning opportunities (Junior Farmers and Climate Nature) and programs.

- ***Racial Justice*** strives to eliminate systemic and institutional racism that leads to disparate health outcomes.
  It is being advanced by the Racial Equity and Justice Grant program with $350,000 to support Black, Indigenous, People of Color (BIPOC) led nonprofits with two-year grants in Massachusetts communities.
  A $1 million grant, to be paid over four years, was awarded to The New Commonwealth Racial Equity and Social Justice Fund founded by a coalition of nineteen prominent Black and Brown business executives. The purpose is to impart community guidance to researchers engaged in clinical trials on how to increase equity and address barriers to participation.

Additional programs aligned with these objectives include the following categories: sustainability, pandemic assistance, food security, youth fitness and safety, and community giving campaigns.

Sustainability efforts reduced wastewater consumption by 31 percent compared to 2015. Electricity was reduced by 56 percent compared to 2015. Landfill waste was reduced by 76 percent compared to 2010. Paper use was reduced by 86 percent since 2010.

Pandemic Support improved access to vaccines through transportation programs that provided free rides to community health centers' patients for vaccination appointments. Grants in the amount of $2,500-$7,500 were made to forty-six Community Health Centers to support transportation needs. A commuter rail train was repurposed as a mobile vaccination site for communities with the lowest vaccination rate in the state. The company's Bluebikes program was expanded to include 1,700 rides as well.

A total of $360,000 was invested with numerous nonprofits to administer seventy-two vaccination clinics in public spaces in fourteen communities across the state.

Food Security during the pandemic was addressed by funding a new South Shore Food Bank, which serves as a distribution center for nutritious food for eighteen communities in the South Shore.

Fitness and Safety programs for low-income youth funded ($45,000) Swim Safety Boston in collaboration with the City of Boston, Boston Public Schools, and YMCA of Greater Boston. The program offers free swimming lessons and the provision of Soul Caps especially designed for natural hair.

Summer Park Fitness was developed in partnership with Worcester Office of Health and Human Services and the YMCA to sponsor a fifteen-week Summer Park Fitness series to promote health and well-being in communities of color. Park fitness programs in Boston and Lowell were likewise supported to enable in-person classes in local parks and virtual workouts.

Annual Service Day (company-wide) in 2021 involved 2,800 employees who virtually volunteered with ninety nonprofit organizations. Seventy-four percent of company leaders served on community boards and strengthened nonprofits through board governance for an estimated value of $730,000. Since Service Day's inception in 2011, Blue Cross has contributed $10 million to the community through the annual volunteer day.

Community investments represented $41.7 million in 2021. Corporate contributions worth $33.7 million went to 413 nonprofit organizations. $3.7M of Foundation grants supported eighty-six community organizations. Volunteer service and pro bono support amounted to $4.3 million. Civic engagement involved 2,797 employees representing 76 percent of company workers that amounted to 29,582 hours dedicated to 303 projects (70 percent virtual and 20 percent in-person).

Health Inequities and Racial Justice

In 2019, health data on 1.3 million members identified racial disparities that, in many cases, represent lower quality care for Black, Asian, and Hispanic members on forty-eight industry-standard measures that are part of ongoing quality assurance operations.

Examples of the company's findings include:

- Asian, Black, and Hispanic members were less likely than White non-Hispanic members to receive screenings for colorectal cancer (67.0 percent for Asian, 63.8 percent for Black, 65.4 percent for Hispanic, versus 70.8 percent for non-Hispanic White members).
- Rates of severe maternal morbidity (life-threatening medical issues during childbirth) for Black commercial

members were more than double that of White non-Hispanic members (2.8 percent versus 1.2 percent).
- Rates of adolescent well-care visits were lower for Black and Hispanic members than for White non-Hispanic members (68.9 percent for Black, 70.3 percent for Hispanic versus 80.2 percent for non-Hispanic White members).
- Black and Hispanic members were 15-20 percent less likely than White non-Hispanic members to receive recommended antidepressant medication management.

The data refers to "Equity Measures and Payment Models" section and can be accessed at https://www.bluecrossma.org/myblue/equity-in-health-care/health-equity-report.

"It has long been known that racial inequities have devastating consequences across American healthcare, and the pandemic has made that clear to all of us in the past year," said Blue Cross president and CEO Andrew Dreyfus. "Measurement is a critical first step in addressing those disparities. We're publishing these results to hold ourselves accountable for progress toward our goal of eliminating racial inequities in the care our members receive."

As part of reducing address racial inequities, an in-house Spanish-language call center was created with a website available in five additional languages: Spanish. Portuguese, Russian, Chinese (Simplified), and Vietnamese.

Blue Cross also supported a variety of statewide efforts to help provide equitable access to COVID-19 vaccines. This includes funding transportation, sponsoring Vax Express, and partnering with Equity Now & Beyond to host vaccine clinics and provide educational outreach in immigrant communities across the state. Vax Express is a commuter rail line that was repurposed as a mobile vaccination clinic for under-served populations.

Data showed significant gaps in vaccination rates among Black and Latino residents compared to White and Asian residents as well as disparities in neighborhoods with large immigrant populations. Blue Cross' $168,000 investment enabled Equity Now & Beyond to scale COVID-19 vaccination education programs by increasing staff and launching new communication tools.

"Our goal is to provide education on the COVID-19 vaccine and create an accessible environment where Boston's African, Haitian, and other Caribbean Black immigrant communities feel safe and don't fear retribution because of their immigrant status." Kevin Whalen, Co-Director of Center to Support Immigrant Organizing and Coordinator of Equity Now & Beyond.

Equity Measures and Payment Models

One of the primary ways Blue Cross addresses inequities in members' care is by incorporating equity measures into its payment models, starting in 2023. Equity measures focus on differences in the quality of care across racial and ethnic groups.

A $25 million investment in physician practices and hospitals will support the medical community's efforts to reduce inequities in access and care. New provider contracts will be designed to give medical organizations a business case for investments aimed at closing care gaps.

Blue Cross and the Institute for Healthcare Improvement recently launched a collaborative to assist physicians and hospitals enrolled in the health plan's value-based payment model. The purpose is to improve the equity of care and prepare providers for equity-based financial incentives linked to improvements in racial inequities in care.

"As a health plan, we have a responsibility to address inequities directly with our members and by supporting the clinicians who serve them," said Dr. Mark Friedberg, senior vice president for performance measurement and improvement at Blue Cross. "Our aim is to produce meaningful, measurable, and sustainable improvements in the equity of care. Payment is necessary but not sufficient to do this. So, starting now, we're sharing data on inequities and engaging our provider network in collaborative efforts to address them."

In addition to sharing detailed data with clinicians on how their practices compare with others on racial inequities in care, employer customers will have the option of receiving similar data for their employees.

Healthy Living Support

Healthy Living is the company's legacy strategy for supporting communities in Massachusetts. It included three pillars: healthy eating, healthy active lifestyles, and healthy environment.

The initiative employed a two-track accelerator program of funding and training support. Track 1 involved a collaborative with multi-year training and facilitation support. Up to five organizations were invited to convene around a promising idea or model in a specific community. Track 2 involved one year of funding and training with individual organizations to jump-start a new idea or scale an existing model in the community.

Healthy Living initiatives promoted easy access to affordable and nutritious food, as well as safe and convenient recreational opportunities. "Dot.Rx" was the first collaboration on how to develop and implement a "prescription for living" program. It was sited in Dorchester at the Codman Square Health Center. With a prescription from their clinician, families can connect with a peer coach for help on healthy eating, outdoor activities, and exercise programs at the Dorchester Y. Clinicians wrote 517 prescriptions that engaged 150 families to date.

The BCBSMA grants supported a full-time program manager to take over all day-to-day responsibilities at the center, including coach referrals. A second collaboration funded the East Boston Neighborhood Health Center's referral program associated with 300,000 primary care visits a year and the development of a new wellness center. The pediatrics department cares for almost every child living in East Boston, which is geographically cut off from the rest of the city.

Healthy Eating

One out of eleven Massachusetts residents do not have enough to eat. Initiatives to support healthy eating addressed food insecurity, youth development, and supplemental programs for low- income residents. Examples include:

- Project Bread addressed food insecurity for students in twelve communities. Technical assistance and grant writing support was given to school districts to access federal funding for food programs.
- Springfield School Backpack Program filled 300 backpacks with food to supplement weekend meals for children.
- World Central Kitchen initiatives (Frontline Foods South Shore, Off Their Plate) provide hospital clinicians with food from local restaurants impacted by COVID-19.
- Larraine's Soup Kitchen and Pantry serves Chicopee residents with food insecurity hard hit by the pandemic.
- Employee Food Assistance Program where company associates can pick up free meal kits once a week for a family of four.
- Springfield School Backpack Program is filled with food to supplement weekend meals for children.
- Boston Area Gleaners' Surplus Community Crop Program addressed hunger and food waste. It connected more than 500 hunger relief programs across eastern Massachusetts by providing economic incentives for fifty farmers to move their crops (820,000 pounds of fresh produce) to local nonprofits rather plowing under their crops.
- GreenRoots helps residents in Chelsea expand its Urban Farming Program to purchase infrastructure equipment to allow storage and delivery, as well as to hire and train a Youth Farm Crew.

- Roots Rising enables forty-three youths in Pittsfield to work on farms, in food pantries, and at the local farmers' market.
- Field to Fork Program supported Chicopee Schools and Franklin Community Development Corporation to provide yearly farm trips for fourth grade students to learn about local agriculture. Local produce is also produced for the K-12 food service market, which provides a financial boost to the local food economy.
- Market Match at the Pittsfield Farmers Market provides locally produced foods throughout the year and accepts SNAP, WIC, and senior food benefits.
- Amherst Farmers' Market hosted a Healthy Living Match program that enables those who qualify for SNAP, EBT, and HIP benefits to receive additional match dollars to purchase produce, meat, eggs, and other goods from market vendors.
- Community Servings provides medically tailored meals to seniors with congestive health failure after discharge from the hospital. Each week ten made-from-scratch meals plus snacks and milk are delivered to program participants.

In 2019, $500,000 was allocated to five non-profits to help launch or scale an existing model to improve access to nutritious meals, fitness opportunities, and healthy environments for local communities in the state. Examples include:

- Food for Free takes leftover prepared food from corporate, university, or hospital dining services and repackages it into single-serving frozen meals for community college students who cannot afford a good meal. 2,000 students have been served.
- Collaborative for Educational Services expanded its Healthy Food Where You Live mobile farmers' market program to reach residents in twelve communities in western Massachusetts. Produce from local farms is brought to communities with limited access to grocery stores. It allows low-income residents to receive financial relief under the SNAP program.
- Massachusetts Farm to School provides technical assistance in Salem and Webster schools to increase student participation and improve nutritional value in the state-mandated Breakfast After the Bell program. The pilot will create a toolkit for schools state-wide.

In addition to healthy eating programs, two corporate gardens are located in Quincy and Hingham. Some of the produce from these gardens are used for the meals program and others donated to nonprofits. When farmers' markets were held at the three sites, CSA food boxes could be picked up by company employees.

Healthy Active Lifestyles

Physical activity grants were directed to overcoming the barriers to regular exercise through partnerships with organizations that reach underserved populations. These include:

- Playworks New England supports coaches in low-income schools to engage students during recess periods. As a result, 98 percent of students were better able to focus, 95 percent reported improved school climate, and 83 percent reported fewer bullying incidents during recess.
- Build Our Kids Success offers before-school physical activity and nutrition program, complete with training and on-going support at no cost to schools.
- Movement Inc. provides a movement program for young women rooted in self-care, reflection, and mindfulness delivered by volunteers to prevent violence.
- Councils on Aging and Senior Centers provide free fitness classes (yoga, tai-chi, strength training) for older adults called Silver Sneakers at twenty-three Council on Aging sites.
- Springfield YMCA supports the Active Older Adults program to increase muscular strength, range of movement, and activities of daily living.
- City of Worcester and Friends of Worcester Senior Center offer evidence-based health education, health screening, and fitness programs. Funding was also provided to support the capital costs of a Fitness/Wellness Center.
- Boston Parks Summer Fitness Series expanded to include Allston. A total of 11,700 youth, teens, adults, and seniors participated in 510 outdoor classes held in twenty-six parks in ninety-seven neighborhoods during summer months. Boston Park's Winter Fitness Series

offers eleven free classes each week held in parks and indoor community centers in seven neighborhoods.

- Camp Harbor View enrolls 900 youths from Boston's underserved neighborhoods in their summer camp at no cost. It also includes summer camp jobs for one hundred teens.
- In 2017, BCBSMA began the Leader in Training program that supports forty students each year to help coach high school students and navigate post-secondary plans. These students also work as camp counselors and peer mentors at Camp Harborview.
- Boston Social Fitness Festival is a one-day event of free fitness activities such as movement, cycling, play, and dance.
- Esplanade Frost Fitness Series involved 400 participants attending a Saturday boot camp (in February) that included running loops and body-weight exercises.
- Greenway Fitness in the Park offers 144 fitness classes from May through September for 3,700 people.
- Lowell Fitness in the Park summer series in newly renovated Kerouac Park offers free yoga, CrossFit, and Zumba.
- Worcester Parks Summer Fitness Series provides a seventeen-week program of free outdoor fitness classes in ten parks, including tai chi, dance, and boot camp in four languages (English, Spanish, Portuguese, and French).

- Trustees of Reservations challenges residents to hike 125 miles from April through December at 116 parklands. Each year, 1,500 participants total 5,000 hikes covering 10,000 miles.

Healthy Environment

Five years ago, Blue Cross Blue Shield of Massachusetts committed to reduce the environmental impact of company operations, based on the United Nations Sustainable Development Goals. From 2010 to 2020, greenhouse gas emissions have been reduced by 34 percent, paper use by 63 percent, waste sent to landfills by 40 percent, and water use by 16 percent. Eliminating food waste from company cafeterias and eliminating toxic chemicals from workplaces are new targets.

- Nineteen percent of local food spend focused on local products because of working with company food service teams.
- The company has committed that 65 percent of overall spend for building renovation and expansion projects be chemical free (including flame retardants) for office furniture, fixtures, and equipment. A "living wall" was installed in the Boston office to improve air quality.
- A comprehensive Community Supported Agriculture program was initiated with an onsite farmers market highlighting local and sustainable food. A community gardening program in Hingham and Quincy, from May

through October, produces 5,000 pounds of produce and herbs each year.

BCBSMA also promotes a healthy environment by addressing incidence of disease including childhood asthma, COPD, autism, neurological diseases, and some cancers. Initiatives include:

- Salem Bike Share Program provides eighty bikes and sixteen docking stations. Riders logged 10,000 in the first two years, replacing hundreds of car trips on local roads.
- Bluebikes is a metropolitan bike-sharing program with stations in Boston, Cambridge, Everett, and Somerville. Twenty-five thousand active members logged 2.3 million trips and grew 29 percent year over year. The program was recently expanded to the underserved communities of Mattapan, Dorchester, and Roslindale with fifty-four additional docking stations.
- Melanoma's Practice Safe Skin program for residents in Lowell provides ten automatic sunscreen dispensers around the city. It provides education about skin cancer prevention to forty-five lifeguards, counselors, and recreational staff.
- East Boston Air Partners improves air quality by developing community strategies to address sources and effects of pollutants in their neighborhoods.

Blue Cross Blue Shield Foundation

The Blue Cross Blue Shield Foundation of Massachusetts has made assessing racial inequities in healthcare one of its three focus areas, along with access to care and mental health. The Foundation works with partners to identify policies that present barriers to equitable access to care and coverage for people of color. There is a compelling need to diversify the workforce and leadership of healthcare organizations. The Foundation launched seven focus groups across the Commonwealth to discuss with BIPOC-led organizations what they see as the solutions to structural racism and racial inequities in healthcare.

The Foundation's thinking and focus evolved during the pandemic. A new emphasis on measurable change emerged on behalf of residents, community-based organizations, and the healthcare system. The organization's recalibrated focus expands access to health coverage and care for the state's most marginalized communities. Three interconnected priorities—food justice, environmental justice, and racial justice—are targeted for funding over the next five years.

In 2021, the Foundation launched a new grant program to help organizations run by and serving people of color to build capacity and strengthen expertise. The objective is to support grantees (up to $100,000) in reaching their community goals rather than a return-on-investment or cost-benefit benchmarks. Grantees are encouraged to decide on metrics and how to evaluate impacts over time.

The Foundation's approach to Social Determinants of Health explicitly acknowledges two important tenets: 1) the role that structural racism plays in creating and maintaining racial inequities in health, and 2) the need to invest in efforts to diversify the behavioral health workforce.

The Foundation supports dozens of other projects that improve access to care:

- Expanding Access to Behavioral Health Urgent Care: $1,200,000
  Three-year grant to support existing Emergency Services Program system and community-based continuum of care strategies that promote treatment and recovery.
- Strengthening the Voice for Access: $715,000
  The program targets vulnerable populations.
- Connecting Consumers with Care: $625,000
  Two-year grant to community-based organizations and health centers to assist with enrolling in publicly subsidized health insurance, decreasing rates of churn, and addressing post-enrollment issues to increase access to care.
- Going Beyond Our Healthcare: $225,000
  Two-year implementation grants to build teams of social service and healthcare organizations to address clinical and non-clinical needs for low-income and vulnerable populations.
- Policy and Research Grants: $205,000
  Grants support research, evaluation, and convenings to

advance public policy and programs that align with the Foundation's strategic focus areas.

- Nick Littlefield Award for Excellence in Community Health: $50,000
  Two-year award to an organization making extraordinary contributions to children's health.
- Network of Care Massachusetts: $122,800
  Funding for development and initial operating costs of a state-wide online database of behavioral health, substance use, and social service resources in the state.
- Special Initiatives: $500,000
  One-year grant to organizations undertaking innovative pilots that expand access to care for low-income consumers and promote synergy between grant making and policy initiatives.
- Catalyst Fund $164,000
  One-year grant to help community-based organizations strengthen their capacity to expand access to healthcare in the state.

Summary

Blue Cross Blue Shield of Massachusetts' corporate citizenship mission is committed to addressing racial inequities and serving marginalized populations throughout the Commonwealth. The company is focused on eliminating physical and societal barriers to health equity. This requires implementing sustainable strategies on three drivers of inequity: food justice, environmental justice, and racial justice. This includes linking financial incentives in provider contracts to improving racial inequities in care.

The Blue Cross Blue Shield Foundation has likewise expanded its mission to address racial inequities and care disparities. Grant awards are directed toward initiatives on racial inequity, access to care, and mental health. In conjunction with community partners, the Foundation is addressing measurable change on behalf of residents, community organizations, and providers. Community building is essential for these efforts to be sustainable.

Chapter 14.

Blue Cross Blue Shield of Massachusetts

Health Plan Consumer Research on Social Determinants of Health Case Study

Blue Cross Blue Shield of Massachusetts conducted focus groups of customers to better understand the challenges that employees face trying to keep healthy. What they found was surprising and shed new light on the barriers to designing Social Determinants of Health programs with employer health plans.

Designing interventions to meet social health needs of employees requires a granular level of detail not generally available through claims histories alone. By including the "voice of the member," health plans can collect valuable information and insight on how to improve health opportunities for employees and their families.

What BCBSMA found was that employees and managers were very open about their health challenges and how often personal ingenuity was required to get around barriers. They commented how helpful it was that health plan representatives conducting the focus groups were very open about their own struggles with health, and this built trust and credibility throughout the focus group process.

While the health plan reviewed available data for each employer, the most impactful and valuable information came from personal stories that recounted the enormous challenges many employees encounter every day, especially workers with chronic illnesses. The most health-challenged employees often worked the hardest to improve their health.

The most pervasive issue was understanding the extent of "surprise costs" and navigating the medical system. Employees simply did not understand why out-of-pocket expenses were so high, what to do about it, or who to turn to. The next most important issue was cultural: how to find a "comfortable" physician. They want a physician who listens well. Just as important was how to find a physician that accepts new patients.

In terms of social determinants, the most frequently mentioned need is finding workable solutions to healthy eating and getting physical activity during the week within very busy lives. The need to access behavioral health services was also a high concern and a source of stress.

Another set of concerns that troubled employee resource groups was financial barriers associated with the health plan. Copays, coinsurance, and deductibles weighed heavily on the minds of employees and their families. This was also a source of worry, especially for lab tests and follow-up visits for chronic medical conditions. Financial challenges posed a significant barrier to access needed medical care.

Most of the requests from focus groups was for more support to understand heath plan benefits and services, improvements to what BCBSMA already does.

Focus Group 1: Insurance

A diverse group of employees in Massachusetts reported numerous barriers. A number of comments related to cultural issues such as cooking, eating, and social patterns that are very difficult to work with, or around when need be. Cultural norms for wellness, weight, and prosperity differ by income, ethnicity, and neighborhood. Focus group participants referred to finding physicians they are "comfortable with" (i.e., culturally sensitive physicians) and finding doctors with open panels. Spanish-speaking clinicians are much preferred and more trusted than language interpreters.

Wait times in physician offices are often too long to take time off from work, making it difficult to bring family members to medical appointments. Moreover, cultural and language barriers keep people from getting the care they need. In some cultures, people tend to visit the doctor only when they are sick. Health is not seen as a priority for people who have other challenges that affect every day living.

Employees do not understand the benefits of screening for cancer and other chronic diseases, nor how to manage chronic conditions through exercise and nutrition. Many communities have limited access to safe walking routes, which reflect the built environment of some underserved communities.

With persistence, a number of employees noted they were able to maintain regular exercise programs. Others were able to educate family members about cancer screening benefits and finding culturally matched physicians. These are examples of personal victories that surfaced during the group discussions.

Several comments identified potential supports that would address barriers to health improvement, including:

- Decreased copays and coinsurance for labs and medications for chronic diseases
- List of culturally matched physicians who speak the patients' language
- Language appropriate and culturally sensitive information for cancer screenings
- Partnership with church leaders in many communities to encourage primary care
- Culturally competent approach to Case Management that "meets patients where they are"

Focus Group 2: Apparel Manufacturer

This focus group represented manufacturing plant managers from across Maine. Participants were very insightful, and knew their employees' struggles as well as their own attempts to maintain healthy behaviors. Barriers to health centered on economic factors such as low wages and whether food costs and gym membership fees were beyond reach. If so, they would not join a gym and would skimp on healthy food if necessary to make ends meet. There is extensive poverty in the state and few good jobs, thus making healthy lifestyles difficult. The only factor that companies can control is a thirty-minute lunch break.

At the same time, personal victories were noted. One of the managers discussed a struggle to quit smoking. Another indicated he was willing to champion weight watchers or a nutritionist due to his own struggles with weight management.

Participants had creative ideas on how to support change at the workplace. One idea from managers was to use the thirty-minute lunch break as an opportunity for a locally produced healthy lunch (free or nearly free). Employees could also go on a fifteen-minute walk with a local trainer and buy extra meals for dinner at a very low price.

Company managers decided to meet among themselves and decide what next steps could be taken to influence better health. This led to a corporate multi-year strategy that now includes regular focus groups to determine approaches that encourage healthy behaviors, motivation to quit tobacco use, group exercise, and more affordable healthy-eating options. A further recommendation is to incentivize plant management to support wellness initiatives.

Focus Group 3: Faith-Based Organizations I

BCBSMA was invited by church leaders to help their community address high rates of cardiometabolic disease by identifying church champions who could be trained as health behavior leaders ("train the trainers"). Focus group participants were very enthusiastic when BCBSMA was represented by a Black physician to talk about disparities in healthcare and knowing the importance of tracking day-to-day disease markers to better manage medication.

Church leaders and members were aware of barriers to better care. They did not generally trust providers and, instead, relied on friends and family referrals when selecting a physician who was familiar with their culture. Another barrier was the cost of buying healthy food groups like fresh fruits and vegetables, especially organic produce.

Some participants with high blood pressure and diabetes did not understand the fact that they had normal weight and eat healthy foods but still had a serious and worrisome diagnosis like diabetes. The BCBSMA physician clarified the impact of genes and the influence of environmental factors in daily life. This led to an easy-to-understand discussion about blood pressure, weight management, diabetes, and misuse of medications.

There were also stories of personal health improvement victories such as exercising with a workout buddy, coworkers, friends or family members. It creates accountability and consistency, which is necessary to maintain an exercise routine. Keeping a journal to track progress was also helpful and pointed out what works and what does not. In sharing information about best practices on fitness and nutrition, some members had lost 10-40 pounds since beginning the regimen. Some worked out regularly with their spouse, others walked regularly on their own, and a few joined a gym.

Church leaders and social services agencies wanted help with health promotional information, especially information on eight topics: diabetes, nutrition, healthy cooking, high blood pressure, nutrition, physical activity, childhood obesity, and depression. They wanted to build relationships with BCBSMA, and the health plan could pursue partnering with community leaders and churches to address healthcare disparity and share resources.

Participants said working with the community and faith leaders on interventions would be welcomed, especially among African American and Latino communities. Employee resource groups would identify and support community champions. Members indicated they would attend BCBSMA-hosted community events focused on how to manage their medical condition. More specifically, when to remain on medications, when to stop, and to avoid sharing prescriptions with others, including family. Having church leaders involved in the discussion make an impact. BCBSMA's physician gave examples on how a patient changed his lifestyle after learning he was pre-diabetes, and how he made changes to a healthier life as a result.

The group's consensus was to continue to work on nutrition and fitness with the health plan and to reduce salt intake as the number-one goal. Eating less was also a priority and that meant consuming less of the "American way" and adhering closer to their Caribbean culture and eating habits involving portion control, grain, vegetables, and protein. The group has a high percentage of Caribbean population. The group also reiterated the need for a more culturally competent Case Management Team to meet members where they are in terms of culture and language.

Focus Group 4: Faith Based Organizations II

This group represented managers and principals of agencies representing twenty-five nursing homes, schools, and local agencies in Massachusetts. A number of barriers were reported related to the sedentary nature of teaching as an occupation, complete with lots of candy brought into the classroom. It extends to after work as well as one participant noted: "We serve God and our students and patients, and when we get home, we're drained and don't serve ourselves." Master's degree training programs do not train teachers about healthy behaviors at school and home.

There were also examples of small steps (and some setbacks) that were encouraging such as one person's comment that it was difficult to lose weight, but they could still "feel better about my health behavior." One participant used to set personal health goals but discarded them over time. Another had a walking group with 4-6 women, and some joined a Zumba class, but the numbers dwindled over time.

The group came up with suggestions on how to change the culture and to find the right life/work balance that was realistic in setting priorities and sustaining healthy habits. These educators were optimistic about learning more healthy habits about nutrition and exercise and that "we all find time to eat, so teachers have the opportunity to teach kids about eating healthy too." The YMCA in town was also seen as a good resource.

The summary impressions of the group were they needed to stop focusing on weight loss and emphasize healthy behaviors and feeling better as the overriding frame of reference. They saw their role as teachers as an opportunity to lead by example and motivate colleagues and students on healthy eating and physical activity.

Focus Group 5: Medical Device Manufacturer

Participants included single moms who identified as Hispanic, African American, and Cambodian. The group was very insightful and resourceful despite an array of social, medical, and financial challenges. Many had Primary Care Physicians, participated in company walking programs, went to the gym, and knew about nutrition. The Human Resources manager had a very strong bond with employees and knew their issues. An external wellness program, Health Advocate, was already in place.

There was not a company cafeteria and nearby food options consisted of fast-food outlets. Weight loss was a continuing challenge to these women ("just can't lose these last five pounds"). One employee acknowledged having a good doctor until they retired. Another mom stopped going to her doctor because they did not acknowledge her medical concerns.

One of the most impactful stories was told by a mom who had developed diabetes during pregnancy and then was diagnosed with tendonitis. She decided to switch to a radically different health diet after working with a dietitian and reversed her diabetes. Health Advocate also really helped a sick employee find a doctor quickly. One mother figured out which gyms had day care so she could go there and get in one to two hours of exercise on a regular basis.

The focus group decided they could help each other out by sharing ideas, supporting each other in walking groups, going to the gym, and recommending good physicians when they were in the lunchroom together. They also decided to stop focusing on weight loss and pay more attention to healthy behaviors and feeling better. Having a supportive and caring HR manager was helpful as well. In fact, the HR manager, who took extensive notes during the focus group, asked BCBSMA to return in six months to monitor the group's progress.

Focus Group 6: Union

A union focus group included twenty-five shop leaders and workers representing a cross-section of race, ethnicity, and genders. Most faced challenging economic conditions.

One of the most frequent barriers was Primary Care Physician access or open panels, not getting an appointment when sick, and then being sent to the ER. Members were not always comfortable with replacement PCPs. Union members were not able to get nutritious lunches near their garment workplaces and had to pack lunches. Several mentioned cooking for the week on weekends, then packing healthy lunches. Walking for exercise inside buildings in winter is not always possible or permitted. A further barrier was anxiety around the perceived costs of cancer screening.

Several personal stories of dealing with complications of diabetes stood out, as well as supporting family members with strokes. A number of members managed to take control of their health and turn things around.

Potential solutions for better health were offered on nutrition, exercise and finding PCPs as demonstrated by shop leaders or those who had accomplished healthy lifestyle change, and were able to personally support others. Further education on health promotion efforts was suggested. Members acknowledged that even broad education on different health practices was not easy to put into everyday practice. One of the most important factors was having the support of shop stewards.

Focus Group 7: Food and Beverage (national franchise)

Participants in the focus group were thirty corporate office workers who were already engaged in their health. Most were in their thirties and young forties, white and a mix of genders. Two individuals had successful gastric bypass surgeries with good results.

It was difficult for these employees to easily access healthcare services due to working full-time and the difficulty of finding a PCP that met their needs and did not entail a long drive. Finding time to exercise was likewise difficult, and employees were not comfortable taking time from workday schedules to exercise. Most did not have the motivation or time to exercise after or before work. Burnout from work was a factor as well as home commitments and parenting demands. People were confused about the requirements of the wellness incentive program and what they could do to qualify for rewards. Not everyone was aware of all the wellness programs offered or support activities like walking groups. Seeing a nutritionist really helped one individual.

Biometric screenings were well received among this group. They liked having a free screening and the ability to earn a large incentive ($500 per year). At the same time, others in the group pointed out that on-site biometric screening was hard to do at a testing lab because it required coordinating with working on weekdays. One person suggested allowing the doctor to send in their measures. Obtaining needles required for venipuncture, as part of biometric screening, was noted as a barrier for some employees.

Many workers were reluctant to use the on-site gym because they were too embarrassed to exercise in front of coworkers. Others did not find food choices at the on-site cafeteria to be very healthy and became bored with the salad bar. A number of participants said they prepared healthy foods at home and shopped strategically for the weeks ahead. Free fruit offered at work was cited as a good company benefit. Seeing a nutritionist helped one individual get her food plan off the ground.

Personal victories were noted by some of the participants in the group. A few get up early to exercise because they recognize it will never happen after work hours. They are more likely to exercise as part of a workout group or with someone else, even their dog, because others are depending on them.

A very practical suggestion was to bring gym clothes to work, change at work, but avoid going home in between. One woman finds time to exercise at her kids' activities and walks around the field before her son's soccer game starts. Some workers have participated in company sponsored activities like 5K events. Wanting to set a good example for kids was a good motivator for one mother and wanting to feel better like she did at a younger age.

Everyone felt that having supervisors and colleagues modeling healthy activities makes a big difference in terms of motivation and setting an example at work. Encouraging middle management and senior management to show visible support for exercising during the workday was strongly suggested by the group. This could be incorporated into their formal goals and performance review. Another suggestion was to offer more healthy food options at on-site cafeterias.

One of the important suggestions of the group was to initiate a company-wide campaign that builds on the "What's Your Why?" premise. The objective is to get people thinking about things that would motivate them to eat better and be healthy, whether it means a healthy retirement, being a good example for their kids, feeling more energized, or supporting their coworker who is trying to lose weight.

Additional health promotions could be developed through training sessions conducted with Optum as well as having more clarity around requirements for wellness incentive programs. Consideration should also be given to new wellness programs and a platform that is easier to navigate and helps people track their healthy habits. Subsidies for registering for a race and participating in Weight Watchers would also be a welcome addition. So would having an on-site nutritionist.

In terms of increasing participation in biometric screening, a finger prick test instead of venipuncture would ease fears of employees afraid of needles.

A summary of next steps was based on impressions by BCBSMA. The focus group was very health-literate, quite knowledgeable on how to be healthy, and tuned into their own motivators and barriers. A lack of time seems to be their biggest barrier to better health, followed by uncertainty about what the company offered in relation to wellness-related offerings. Overall, senior and middle management support for exercising and adopting healthy behaviors is an important motivator.

Managers and leaders thought several next steps could be taken by working with the company's HR worksite director to consider the following:

- Work with cafeteria vendor to find ways to offer better and healthier foods.
- Explore new vendors for on-site screenings and an improved wellness platform.
- Consider new ways of communicating to employees and motivating them to adopt healthy behaviors.
- Work on getting more senior and middle management buy-in and visible support for encouraging exercise and other health-related behaviors during the workday.
- Meet with the insurance broker and the company's corporate HR team to discuss additional next steps in greater detail.

Key Takeaways

- Language, cost, and time (i.e., member convenience) were the key issues across all groups.
- The importance (and challenge) of developing culturally sensitive screening for diabetes and cancer should be among the top priorities.
- Surface-level impressions of member and provider relations can mask underlying cultural issues and disconnects that undermine care.
- Low wage workers cannot afford health plans with large out-of-pocket costs, copays, and coinsurance requirements.
- Personal stories of members are especially valuable in assessing health plan design and strategies intended to promote healthy behavior.
- Many members are resourceful and motivated to practice healthy living habits amid busy lives and demanding work schedules.
- The most health-challenged employees often worked the hardest to improve their health.

Executive Comments

Thomas Hawkins, MD, Medical Director, Health Informatics

Important demographic data is often missing to design specific employer interventions.

Claims data is essential to understand what drives healthcare costs and disease trends, but it doesn't generate insight into what influences the behavior of consumers in selecting providers, avoiding treatment, and instead turning to medical advice from friends and family.

Our focus group comments uncovered cultural misalignment and unconscious bias among providers toward patients with diverse income, racial, ethnic, and gender identities.

Gaps in care may be indicated by claims data and electronic health records, but not the underlying reasons. Many of the reasons why members didn't receive appropriate care, as intended by their employers, was unknown to the health plan.

Based on focus group feedback, BCBSMA is in a better position to reassess and redesign health plan features to close gaps in care, address cultural misalignment issues, and weed out providers in the network whose values are not in sync with those of the employer, member, or health plan.

One of the underlying issues of some employees was low wages, compelling many workers to hold two jobs, juggle home and work responsibilities, and do without adequate nutrition, exercise, or sleep—all factors that contribute to poor health.

The health plan can devise ways to address these barriers through benefits redesign, but it's up to the employer what level of investment the company can make in its workforce to address income inequality issues inherent in service industry jobs and at many manufacturing sites.

Factors that influence an individual's health are closely tied to numerous barriers associated with working conditions as well as home life, neighborhood characteristics, and exposure to environmental harms.

Chapter 15.

Robert Galvin Executive Interview

Robert Galvin, MD, MBA

Bob was an Operating Partner at Blackstone and served as CEO of Equity Healthcare, a Blackstone-owned LLC that managed healthcare costs and benefits for companies invested in by Blackstone and selected other private equity firms. This represented $1.5 billion of annual spending for 250,000 employees and families in seventy-plus companies. From 2020-22 he also served as Chief Medical Officer and managed Blackstone's 150 companies through the COVID-19 pandemic. Before joining Blackstone, he was a Senior Executive at General Electric where he managed healthcare costs ($2.5 billion, 230 medical clinics in fifteen countries, 800 physicians and nurses) and served as Chief Medical Officer for fifteen years.

Dr. Galvin is a nationally recognized leader in the areas of employer-sponsored insurance, quality measurement, and payment reform. He was co-founder of the Leapfrog Group and founder of Bridges to Excellence and Catalyze Payment Reform (currently CPR Board Chair). These organizations have helped define and accelerate value-based purchasing. He is a member of the National Academy of Medicine and Professor Adjunct of Medicine and Health Policy at Yale.

You were the top healthcare executive of GE's health program, $1.5 billion annually in US and $2.5 billion outside the US. What did you learn that applies to current employer efforts to reduce spending?

Well, in my mind, there's a fallacy that the value-based purchasing approach used successfully by a small number of jumbo employers will scale throughout large and mid-market employers. There are shining examples of when this works—the two or three dozen biggest companies like Amazon, IBM, and Walmart—but for the remainder of the several million firms that sponsor health benefits, this is simply not the case. Employers don't approach healthcare in the same way a rational purchaser does.

For the vast majority of the 150 or more companies I've worked with, at GE and Blackstone, what it takes to have a vibrant buy side in a market-based system simply doesn't scale. There aren't the right incentives to make it work. In fact, any momentum that was building for change twenty to thirty years ago has regressed. Cost has been addressed in a "good enough" way by shifting the increases to employees, which though it flattens their wages, has become the stable paradigm so cost is not as burning a platform as it was in the past. We used to say that this approach could only last so long, but the truth is that it has stood the test of time. Even in the face of increasing personal bankruptcies due to medical costs, employers have not been willing to make the hard choices to truly lower costs. It kind of defies logic, but the US healthcare system is a world of its own.

Can you say more about that?

For employers to be effective buyers of healthcare, they need to apply standard purchasing principles; the most important of which is choosing the supplier with the highest quality at the lowest cost. In healthcare, this could mean that the most popular hospital or doctor group in an area, which it turns out is not the highest quality and is high cost, could be excluded from a network or become much more costly to the employee. However, this inevitably causes some employees to be unhappy. There has been little tolerance for this "employee friction" for what I consider to be the urban myth that people will leave jobs they like because their doctor is no longer available to them at a low cost. This has never been substantiated. Nonetheless, the human resource employees who manage health benefits at firms are chastised for employee dissatisfaction with benefits even if it is very few people. It's their bosses, the C-suites, that incentivize them to favor almost perfect satisfaction over higher value care.

It also appears at first blush that employers should invest deeply in wellness and condition management programs.

However, since there is a considerable lag between when a person improves their lifestyle habits and when this is reflected in lower costs, employers have under-invested in this area. As one CEO said to me, "twenty percent of my employees turn over every year, so there is little return on this investment. Plus, the average tenure of a CEO is around five years so neither the employee nor I will be around to benefit from this use of resources." Also, it should be noted that there is scant evidence that these types of programs produce better outcomes.

You founded The Leapfgrog Group in 2000 to advocate safety and quality. Is quality still a focus for employers?

Employers still care about quality, though they are less focused on the delivery system than they used to be. When a few employers started Leapfrog twenty-three years ago, I was more optimistic employers would be proactive about backing quality and patient safety initiatives. Times have changed. In the end, most employers are unwilling to do what good buyers do, which is to continuously cull their supply chains to preferentially use those suppliers that provide the highest quality at the lowest cost. Employers are, in my mind, overly concerned about not having a single unhappy employee—which can happen if a lesser quality option is culled from the network—and continuously cost shifting excess costs to employees. It turns out that it's easier to neutralize high health costs savings and growth initiatives in other parts of the firm, e.g., globalization, technology, etc., than by becoming value purchasers.

Is quality ripe for a change?

I think so. Despite the best intentions, we have created a "quality-industrial complex" with too little to show for it. While there have been some notable improvements, inpatient hospital safety is still way below where it should be, and we have not found measures that patients can use, and which providers find relevant. Clinicians are overly burdened by senseless tasks. I think when the two main players in quality—providers and patients—do not find value in the metrics, it's time for an overhaul.

Quality metrics will never be useful if physicians and patients see no value in them. CMMI recognizes that quality terminology and mandates are too confusing. It's time to begin again with a clean slate about what constitutes quality and how to measure it.

What other structural barriers do you see facing employers?

Employers almost always lack the volume to meaningfully impact health plan or provider revenue in their local markets. And employers have had little success in combining purchasing power. Healthcare is local, and other than in select regions, employer workforces have decreased due to globalization and now a workforce that can be physically remote from the worksite. An equally big structural barrier is how employers think about healthcare costs. They see them as part of employee compensation and ask the Human Resources team to manage health benefits. The HR teams are evaluated on the satisfaction of the workforce and their ability to recruit and retain the best employees. The moves you need to make to manage costs do not always make every employee happy. These are incentives that are impossible to reconcile.

What can employers do to improve healthcare for employees?

Employers have invested in wellness and condition management programs for employees, and while the impact on cost is small, employees like these programs and a small number of them benefit. These programs are particularly helpful in the field of mental health, where digital initiatives are helping solve the access problem. Also, I think employers are backing away from high deductible plans because they realized that having employees avoid care was not helpful in the long run.

You recently ran Equity Healthcare, LLC, for Blackstone and reported decreased healthcare costs and improved quality in its employer customers. Given all the constraints you listed, how did this get accomplished?

I was responsible for healthcare-related operations at over one hundred Blackstone companies. These were mid-sized employers—the average firm has around 2000 employees—and we were able to apply some basic purchasing tactics to improve value. The portfolio companies, though majority owned by Blackstone in most cases, remained independent companies and could choose to join Equity Healthcare or not.

First, we learned that managing health benefits was tied to HR, and they in turn relied on insurance brokers. The latter's compensation was tied to how much was spent, not on how much was saved or even quality. We needed to intervene in the annual RFP process and change how that part of the business played out. We built in strict requirements for choosing brokers, and renewals would be based in part on results and service, which included full access to collected data. This interrupted long-standing broker relationships and eliminated most of them.

Second, we used our collective volume to get 10-15 percent discounts off insurer ASO fees.

Third, benefits were redesigned to give clear choices to employees: We set the highest quality, low costs health plan as the benchmark and had employees pay more if they wanted to access a higher-cost option. This led to a big migration into the benchmark plan and resulted in few complaints from employees because they had choice.

Fourth, and in some ways the most important change we made was to reinvent customer service. We had our health insurers scrap their typical customer service approach and set up a concierge experience. This meant that the person who answered the phone had to solve the caller's problem—there were no transfers to PBMs or provider offices. The health insurers hired different types of people to do this—sometimes retired teachers or ombudsmen in prior careers—anyone who had a maniacal commitment to solving problems. These concierge agents were given power to solve problems, and they were responsible for calling the employee back with the outcome. There were measurements in place to monitor quality. One thing we insisted on was that the customer service agents were not measured on how many calls they answered—a typical measure—but instead on whether the problem got solved to the employee's satisfaction. Not surprisingly, our NPS scores were in the high eighties. Compare that to the typical experience of long waits, getting transferred from agent to agent, and finally having someone not be able to solve your problem. Employees were so delighted with this experience that the change in their health benefits and sometimes their providers was an acceptable tradeoff.

What is the broader context that employers face, regardless of size?

The healthcare system is simply too dysfunctional for everyone, especially consumers.

To makes matters worse, the US has become a nation of illness. Eighty percent of spend is for 10-20 percent of the population, and we haven't come to terms with that. Doing more of the same will generate even more lopsided spending with the same outcome. The primary care system, which is the most important component, is in tatters today. And customers are simply at a loss about how to navigate it.

Advances in life sciences are widely promoted as an answer to healthcare challenges. Do you agree?

That's a complicated question with no easy answer. From a medical perspective, I couldn't be more positive and excited about the breakthroughs ahead from cell and gene therapies. We've waited a long time from the initial mapping of the genome twenty-five years ago to translate that astounding scientific advance into usable therapies and now here we are. Fantastic. And I think the recent breakthroughs in AI will accelerate new treatments and cures.

But the idea that these therapies will result in lower healthcare costs is unlikely. The therapies are expensive, require expensive technology infrastructure costs and there will be little competition for a long time to come. Medicare will set fees for these treatments which means, as always, the costs will get shifted to the private sector, which in the end, means employers.

The initial beneficiary of a host of gene and cell therapies will be individual patients with rare medical conditions. For example, the company I recently started (Right Doctor) had a patient that was recently treated for recurrent lymphoma at a leading cancer center of excellence. The cost was $1.5 million. It saved her life, but the price tag is unsustainable. These therapies today address mostly rare conditions—but it's only a matter of time before therapeutics like CRISPR get applied to common cancers and other conditions.

What is the expected timing of this development?

Over 2,500 clinical trials are already underway on gene and cell therapeutics. More widespread applications will likely hit by 2028-2030. We have already cracked the DNA code, just as the Wright Brothers cracked the barriers to flight aviation in 1903. No one could have imagined the consequences of their discovery back then.

Will this likely become an enormous cost shift issue?

Yes.

What I'm trying to say is that a fundamental paradigm shift is underway where advances in life science will overwhelm our current ability to pay for worthwhile care, in stark contrast to paying for so much low-value care today (30 percent by many estimates).

We need to grapple now with what lies ahead in terms of rapid advances in life sciences.

Are you saying advances in life sciences pose not only a cost dilemma but also a question of what society is willing to pay as a social value?

As a cultural value, we can't say "no" to such progress that greatly enhances life and greatly reduces suffering. It will turn current healthcare industry practices on its head, including reinsurers and actuaries. In the end, we will need a reinsurance pool backed by the federal government.

But let's be clear: The cost increases we fight are due to inefficiency, poor quality, or lack of competition and poor purchasing processes. The costs from breakthroughs like gene and cell therapies should continue to increase. If you want to pay for value, what is more valuable than curing disease or relieving suffering?

What should or can employers focus on?

Right now, we focus too much on what self-insured employer can do, given limited incentives to change employee behavior (benefit design) or provider performance (better outcomes). And we tend to look to the federal government for solutions. That too is likely to be the wrong place to focus our attention.

Where should the focus be?

The best bet is probably at the state level, and particularly state employee insurance programs. They tend to be the most efficient and effective purchasers in the market. They have clout and they have budget limits to work within. They can't raise taxes each year to cover costs.

Maryland and Massachusetts have worked with budget caps on health expenditure with some success. Oregon has instituted a powerful commission that makes sure that competition is occurring. North Carolina and Rhode Island have implemented new approaches, and California is moving in that direction.

Will government play a larger role regulating cost going forward?

I think so. And it may be inevitable, given what lies ahead and the resistance of the healthcare industry to do the right thing.

Can you say more?

Some form of "managed regulation" may be necessary at the federal *and* state level to deal with the magnitude of health expenditures within the decade, including the bolus of life sciences breakthroughs coming through the system.

At the same time, regulatory approaches are not usually embraced by employers. But this may be different. It's now in everyone's interest to establish a reasonable framework to rein in costs. But the type of government intervention and regulation is very important. It will have to be different than what has turned off the private sector in the past.

For example, a cap on the increase of expenditures—not price controls—would motivate every player in the system to become more efficient and increase their focus on what represents real value. Paying for low value interventions will no longer be afforded the luxury of crowding out necessary life-saving treatments that increase *justifiable* spending.

In the end, paying for low value can be seen as harmful.

What is The Right Doctor, your current focus?

It's a concierge triage service for employees. We help sick people find the right doctor for their serious illness and at the best facility. It's based on my work at GE and the emphasis on Centers of Excellence. Jack Welch always insisted on getting employees to the best facility anywhere in the world.

In addition to my personalized network of facilities, I comb through public and private data sources to see who produces the best outcomes for specific conditions and treatments. I already know many of the CEOs and CMOs in top management who can be helpful in offering me their personal experience. As healthcare "insiders," a lot is known about quality that simply doesn't get measured.

In essence, I provide a triage service that fills an essential need to patients caught up in a broken system they don't understand and at a time when they most need to. There are significant variations in quality, within communities, and within provider organizations. People want the best. Their life often depends on it.

I listen to a patient, understand what their need is, and fill a gap that shouldn't even exist. I wish we had a primary care system or less variation in quality so an independent company would not need to fill this gap. But I don't see primary care getting better. And it is still a privilege and a joy to help people in need.

Chapter 16.

Blue Cross Blue Shield of Minnesota Case Study

Introduction

Blue Cross and Blue Shield of Minnesota has a long history of advocacy for health improvement and health equity. Beginning in the 1990s, Blue Cross was part of a historic lawsuit with the tobacco industry and advocated for elimination of tobacco when it led the statewide campaign against tobacco advertising that targeted youth. The advocacy role became a cornerstone of the organization's DNA.

The Center for Prevention was established in 2006 out of BCBSMN's settlement with the tobacco industry ($241 million). The Center's mission is to advance racial and health equity to transform communities for a healthier Minnesota. The focus is increasing access to healthy, affordable, culturally relevant foods and to eliminate the use of commercial tobacco.

The organization emphasizes a comprehensive approach to advocacy that includes policies, systems, and environmental change. It also stresses targeted universalism for communities most impacted by inequities. It means being a strong community partner, listening to communities, letting them lead, and ensuring that equity principles are at the heart of decision making throughout the organization.

Funding initiatives are primarily evaluated by the strength of community engagement; policies, systems, and environments that have changed; as well as other community-driven measures of success. This approach is not limited by a short-term return on investment yardstick. While the health outcomes related to these investments may take decades to assess, other indicators give important feedback that the investments are making a difference in building more healthy and equitable communities.

Commercial Tobacco Use

While the overall smoking rate in Minnesota has dramatically decreased, marginalized communities have been disproportionately targeted by Big Tobacco and have higher rates of commercial tobacco use and exposure to secondhand smoke. Smoking rates are higher among Black, Indigenous, communities of color, and LGBTQ+ communities, as well as people experiencing mental illness and substance use disorders. This has led to significant inequities in smoking-related disease and death.

Center funding aims to reduce commercial tobacco use in communities by supporting community-driven, culturally specific efforts that raise awareness, shift cultural and social norms, and influence organizational and local public policy. The

Center funded five local community organizations to advance policies that reduce the availability of commercial tobacco.

The Association for Nonsmokers–Minnesota (ANSR), North Point and Lincoln Park Children and Families Collaborative advocated for local commercial tobacco policies in the cities of St. Paul, Roseville, Lauderdale, Duluth, Shoreview, Bloomington, Dilworth, Clay County, and Columbia Heights. This resulted in twelve local policy successes in 2021, including many that prohibit sales of flavored or menthol products.

Twin Cities Medical Society engaged Minnesota physicians, medical students, and healthcare professionals by providing educational resources and preparing those interested in serving as advocates for commercial tobacco policies.

ANSR researched online sales regulation of e-cigarette retailers by the FDA's Center for Tobacco Products. This is part of an ongoing surveillance project that allows the field to stay abreast of an evolving industry and is essential to creating effective tobacco control policies.

The Center offered additional assistance to the following projects and coalitions:

Supported the American Lung Association (ALA) to fund supply needs related to commercial tobacco treatment for mental health and substance use treatment providers. Providers received funds for nicotine replacement therapy (FDA approved products) and carbon monoxide monitors.

Implemented Behind the Haze and Quit the Hit, two behavioral change communications campaigns designed to increase knowledge and decrease tobacco use among communities most impacted by commercial tobacco including teens and LGBTQ young adults. More than 53,000 Minnesotans engaged in these campaigns.

Minnesotans for a Smoke-Free Generation coalition is co-chaired by Blue Cross and made up of more than sixty organizations that share a common goal of saving Minnesota youth from a lifetime of addiction to commercial tobacco. This coalition played a significant role advocating for the legislature to dedicate funding to commercial tobacco prevention, which resulted in a $4 million per year allocation to the Minnesota Department of Health.

ALA led the Lung Mind Alliance, a statewide coalition committed to reducing commercial tobacco disparities among people experiencing mental illness and/or substance use disorders. In 2021, the Lung Mind Alliance Statewide Policy Design team developed eight policy recommendations, which were included in the MSFG 2022 legislative agenda. They also trained 535 behavioral health professionals on tobacco use and recovery among individuals with mental illness or addiction.

Physical Activity

Blue Cross believes that people are happier and more active in communities that are welcoming and offer convenient opportunities for them to walk, bike, and play. People are more active when their communities have:

- A sense of belonging and safety for all people.

- Access to housing, schools, jobs, grocery stores, and other services located near each other.
- A connected network of sidewalks, trails, bike lanes, and parks.

This work supports community-level change that makes it possible for people to have what is needed in their communities to be active and well, including access to secure and livable housing. The Center works with a variety of community partners to provide people of all ages and abilities with opportunities for physical activity.

Some of The Center's early accomplishments include convening the Safe Routes to School (SRTS) coalition, that reduces pedestrian and bicycle deaths and injuries. It also improves kids' health, reduces traffic congestion, and improves air quality. To make it safer for kids to walk or bike to school, it required advocacy and then coordination with Minnesota Department of Transportation (program management) and state Departments of Health and Education. It also meant developing SRTS plans with municipalities, parents, and students. A steering committee identified barriers and opportunities as well as determining priorities to address the most pressing concerns.

Complete Streets was supported by Blue Cross Blue Shield of Minnesota because it makes mobility easier for everyone and it contributes to better health. This applies to pedestrians, cyclists, public transit, and motorists. It requires transportation agencies to identify the best transportation solutions for individuals of any age. Elements include wide sidewalks, well-marked or raised crosswalks, protected bike lanes, and safety islands for pedestrians. The Center played a key role in passage of the Complete Streets law and worked with a broad coalition of diverse stakeholders in the state.

Nice Ride Minnesota is part of the effort to change how residents view transportation. In 2009 the Center for Prevention became the sponsor of the first bike-sharing program in the state, which now includes 3,000 bikes and 400 stations. Blue Cross' title sponsorship of Nice Ride will conclude at the end of 2023.

Recent work of the Center includes:

- The Alliance, focused on keeping renters in place during the pandemic's public health and economic crisis. They worked with partner organizations to advocate for the extension of the statewide eviction moratorium, increased financial assistance to address housing instability, and worked with local elected officials on policies and advocacy efforts.
- Trust for Public Land developed the Healthy Schoolyard Prioritization map to identify gaps in access to healthy school yards. This will help guide resource allocation decisions and is a tool that can be replicated in other states. The Center also supported coalitions that aim to increase active living opportunities for people of all abilities.
- The Safe Routes to School Network supports practitioners to plan and implement equitable safe routes initiatives at the state, regional, and local level.

Healthy Eating Initiatives

Food is a major focus of the Center for Prevention because in many communities, the foods and drinks that are most affordable and available are also the ones that are the least nutritious.

Too often, healthy foods cost more money and are harder to find, or in many communities simply not available. Also, a lack of full-service grocery stores or a high prevalence of convenience foods creates an environment that results in higher rates of chronic diseases.

In Minnesota, before the COVID-19 pandemic, 8.3 percent of Minnesota households were food insecure, meaning they had limited access to healthy, affordable food. That number has grown since the pandemic, and disproportionately impacted BIPOC Minnesotans. One in three Native American new mothers report being food insecure. Black and Latine Minnesotans report food insecurity at more than double the rate of white residents.

The Center funded eleven community organizations across the state to lead community-identified solutions that increase access to healthy, affordable, and culturally appropriate food.

- The Community Voice Funding Initiative is designed to support BIPOC leaders and communities in creating equitable food systems and advancing food justice. In 2021 the Center for Prevention began funding four Black, Indigenous, East African, and multiracial-led organizations as part of the Community Voice Funding

Initiative, which continued through 2022. BIPOC voices have historically been marginalized or omitted when it comes to decision-making about food systems, public policy, or coalition building. Community Voice funding amplifies community voices and supports greater participation of BIPOC leaders in decision making on policies related to healthy food access.

- East Side Table was able to extend their Community Cooks Meal Box program for an additional sixteen weeks (resulting in a total of thirty weeks) for fifty participating households from the East Side of Saint Paul.
- Hunger Solutions supported forty different food shelves and other programs that address food insecurity in Minnesota.
- The Food Group added more than forty new partnerships to distribute essential food to people experiencing food insecurity in 2020-21. They focused on partnering with food shelves that have deep relationships in key demographics such as Hmong, Somali, Oromo, Latino, Cambodian, and the West African community, serving more than 1,000 clients per week.
- The Food Group successfully advocated to maintain state funding for the Market Bucks program, after a serious threat to eliminate it was made by the Senate's Agriculture Committee chair.

Minnesota Food Charter is organized around four main food tenets: food skills, food affordability, food availability, food accessibility, and food infrastructure.

The Food Charter was launched in 2015 to address health disparities by advocating for changes to ninety-nine policies from farm to fork. It started with nine months of community engagement through extensive social media, online workshops, local educational events (103,117 site visits), guidebooks, and toolkits. Statewide outreach and collaboration involved nonprofits, businesses, communities, government agencies, and healthcare systems.

Advocacy and organizing efforts by the Center for Prevention also resulted in a Healthy Food Financing Initiative (2017), Farm to School Funding, Urban Agriculture Funding, Farm to Food Shelf Funding, New Farmer Tax Credit, and Statewide Health Improvement Program.

Key Takeaways

- Creating and implementing effective solutions to health inequities requires working together with marginalized communities over a period of years and even decades.
- Sustainable change requires dedicated advocacy work on policies, systems, and environments to be successful.
- Systems change requires not only advocacy but also working across sectors to build support on behalf of communities.

Chapter 17.

Wisdo Health Executive Interview

Boaz Gaon is Founder and CEO

Wisdo Health is a social health platform that addresses the impact of loneliness, social isolation, and other social determinants on mental health, medical costs, and engagement of health plan members and employees.

What sparked your interest in peer counseling?

It began in 2008 with my father's terminal illness. I was an investigative reporter and journalist in Europe then. I began writing about his death, and many readers understood and empathized because they too lost loved ones. And like me, they had no ready connection with others going through the same experience.

That experience led to creating Wisdo with a team of friends, entrepreneurs, and mentors who shared a common vision of peer-to-peer community support.

Question: Wisdo recently conducted a twelve-month pilot study in collaboration with a national Medicare Advantage plan. What was the target population?

The Medicare Advantage members were aged 65-80, had one or more chronic conditions, one or more ER visits, or inpatient admissions in the prior twelve months, and screened positive for loneliness using the UCLA-3 Scale. The scale measures three dimensions of loneliness: relational connectedness, social connectedness, and self-perceived isolation on a scale of 3-9.

A total of 1,374 members met the study criteria. The average age was seventy-one. Seventy-four percent were female, 51 percent low-income subsidy, and 40 percent dual eligible. Seventy-four percent of participants were White, 23 percent Black, and 3 percent Other.

Question: What did participant screening indicate?

Seventy-five percent had two or more chronic conditions, including coronary artery disease, congestive heart failure, diabetes, depression, and hypertension.

Fifty-seven percent screened as severely lonely (7-9 on the UCLA scale). Forty-three percent screened as lonely (4-6 on the UCLA scale. Fifty-five percent reported having twenty-six or more mentally and physically unhealthy days in the prior month as measured by the CDC Health-Related Quality of Life scale (HRQOL-2).

Question: How did these scores change during the twelve-month study?

There was a dramatic change.

In the first month, participants reported an average decrease of 6.5 days in the number of mentally and physically unhealthy days (n=517).

At six months, 58 percent of participants reported an average decrease of 3.6 days in the number of unhealthy days in the prior thirty days (n=212). Also at six months, the same group reported an average decrease of 6.1 days (69 percent higher reduction) in the number of unhealthy days compared to the average decrease during the same period (n=201).

Question: How did participants fare on loneliness?

At three months, 58 percent of participants reported lower rates of loneliness compared to baseline (n=336). Also at three months, 19 percent fewer participants reported levels of severe loneliness compared to baseline (n=336). Likewise at three months, 13 percent of participants no longer screened positive for loneliness (n=336).

Further analysis suggests that Wisdo has the largest opportunities to decrease loneliness and unhealthy days among female or Black participants in the program.

Question: Were there impacts in addiction to loneliness?

Yes, participants reported an average of twenty-two gaps in care, obstacles, and goals. The top ones were sleep problems, nutrition, financial worries, and depressive symptoms.

To be more specific: 3 percent experienced side effects of medication and surgery, 8 percent had challenges with diabetes care, 17 percent noted depressive symptoms, 18 percent experienced grief, 21 percent had nutrition and financial concerns, and 22 percent experienced sleep problems.

These findings could be applied to improve STARS ratings or trigger additional referrals to clinical or SDOH programs in the community.

Question: Can you say more about the impact of connecting these members with clinical services?

In addition to creating personalized peer networks around every new member, Wisdo also sent messages to participants that identified as ones who could benefit from therapy.

A total of 484 users received the message, and 120 clicked on the link in the message to schedule an appointment on the portal. Another 77 percent of a subset of participants completed an additional survey and said getting recommendations and reminders for clinical and community services would have a positive impact on their decision to follow through with the recommendation.

The referral rate success to teletherapy services was 25 percent. Participants averaged seven monthly visits to the Wisdo app. That's very high.

Question: How about the impact on service utilization and medical costs?

There was a 10 percent reduction of inpatient visits, 4 percent reduction of ER visits, and a 6 percent reduction in urgent care visits. We will require a larger sample to increase the significance of these trends—but directionally, these are very positive trends especially when considering that the form of the intervention was peer support, rather than clinical, mental, or physical therapy.

As for medical costs, we now have more internal data showing equally positive trends. Our goal is to create a five-time ROI for plans who are considering integrating a peer solution component their members can access to address social health. Based on what we've seen so far, I believe that's an attainable goal.

Question: What are the main takeaways from this pilot?

Our digital platform uses peer support methodology as the social care vehicle to enhance members' lives. It reduces loneliness while increasing member experience and health-related quality of life.

These findings showed the positive impact of how a supportive peer community can work with Medicare Advantage members with multiple chronic conditions.

Question: Can you cite another example of how peer support can be applied in a community?

Peer Assistance Services (PAS), a Colorado nonprofit, wanted to see whether our program could offer a scalable and cost-effective approach to address the impact of loneliness and social isolation on mental health and substance use of vulnerable adults in the state. Wisdo recruited 815 Colorado residents to join Wisdo's peer support and clinical referral platform. We analyzed changes in health measures.

After ninety days, there was a statistically and clinically significant reductions in loneliness, depression, anxiety, and number of mentally and physically unhealthy days. A peer-reviewed paper published at JMIR Formative Research with additional results can be viewed at: https://formative.jmir.org/2023/1/e48864/

Question: What was the approach?

We provided a six-week open enrollment period at no cost for a year. Enrollees were asked to complete monthly surveys during the first ninety days. Participants could access the Wisdo platform on mobile phones or by personal computers.

Participants had the option to join weekly group coaching sessions led by Wisdo's certified coaches. Sessions covered topics such as resilience, self-care, mindfulness, and social skills.

Question: What gaps in quality of life came up during the pilot?

The most common user gaps and challenges were behavioral health (71 percent), sleep (32 percent), and nutrition (13 percent). 14 users joined each coaching session, with a total of 3.3 sessions for each participant.

The survey was administered on days thirty, sixty, and ninety. Questions assessed depression, anxiety, alcohol or other substance use, quality of life, loneliness, and overall satisfaction. Thirty-one percent of active users completed the survey.

Question: What were the specific measures?

Each of the study categories indicated important findings:

Statistically significant improvements in all clinical outcomes, including loneliness (15 percent), depression (50 percent), anxiety (29 percent), and quality of life/unhealthy days (13 percent).

An average decrease in self-reported unhealthy days by more than three days per month—the equivalent of $615 reduction in the overall cost of care per participant per year.

Eighty-six percent of participants engaged ninety days after joining the platform (4.5 times the industry average engagement rate).

Eighty-eight percent of participants reported that they would recommend Wisdo to others.

- *Loneliness and social isolation* showed a 15 percent reduction in loneliness rates within ninety days.
- *Depression and anxiety* indicated a 50 percent reduction in depression rates and 29 percent reduction in anxiety rates within ninety days.
- *Quality of life* showed a reduction of 13 percent in number of mentally and physically unhealthy days a month.

- *Healthcare costs* indicated a reduction if $615 in medical costs per member per year.

Question: How large a factor was depression?

Sixty-three percent of participants scored positive for depression on PHQ-2 when joining Wisdo. After thirty days, a reduction of 33 percent was found. A ninety-day follow-up survey indicated a reduction of 50 percent in the levels of depression.

Question: How about anxiety?

Participants were asked at the beginning of the program how often they had been bothered with feeling nervous, anxious, or on edge. Eighty-eight percent reported such feelings for at least several days over the past two weeks when joining Wisdo. At day ninety the average anxiety score was statistically significantly lower by 29 percent.

Question: And substance use?

Nineteen percent reduction in alcohol consumption.

This is important because 41 percent of men and 34 percent of women screened positive for hazardous drinking or active alcohol use disorder, based on the screening tool.

Follow-up surveys found that 36 percent of women and 21 percent of men who screened at risk for hazardous drinking or active alcohol use disorders reduced their risk level within thirty to ninety days.

Question: How successful were referrals to behavioral health counselors?

In this engagement, our partner strategy was to refer relevant participants to mental health educational resources that they had available. In total, 27 percent percent of participants clicked the link to access an educational module about how to support peers experiencing alcohol misuse or psychological distress. Additionally, 15 percent of all female members clicked the link to access an educational module on the risks of excessive alcohol consumption for women.

Question: What was the member satisfaction score for this pilot program?

Eighty-eight percent said they would recommend Wisdo to others, and 98 percent recommended that it be made available to everyone in the state.

Question: What conclusion did you draw from this study?

Wisdo is effective in engaging health plan members who are at risk for mental health and substance use disorders. Our service shows significant reductions in depression, anxiety, social isolation, and substance use consumption.

What participants liked most was being able to connect and talk with others who have shared lived experiences. This support was provided in a safe, judgment-free, and supportive environment.

Question: Why is loneliness such an important issue?

It's an issue that impacts most of us.

Loneliness affects 40 percent of Americans over 65 and 60 percent between 18 and 65. It's growing 5 percent to 9 percent a year. Forty-five percent report not finding the social and emotional support they need.

Question: What is the answer to this unmet need?

I believe the answer is providing connections with people who have the lived experience ("been in one's shoes") and offer sincere understanding and encouragement. In two words, Social Health.

That's the crux of what Wisdo does.

Question: How many members have used your services to date?

More than 500,000 members aged eighteen to eighty.

Question: What is the impact of social isolation on medical costs?

Loneliness and social isolation add an additional $6.7 billion in Medicare costs a year. Employers spend $154 billion every year in additional workdays lost due to loneliness.

In terms of healthcare services, loneliness reduces engagement in self-care and clinical services by 50 percent. As far as healthcare delivery is concerned, it's not surprising that loneliness is the largest predictor of dissatisfaction with health plans and medical care.

People are 29 percent more susceptible to premature death and increased risk for cardiovascular disease, stroke, and suicide.

It likewise affects health equity. Loneliness makes a 21 percent contribution to health disparities among socioeconomic groups coping with chronic disease. In fact, each increased point in a person's loneliness score doubles the risk for depression.

Question: What is the evidence that peer support is effective?

There is a volume of evidence on effectiveness. To name a few:

- Reducing hospital admission rates
- Decreasing substance use and depression
- Decreasing costs to the mental health system
- Increasing engagement in self-care and wellness
- Increasing sense of control and ability to bring about life changes
- Increasing quality of life

What makes peer support widely available today?

Online chat and social networking exploded in recent years, as well as smartphone adoption including in older adults. This makes peer-to-peer possible—and at scale.

Digital health solutions are particularly appropriate for older adults and for people coping with mental health issues. Seventy-two percent of adults over age seventy have smartphones or use tech devices in daily life.

Question: How does peer support relate to Social Determinants of Health?

Social health services improve mental and physical health outcomes as well as preventing deterioration in health across the acuity spectrum. That points to adopting peer-to-peer support services as a core SDOH strategy. It's a key to engagement, especially for vulnerable populations and for those lacking access to care.

Question: How does current technology improve peer support?

We now have the capacity to monitor key words and phrases, analyze sentiment, and provide support in a safe social setting, such as at home.

This allows us to provide emotional support, companionship, and empathy when it's needed.

Question: Can you say more about the safety aspect?

A self-moderating community will not produce the appropriate outcome for a person wanting emotional support. There aren't safety guidelines built into free-wheeling social networks.

Rigorous safety guidelines are a must as well as artificial intelligence that rigorously flags "watch listed" content and triggers already created scripts and escalation policies as needed.

Question: How is this different from other popular social networks?

Ad-driven social media networks increase mental illness for heavy users. Just the opposite of what is needed today. Those networks do not consistently offer and measure peer support—nor measure whether the connections that are provided and made increase or reduce health. That's not Social Health.

Question: What type of training is involved for Wisdo counselors?

Peers are trained to effectively offer emotional and social support, through a program co-designed and vetted co-developers of the UCLA loneliness scale. These peer "Helpers" are drawn from the community that demonstrate a sense of altruism and a consistent commitment to helping others, as well as a pattern of 100 percent safety adherence.

Question: How does peer counseling affect ROI and STAR ratings for Medicare?

Buy-in from commercial insurance carriers and employers is necessary for widespread adoption. Peer support solutions have shown a three-to-seven-time return on investment. It's a necessary building block of strategies to reduce costs while improving outcomes and member satisfaction.

Question: Any final thoughts on this subject?

The loneliness epidemic can be cured. I look forward to joining like-minded partners in changing social health in America.

References

Larry Davidson, Chyrell Bellamy, Kimberly Guy, and Rebecca Miller. "Peer support among persons with severe mental illnesses: a review of evidence and experience." *World Psychiatry*, 11(2), 123-128. 2012.

Michael Bologna and Richard Pulice. "Evaluation of a peer-run hospital diversion program: A descriptive study." *American Journal of Psychiatric Rehabilitation*, 14, 272-286. 2011.

Maria Trachtenberg, Michael Parsonage, Geoff Shepherd, and Jed Boardman. "Peer Support in mental health: Is it good value for money?" *London Centre for Mental Health*. 2013.

Chapter 18.

Blue Cross and Blue Shield of North Carolina Case Study

Introduction

The purpose of Blue Cross and Blue Shield of North Carolina (Blue Cross NC) is to improve the health and well-being of its customers and communities. The company's commitment to building a healthier state goes far beyond health insurance. North Carolina communities face a host of non-medical factors that have a profound impact on health. Financial stability, housing, education, and access to healthcare and healthy foods—all play a role in the overall health of communities throughout the state.

More than half the population has an unmet need relating to social, economic, or environmental factors. When these social needs are not met, they lead to more illness, emergency room visits, and hospital admissions. This cycle of illness impacts healthcare costs for everyone. Blue Cross NC is intervening sooner in the illness cycle ("upstream") with several prevention strategies and programs.

For example, in North Carolina every $1 spent on:

- Tobacco prevention saves up to $55 in tobacco-related healthcare costs.[1]
- Diabetes prevention programs save $25.63 in healthcare costs.[2]
- Nurse home visits for newborns can save $3 in healthcare costs.[3]
- Community water fluoridation saves $38 in dental treatment costs[4].
- Biking and walking trails save nearly $3 in medical costs.[5]

Blue Cross NC believes every North Carolinian deserves an opportunity to live their healthiest life. To improve healthcare in North Carolina, the underlying drivers of health that most impact communities must be examined. From 2018 through 2020, Blue Cross NC made more than $77 million in strategic community investments to help address drivers of health with a high priority in five areas: food security, access to care, early childhood development, safe housing, and education.

In April 2021, Blue Cross NC announced a new long-term plan to address non-medical drivers of health and promote health equity. The approach focuses on four drivers of health: food security, housing, transportation, and social isolation. The impact of each program will be measured to determine which interventions will be effective long-term strategies for eliminating health disparities, strengthening communities, and reducing healthcare costs for North Carolinians. This work builds on the company's ongoing philanthropic efforts to improve individual outcomes and community health status.

John Lumpkin, MD, MPH, Vice President of Drivers of Health Strategy for Blue Cross NC, believes the company is moving quickly to improve the health and well-being of its 4.2 million members as well as all North Carolinians. "Blue Cross NC is committed to improving the health and well-being of our customers and communities, and we're determined to make healthcare better for all. We understand that access to basic needs beyond traditional medical care is the foundation for good health, but everyone doesn't have access to the same resources to meet basic needs. In 2020 alone, Blue Cross NC invested $7.1 million to help underserved individuals get better access to nutritious food and to help communities and farmers bring structural change to North Carolina's food system. Our work extends well beyond traditional philanthropic efforts."[6]

Dr. Lumpkin continued, "We are also implementing innovative new models to enhance access to the resources that can improve health. Just as importantly, we are rigorously measuring the impact these models have on well-being. If the data shows that these initiatives improve health and well-being, we'll have an informed incentive to scale up these models. We certainly hope to see evidence that these investments help members establish habits for good health that stick, and if these habits ultimately reduce the need for expensive medical interventions. We'll use the information we gather to scale up the programs that prove effective."

Blue Cross NC cites research showing that food security is the most reported unmet social need. Healthy food impacts overall health and promoting food security can play a significant role in improving both individual and community health. North Carolina is considered the tenth hungriest state in the U.S. with an estimated 600,000 residents struggling to put food on the table.[7] As a result, Blue Cross NC is strengthening its focus on food security. This effort includes improving health and reversing chronic conditions through increasing access to healthier food in the following areas:

- Supporting members and communities experiencing food insecurity
- Improving health for members with chronic conditions
- Expanding philanthropic support, capacity building, and investments.

Collaborations with two of the leading food banks in North Carolina help illustrate the impact of Blue Cross NC's $77 million in community investments during the 2018-20. Highlights of these collaborations to improve food security are as follows:

Partner: Food Bank of Central & Eastern NC (FBCENC) and Mountain Area Nutritional Needs Alliance (MANNA Food Bank)
Investment Amount: $1,420,862 (three-year commitment, 2018-20)

Geographic Impact: Thirty-nine counties

Program Description: FBCENC and MANNA Food Bank are creating innovative partnerships in the community to reach potentially unserved families with needed food assistance. Blue Cross NC funding supports expanding access to nutrition-dense fresh produce through partnership pilot programs across the state. These programs include:

Healthy Meals for NC Families—Expanding Access ($676,991, began 2018)

FBCENC: Through partnerships with local farmers and growers and investments in transporting and distributing fresh fruits and vegetables, produce has become a staple at the food bank. After moving into the new Raleigh headquarters in late 2016, FBCENC significantly increased its capacity to handle more produce, distributing 70 million pounds of food in its thirty-four-county region. Produce flows from the Raleigh branch to the food bank's five branches in central and eastern NC, including Wilmington. Funding supported a new refrigerated truck at a cost of $152,500 over a three-year period, including purchase and maintenance costs. When FBCENC began its Community Health & Engagement department, Blue Cross NC funding supported a Nutrition Education Coordinator to offer cooking classes, nutrition education, healthy recipes, food storage, and preparation tips, throughout the counties.

MANNA Food Bank: Since 2015, MANNA has tripled its local produce sources and now works with more than sixty local farms. Blue Cross NC funding from 2018 through 2020 enabled the food bank to increase its cold storage capacity by more than 400 percent through a donation of $1 million for refrigerators and freezers for perishable foods. Utilizing a refrigerated box truck already owned by the food bank, MANNA Express is an innovative and cost-effective method of getting the products with the shortest shelf life, such as dairy and produce, delivered to partners.

Despite these efforts, MANNA cannot meet the food needs of local counties through brick-and-mortar pantry locations. Overlaying a map of areas of highest need with a map of its partner agencies, MANNA identified pockets of extreme need (pantry deserts) or areas that do not have MANNA partner agencies within a reasonable driving distance. Blue Cross NC funding now supports ($262,631) a Mobile Resource Center/ Pantry staff, supplies and travel for a three-year period to bring food to these food-insecure populations over a 6,434 square mile service area.

Food As Medicine—Building Healthcare Partnerships (2018-2020)

FBCENC: In 2017-2018, FBCENC partnered with Vidant Medical Center to develop an outpatient food pantry where patients are screened for food insecurity. Patients are then “prescribed” a pre-packed box of nutritious food to take home. The goal of the collaboration is to improve overall health outcomes for food-insecure patients by improving the nutrition of individuals affected by malnutrition, those required to take medication with food, and patients who need a healthier diet to improve diet-related conditions such as diabetes, heart disease, hypertension, and obesity. Funds supported this program's expansion through partnerships with Rex Healthcare, Duke Health, and New Hanover Medical Center.

Funds also support *Food for a Healthy Start,* which is a partnership with Urban Ministries. It combines the latter's medical and clinical resources with FBCENC's experience in food sourcing and delivery. The joint effort creates a network of referring pediatric healthcare providers, outreach partners (including early childhood care centers), Smart Start, CDSA (early childhood intervention services), and WIC to "prescribe" food for young children. Food source partners include local growers and farmers to provide fresh produce.

MANNA Food Bank: For two years, MANNA and its local clinical partners and community-based partner network have piloted a three-pronged initiative: 1) identify food-insecure individuals at health clinics, 2) match individuals in need with community resources, and 3) build capacity, as determined by MANNA to provide more nutritious food choices.

MANNA works with eight health clinics and Mission Health's Pathways HUB, in conjunction with eighty-one clinics, to identify food insecure individuals. Referrals are then made via MANNA's confidential 1-800-Food HelpLine. Individuals are also referred to partners that provide healthy food and clinical evidence-based meals, nutrition-related cooking demonstrations, recipes cards with storage tips, and further nutrition education.

This work supports a culture of health and nutrition throughout MANNA's service area with an emphasis on becoming independent and sustainable. Nutrition lead partners will continue to provide peer support to other MANNA partner agencies.

MANNA and its partners see potential to expand this effort to develop multi-sector collaborations to address food insecurity. MANNA has selected the Toe River District of Avery, Mitchell, and Yancey counties to address the unique health disparities in rural communities. Like much of MANNA's service area, the Toe River District has pockets of social need with high levels of poverty, unemployment, and food insecurity. Geographic isolation, lack of resources, and lack of employment opportunities contribute to the economic health challenges in these communities.

Funds will support the expansion of a more formalized model determined by MANNA and partners for building community collaborations at food distribution sites in the Toe River District with a goal of replicating this model across MANNA's sixteen-county service area.

In addition to working with the two food banks, Blue Cross NC provided a $1.2 million investment in Meals on Wheels of North Carolina to address food security in forty of the state's one hundred counties. Blue Cross NC funding supported a home-delivered meal service in the forty counties to ensure seniors have access to food. A total of 4,013 home-delivered meal clients have been served as of August 2020. Funding covers the cost of meals and equipment for food delivery.

To address other non-medical drivers of health during 2018-2020, Blue Cross NC made the following seven community investments focused on one of the company's other priority areas for community investments during the three-year period: access to care, early childhood development, safe housing, and education.

Access to Care

Partner: Atrium Health Foundation (2019-2021)
Investment Amount: $750,000 (three-year commitment)
Geographic Impact: Cleveland County
Program Description: The communities surrounding Graham Elementary School in Shelby, North Carolina, face high rates of poverty and unemployment, lack of insurance, and lack of access to primary care and a medical home. They encounter barriers to medical care, including lack of transportation, difficulty navigating the healthcare system, and parental job commitments that conflict with routine physician office hours. Because of these barriers, many students at Graham Elementary School experience delayed medical care, increased school absences, and inappropriate utilization of the emergency department for routine primary care needs.

To improve access to high quality medical care for Graham Elementary students, a virtual care clinic was piloted by a consortium of local providers: Cleveland County Public Health Center, Cleveland County School System, Atrium Health's Shelby Children's Clinic and pediatricians in

Atrium Health's Community Health division. The students acquired virtual access to pediatricians, who provided 1,754 telemedicine visits for 1,115 patients. Treatment plans are developed, and treatment is monitored while students remain in school. Atrium Health Foundation data showed a 77 percent decrease in emergency department use, 52 percent reduction in early school dismissal (due to health concerns) among school children seen via a telehealth encounter, and more contact with a primary medical home.

Funding from Blue Cross NC expanded the program to include other Cleveland County schools with high percentages of low-income, at-risk students. The original pilot program at Graham Elementary saw ninety-five telehealth visits during the school year. Through mid-January 2021, there were 228 visits for 200 students.

Partner: American Heart Association (2019)
Investment Amount: $750,000 (three-year commitment)
Geographic Impact: Mecklenburg, Wake, Durham, Guilford, and Forsyth counties
Program Description: In communities across the state, AHA led a community impact initiative that reviews needs assessments and interviews community stakeholders. AHA prioritized the policies, systems, and environmental changes that are equity-focused, community-driven, and shown to be effective. Three geographic areas were prioritized in conjunction with community objectives to address health equity.

In Charlotte, Raleigh, and Durham, the *Promotores de Salud* program engaged the Spanish-speaking community in heart health behaviors through highly trained volunteers and culturally specific outreach strategies. AHA is currently sponsoring these activities:

- Working with community centers to identify, empower, equip, and sustain Spanish-speaking community ambassadors, with an initial goal of training sixty Community Health Workers.
- Customizing and translating a four-part heart health curriculum and developing new and culturally appropriate Spanish language educational materials.
- Developing meaningful incentives for individual participation to distribute at community events.
- Training ambassadors through a four-part heart health curriculum (overall heart health, CPR, blood pressure, healthy eating). It shares best practices, reviews results, and sustains momentum.
- Training community ambassadors to increase community engagement through educational materials and the use of scales and blood pressure cuffs.
- Helping partners such as El Puente, Camino Community Center, Compare Foods, and YMCA to systematically integrate community ambassador programming into existing services.

In Greensboro and Winston-Salem, the *Hair, Heart & Health* program engages neighborhoods in heart health behaviors through Community Health Workers and selected barber shops and beauty salons. The goal of the program is to equip community leaders with practical information on how to manage blood pressure, increase physical activity, develop healthy eating habits, and identify risk factors for heart disease. Staff at seven barbershops and salons are being trained by AHA to have ongoing conversations with their clients about heart-healthy practices and the importance of regular blood pressure checks. The barbershops and beauty salons were identified by local universities, health departments, healthcare systems, and community centers. AHA is working with partners to identify three more barbershops and three more beauty salons to participate as *Hair, Heart & Health* ambassadors.

AHA is also working with Healthy Blue (Blue Cross NC's Medicaid managed care plan) to fund a program that engages and trains community members in targeted communities in the Simple Cooking with Heart series. Up to 600 community members will be recruited through ambassador outreach.

These community efforts will be supported by statewide strategies that highlight best practices and lessons learned. Blue Cross NC and AHA plan to continue funding community partners engaged in these initiatives.

Early Childhood Development

Partner: SAFEchild
Investment Amount: $300,000 (2018-2019 school year)
County of Impact: Wake County
Program Description: Funny Tummy Feelings (FTF), SAFEchild's school-based child abuse prevention program, helps protect children from sexual and physical abuse, teaches them ways to distinguish between pleasant and unpleasant emotions, and presents concepts to first graders to help them recognize situations that could pose harm. SAFEchild has presented the FTF program in fifty Wake County elementary schools annually (226 classrooms with more than 5,000 first-grade children).

Wake County Public School System (WCPSS) is the largest school district in the state and the fifteenth largest school system in the United States. SAFEchild has the potential to reach 13,000 first graders in 113 elementary schools.

Blue Cross NC funding supported expansion of FTF in Wake County's eighty private and twenty charter schools.

The expansion allowed for kits to be distributed to 115 WCPSS public schools and an additional eighty-five private and charter schools. A total of 270 WCPSS elementary school mental health professionals were trained to become Funny Tummy Feelings professionals.

Safe Housing

Partner: North Carolina Community Action Association (NCCAA)
Investment Amount: $2,000,000 (2-year commitment begun in 2018)
Geographic Impact: Fifty-six counties
Program Description: NCCAA is the statewide association of North Carolina's thirty-four Community Action Agencies, the only nonprofits mandated by federal legislation to serve the poor and disadvantaged. One of the core programs implemented by NCCAA agencies is the North Carolina State Weatherization Assistance Program (NC WAP), designed to help low-income individuals save energy and reduce expenses through the installation of energy conservation materials. A total of 1,600 North Carolina families benefit from the program annually. One of the by-products of weatherization programs is a positive impact on health. However, the program is limited since a number of repairs are ineligible (see list below) for NC WAP funding, leaving important health-related concerns untouched.
Blue Cross NC's funding helps fill these gaps, enabling North Carolina's most underserved communities to make those additional repairs for families and improve overall health outcomes. Eligible repairs that focus on health and safety include:

- Replacement of carpet with hard surface flooring (includes floor repair and clean-up service)
- Interior pest control
- General cleaning of home, including debris removal

- Interior ventilation issues, including venting and replacement of unvented heat outlets for cooking
- Air purifiers carbon monoxide and smoke detectors (including battery change-out)
- Handicap accessibility and fall prevention
- Moisture control
- Duct cleaning
- Filter change out, plus one-year replacement supply

This area would benefit from further Blue Cross NC funding for safe housing initiatives. According to the U.S. Census, 300,896 households live in poverty in the fifty-six-county region. The total number of NC households living in poverty is 655,131. Thus, 46 percent of NC households living in poverty would be eligible to participate in the Blue Cross NC program.

Partner: Habitat for Humanity
Investment Amount: $1,260,000 (begun in 2019) with a goal of reaching one hundred families. Almost Home program engaged seventy families as of 2021.
Geographic Impact: Wake, Johnston, Durham, Mecklenburg, and Orange counties
Program Description: Blue Cross NC funds support four Habitat for Humanity affiliates, representing four projects.

Habitat for Humanity of Wake County: The initiative seeks to increase Habitat Wake's pipeline of qualified homeowners by launching Almost Home, a program to help people qualify for a mortgage and prepare for the responsibilities of purchasing a home. Almost Home is led by a professional housing counselor, with support from an AmeriCorps member serving with Habitat Wake. Trained volunteer coaches mentor prospective homeowners. In its first year, Almost Home sought to address the needs of one hundred families who lack the income, financial stability, and acceptable credit to become homeowners. Almost Home supports prospective homeowners with the following services:

- Teach financial literacy, including developing a budget designed for the specific family
- Help the family reduce debt and establish good credit
- Assist the homeowner in seeking better jobs or improving job performance
- Help the family set goals for their personal success
- Monitor each family's progress and keep them on track

Habitat for Humanity of Durham: The program used Blue Cross NC funds to expand four project areas in 2019 and 2020: Homeowner Assistance Program, Repairs Program, Homeowner Incubation Program Accessory Dwelling Units Pilot, and Playhouse Build Program.

- **Homeowner Assistance Program (fourteen families):** Funds provided homeowners with a subsidy to keep their mortgage affordable and less than 30 percent of their monthly income, helping fourteen families achieve home ownership.

- **Repairs Program (160 repair projects for 300 individuals):** Provides critical repairs to elderly and disabled homeowners, helping them age in place with dignity. Projects include roof replacements, plumbing solutions, siding repairs, and accessibility add-ons.
- **Homeowner Incubation Program (HIP) Accessory Dwelling Units (ADU) Pilot Program:** HIP is a rental pathway to home ownership for people who are not yet homebuyer-ready but could be within 12-18 months through the addition of an affordable rental unit. With the HIP ADU pilot program, an accessory dwelling unit can be built on a Habitat homeowner's property, which would generate an additional source of income and provides a safe affordable rental for a future Habitat home buyer.
- **Playhouse Program:** This program is an indoor team-building opportunity where volunteers are led through one day of building and decorating a four-by-five-by-five playhouse that can then be donated to a non-profit partner.

Habitat for Humanity of Charlotte: The Critical Home Repair (CHR) program is working to meet the needs of low-income families in Charlotte and Pineville who own non-Habitat homes, but do not have the financial means to fund critical repairs. As one of the only affordable housing providers to offer this type of program, CHR conducts comprehensive repairs focusing on four basic health and safety issues: unsafe roofs or floors, lack of heat, electrical system hazards, and plumbing hazards. While the City of Charlotte has an urgent repair program, they are unable to handle the volume of needed repairs and will refer homeowners to Habitat Charlotte. In 2017, 618 homeowners requested applications for the CHR program, yet it was only able to serve seventy-five families in need. The average age of a homeowner was sixty-eight years old with a monthly income of $1,764. Blue Cross NC funding will support CHR projects, including labor costs and indirect project costs.

Habitat for Humanity of Orange County (twenty-five families): Funding supports the first Habitat development in the nation focused exclusively on affordable home ownership for seniors fifty-five-plus. Crescent Magnolia includes access to UNC Health Care, public transportation, and shared green communal spaces.

Education

Partner: NC A&T University, Winston-Salem State University, Fayetteville State University and North Carolina Central University

Investment Amount: $4,000,000 ($1,000,000 per institution) begun 2018

Geographic Impact: Guilford, Forsyth, Cumberland, Durham (student beneficiaries represent a larger geographic impact) counties

Program Description: The goal is increasing the number of under-represented students (African American, low-income, and rural) graduating from nursing programs at four of North Carolina's

Historically Black Colleges and Universities. Blue Cross NC funding supports nursing programs at each institution. Funding supports seven areas: technology and equipment upgrades, student and faculty development, exam prep workshops and tutoring, RN to BSN pipeline programs in partnership with community colleges, retention programs, and scholarships and financial aid for low-income students and students from rural areas.

Partner: University of North Carolina at Pembroke (UNCP), begun 2019
Investment Amount: $525,000
Geographic Impact: Robeson County (student beneficiaries represent a larger geographic impact)
Program Description: The county is one of the most rural areas in North Carolina, which is the second-most rural state in the country. UNCP's primary service area faces staggering conditions of obesity, heart disease, diabetes, cancer, infant mortality, and death rates for minors. Residents have less access to healthcare providers in every health profession. Most counties in the service area are designated as Health Professional Shortage Areas by the North Carolina Department of Health and Human Services. The health professions workforce in southeastern North Carolina does not reflect the population's diversity.

Health factors and outcomes have proven resistant to change for generations. Robeson and neighboring counties rank in the bottom 10 percent of North Carolina health outcomes and health status. A child born in Robeson County lives seven to eight years less than a child born in Wake County.

In 2017, the North Carolina General Assembly directed the UNC Board of Governors to assess what health science programs would best serve the region to meet its needs. The findings led to the creation of the College of Health Sciences, the first degree-granting program added to the university's academic inventory since 1999. The college is dedicated to improving health outcomes and preparing a diverse workforce for twenty-first-century employment.

Blue Cross NC supports the College of Health and Sciences' goal to improve rural health disparities, diversify the regional workforce, and improve health outcomes. Funding is focused in eight areas:

- **Coalition for Health:** The program matches UNCP faculty, staff, and students with community-based partners to provide enhanced outreach services to rural communities.
- **Makerspace:** A studio environment was created from transforming existing space into a lab for innovation so that faculty and students can develop new ideas and collaborate with each other and professionals on solutions to complex health problems.
- **Careers in Wellness:** UNCP students engage with students in junior high, high schools, and the Lumbee Tribe Boys and Girls Club to participate in health and wellness programs.
- **Life Skills Development Curriculum in Public Schools:** The initiative aims is to develop a volunteer-

based life skills curriculum for high schools across the county. The collaborative effort includes Public Schools of Robeson County, Robeson Community College, Lumbee Tribe of NC, and UNCP's Office for Community and Civic Engagement.

- **Speaker Series:** UNCP offers a speaker series about inter-professional education throughout the academic year featuring nationally recognized experts in team-based care, technology, and healthcare, and Social Determinants of Health. It culminates in an annual symposium that highlights students, faculty, and regional excellence in healthcare and inter-professional education.
- **Academic Service-Learning Opportunities Unique to College of Health Sciences:** The program is a teaching and learning strategy that incorporates meaningful service into course curriculum to enhance student learning and community engagement.
- **CARE Resource Center Expansion:** The on-campus food pantry and professional clothing closet is open to students, faculty, staff, and community.
- **Collaboration to Address Mental Health in Robeson County:** The objective is to reduce mental health disparities and gaps in service among communities of color in Robeson County.

Addressing Additional Needs in North Carolina

Blue Cross NC's commitment to improving the health and well-being of its communities extends to addressing additional needs as they arise throughout the state. Two examples are the company's work to address the opioid epidemic and the ongoing, critical needs in health equity.

Opioid Epidemic

Blue Cross NC awarded $2 million in 2019 to five non-profit organizations helping to prevent addiction and treat opioid dependency, as part of a $10 million investment to address the opioid epidemic.

- Duke University Health System's mobile health tool standardizes opioid screening, prescribing, and monitoring. The platform and a web-based clinician dashboard enable patients to learn about appropriate prescription usage and how to track home opioid use. Clinicians are given tips on how to spot potential misuse patterns before opioid misuse begins.
- University of North Carolina at Chapel Hill School of Medicine sponsors a Rural Primary Care Medical Assisted Treatment program that enables providers to incorporate evidence-based treatment for opioid use disorder in their practices. The initiative's Group Visit Project integrates primary care, behavioral and group therapy.

- Rowan County Health Department created a Post-Overdose Response Team (PORT) as part of a coordinated effort with County Health Department, Center for Prevention Services, and Rowan County Emergency Medical Services. Through the PORT model, Rowan County offers coordinated support beyond initial intervention by providing supportive outreach to opioid users and high-risk communities. Clients are also provided Naloxone kits and information on safe usage and storage.
- Pacific Institute for Research and Evaluation in partnership with Stanly County Emergency Medical Services focuses on enabling first-responders to offer overdose survivors treatment beyond immediate resuscitation. The county trains community paramedics to administer buprenorphine to opioid overdose survivors and assist in getting survivors into a long-term Medical-Assisted Treatment program to prevent overdose deaths and expand access to care.
- Treatment for Resilient Youth (TRY) is based in Durham and works to prevent substance use among youth and adults by reducing community risk factors through education, mobilization, and collaborative action. TRY is also training partners, families, and community peer supports in five counties.

Health Equity

A commitment to diversity is important for an insurance company for customers to feel their needs are understood. What matters to members is *health* and *care*. Blue Cross NC recognizes that racism and discrimination lead to health disparities that impact the health and safety of employees, members and the community. North Carolina's health system ranks forty-sixth out of fifty states for disparities. Lack of diversity, equity, and inclusion affects all North Carolinians.

The leadership of the company recognizes that people of color have historically been at a health disadvantage that cannot be explained away by genetics or heredity. It is due to systemic racism. Health inequities are a threat to everyone regardless of race or ethnicity.

Blue Cross NC explicitly recognizes that race and racism factor into healthcare. A specialized team was created to address the impacts of structural racism and equity, and to better understand past and present policies such as redlining, voter suppression, and disinvestment in low-income communities in the state. The Racial Equity Task Force is charged with partnering with non-profits to broaden their reach and investment in communities throughout North Carolina.

The Task Force complements the long-standing work of the Community Diversity and Engagement team and the Diversity and Inclusion Council (DIC). The Council has three focus areas:

- **People and Culture:** Increasing employee representation of senior professionals and above
- **Health Equity:** Advancing healthcare equity for members and communities to promote equal opportunities for coverage, access, and quality
- **Community:** Investing in and partnering with historically underserved communities.

Blue Cross NC made its diversity, equity, and inclusion resources available to internal and external audiences through the Blue Cross NC 21-Day Equity Challenge education program. It has been shown to form lasting anti-racist behaviors and habits by understanding how racism is embedded in everyday life. Materials are available to everyone, including family and friends of employees.

Diverse employee networks are consulted by marketing teams to provide feedback on the images and language used in external marketing campaigns. To further across-the-board diversity in communication, the company's corporate panel policy commits to only participate in panel discussions (three or more people) that represent gender, racial, and ethnic diversity. The company's Point of Blue blog addresses diversity and inclusion topics as well. For example: "Why Diversity in Business Matters" and "3 Ways to Change Behaviors to Foster Inclusion."

Key Takeaways

- Addressing the underlying causes of illness is required to improve the health of all North Carolinians.

- Social sector partnerships are needed to sufficiently scale "upstream" health-related interventions in underserved communities.
- Gaining the support of clinicians and allied health professionals is essential to changing how healthcare is delivered in the community.
- Training under-represented health professionals is critical to addressing gaps in rural healthcare.
- Structural racism and historical under-investment in low-income communities must be reversed to reduce disparities and improve health status of marginalized populations.

Endnotes

1. Centers for Disease Control and Prevention: https://www.cdc.gov/tobacco/about/osh/state-fact-sheets/north-carolina/index.html
2. North Carolina Office of State Budget and Management: https://files.nc.gov/ncosbm/documents/files/ResultsFirst_CFH_FinalReport_20190531.pdf
3. MedicalXPress: https://medicalxpress.com/news/2013-12-dollars-babies-nurse-home-infants.html
4. North Carolina Department of Health and Human Services: https://publichealth.nc.gov/oralhealth/services/fluoride.htm
5. North Carolina Department of Transportation: https://www.ncdot.gov/divisions/bike-ped/great-trails-state/Documents/great-trails-booklet.pdf

6. *Authority Magazine*, July 2021: https://medium.com/authority-magazine/food-deserts-john-lumpkin-of-blue-cross-and-blue-shield-of-north-carolina-foundation-on-how-they-3279ea63f32a
7. *Health Services Research*, Volume 55, Issue S2: https://doi.org/10.1111/1475-6773.13555
8. Inter-Faith Food Shuttle, Raleigh, N.C.: Hunger in NC—Inter-Faith Food Shuttle

Chapter 19.

Socially Determined Executive Interview

Trenor Williams is Co-Founder and CEO

Introduction

Socially Determined was founded in 2017 and is based in Washington, DC. The company provides social risk data, analytics, and expertise to health plans, health systems, life science companies, and other healthcare organizations seeking to understand how Social Determinants of Health (SDOH) and social risk factors impact the communities they serve, the populations they bear risk for, and the business performance of their organization.

Socially Determined's analytics platform, SocialScape, provides actionable insights into community-level SDOH risk exposure and individual-level social risk factors, and their impact on healthcare utilization, cost, outcomes, and equity. The company's customers use these insights to tailor investments in evidence-based social care programs, partnerships, and organization performance.

What is your role in the organization?

I'm proud to be the co-founder and CEO of Socially Determined. I started working on the idea of Socially Determined two years before we launched the company in 2017, and my first role was to bring on co-founders. Together with our early employees, we helped develop our social risk methodology, product, and solutions. I focus on a range of externally facing activities related to business development, content creation, customer success, public relations, partnerships, strategy, policy/advocacy, fundraising, and thought leadership.

Question: How big is the market opportunity around addressing SDOH and social risk factors?

Massive. Five to ten years ago, safety net health systems and some health plans—specifically in Medicaid—began focusing on social risk. Social Determinants of Health contribute up to 80 percent of healthcare outcomes and impact almost every healthcare decision for a person, a family, or a population. Historically, the healthcare industry has been blind to that information when making decisions or supporting an individual.

Over the last seven years, the opportunity has expanded. Every health plan—government-sponsored, commercial, or self-funded by an employer—is now focusing on social risk. For example, total spending in the managed care market will exceed $3.9 trillion by 2026, and there's an increasing federal and state mandate to incorporate social care benefits and programs in care models. In 2022, 75 percent of state Medicaid agencies reported that they planned to increase SDOH and social risk requirements for Managed Care Organizations (MCOs) operating in their state.

Every life science company has some effort to focus on social risk too. There are several areas where it can play a role for life sciences, including clinical trial participation and retention, prelaunch and launch of new drugs, and medication adherence so they can better understand how social risk is impacting somebody's ability to get diagnosed, get treated, and stay on treatment.

Employers are also thinking about the impact of social risk. Self-insured employers want to understand social risk better to help them manage escalating healthcare costs. They know it can help them improve other important metrics too, like absenteeism, presenteeism productivity, recruitment, and retention. But it's not just self-insured employers. Those offering benefits through a health plan are pressuring their carriers to help them better understand and address social risk as well.

Like I said, the market opportunity is massive. It affects every single sector that touches healthcare.

Question: Focusing specifically on the health plan segment of the market, what are organizations looking for in terms of SDOH and social risk data and analytics?

Health plans carry the most financial risk, which arguably makes them the most interested in social risk data. We consistently see them interested in member-level insight. At best, health plans have ZIP code level information. Whether that's at the community level through the CDC's Social Vulnerability Index or through the University of Wisconsin's Area Deprivation Index, the data isn't granular enough to drive decision making and healthcare outcomes.

Health plans want to know what social risk looks like for every person at a member level and have partners like us combine that with traditional healthcare data—disease, cost, utilization, and quality measurement data. Once health plans integrate social risk data with healthcare data, they can identify cohorts of individuals who share specific characteristics. An example might be individuals who have diabetes that also have transportation barriers and financial strain. Once you identify a group of people that have common challenges, you can start to analyze variations in healthcare outcomes. Maybe some people have higher levels of avoidable utilization or lower quality measure score attainment, for example. After identifying groups of individuals who share certain clinical and social characteristics, you can begin to design and deploy focused interventions to address them.

Finally, health plans want partners that can help them address the social risks they've identified. That might include helping them with better internal care management for individuals so they can understand a person's social risk and challenges and connect them with partners in their community that can help mitigate those risks.

Question: Why are health plans taking an analytics-first approach to this work?

With limited time, money and people, health plans must be thoughtful and purposeful about how they apply their resources. Addressing SDOH requires a data-driven, analytics-first approach so they can understand where they have the biggest needs and what solutions they can implement to address them. So, it's that combination of knowing there's a need that has real impact on healthcare metrics and outcomes and knowing that a solution exists to help mitigate those risks and improve outcomes.

Health plans haven't been able to figure out scalable, repeatable methods for doing this because they've been working with a subset of the information required to make those important data-driven decisions. A comprehensive, integrated approach that takes both healthcare data and social risk data into account, allows them to see the full picture and act with precision and confidence.

Question: How does SocialScape quantify SDOH and social risk?

At Socially Determined, we continuously evaluate and curate datasets from hundreds of different sources. We start with more than forty different sources of deidentified, publicly available data from sources like the CDC, USDA, and American Community Survey. We combine that with licensed data about every US business in the country to help us understand what resources are available to people. For example, we know where every pharmacy, FQHC, dialysis center, and hospital is in the country, and we know where every full-service grocery store, fast food restaurant, and convenience store that takes SNAP benefits is located.

We combine all that with licensed identified data of about 250 million people in the US, including income, house and car ownership, and the language spoken at home. Altogether, this encompasses about 800 to 1,000 data elements per person. We take that public, place, and person level data and run that through algorithms that we've developed over the last seven years to quantify, characterize, and then ultimately visualize social risk. We can look at this data in two ways—at a community level or individual level. Our community-level indices give clients a comprehensive view of the concentrations and contours of social risk in the communities they serve. The individual level obviously gets more granular and specific to people, whether an organization thinks of them as a member, patient, or employee.

What specific SDOH and social risk area, or as you call them, "domains," does Socially Determined assess?

Rather than creating a summary rollup index score, we made the early decision to quantify social risk across seven different domains. Our individual-level social risk factor scores include Food Insecurity, Housing Instability, Financial Strain, Transportation Barriers, and Health Literacy Challenges. Our community-level SDoH risk scores include those same five domains, plus Digital Landscape and Social Isolation.

We use a 1–5-point scale to assess relative risk, where 1 is little to no risk, 4 is high risk, and 5 indicates severe risk. These scores give our clients a starting point to better understand where risk exists, but we've found that the data and information being analyzed to create those scores is what's helpful in enabling the action our customers ultimately take.

Using food insecurity as an example, after identifying someone with high or severe risk, you want to know what's contributing to that high risk so you can begin to address it. Is it affordability issues, accessibility to healthy food, food literacy, or something else? Using our data, we can discern the likely primary, secondary, and tertiary drivers so organizations can use that data to identify the right intervention. The solution for accessibility to healthy food options might be different than the solution for affordability issues. At an individual level, we can also provide additional contextual information that helps paint a picture of the whole person. That can be extremely helpful in determining a path for action.

Question: Can you provide an example of a specific domain and typical data elements?

Let's talk about transportation.

We not only think about whether somebody owns a car, but also whether they live in an area that has access to public transport and what that public transport looks like. We consider financial elements. For example, if someone blows a tire, will that massively disrupt their ability for access and transportation?

We also look at proximity to available health resources—such as pharmacies, primary care offices, and hospitals—which has become especially relevant for our health plan, health system, and employer customers. We do this so we're able to look at transportation when measuring whether somebody lives in a provider or pharmacy desert, for example. That information helps us discern not only if transportation is a challenge, but if it's impacting somebody's healthcare. We recently partnered with Uber Health, which provides services like transportation to healthcare sites, and same-day prescription or grocery delivery. Through this partnership, Socially Determined can help a health plan or other client see where transportation barriers might be preventing someone from getting to their doctor's appointments or accessing prescriptions or healthy food. This visibility enables a care team to connect that person with Uber Health to directly address their needs.

Question: How do health plans use data like your community-level Food Landscape risk index or the member-level Food Insecurity social risk factor score?

Health plans not only want to understand if someone is at risk for Food Insecurity, but they also want to know what's driving that risk. There is a relationship between food and many clinical diseases like diabetes, congestive heart failure, and chronic kidney disease. Health plans are thinking about their existing programmatic efforts or partnerships and how they can utilize them to better support individuals with specific diseases. Knowing the link to food insecurity, they can devise intervention strategies or partnerships to help mitigate those risks.

Perhaps there is an individual who has chronic kidney disease, requires dialysis, and lives in a food desert. A health plan might provide healthy food options tailored to that person's disease set. Another example could be that there are available food options for a population with Medicaid as their primary insurance, and they can't afford the options available. The deployment of a produce prescription program, food bank, or food market vouchers allows people who already have access to healthy food options to be able to afford them. Health plans need that level of precision to not only understand if somebody is food insecure, but to tie that to their healthcare data and then determine the best potential solution that fits the needs of that person.

Question: That is very interesting from a community investment perspective. How are SDOH opportunities quantified at the member or population level?

Social risk data and healthcare data are more valuable as a combined data set, than they are alone. For example, we analyzed the social risk of a regional health plan population with more than 150,000 members with diabetes. We looked at where people live and the resources in that community, and we combined that with claims level data across multiple regions. In one region, we found that individuals with diabetes and elevated risk for both food insecurity and health literacy had more than a $3,500 increase in their per member per year cost (PMPY), compared to members who had diabetes and lived in the same area but had low risk in food insecurity and health literacy.

In another part of this client's market, individuals with elevated transportation risk had a $2,500 per member per year difference. And in another part of their market, it was housing and a $3,200 difference in PMPY. In just one of those regions alone, that's more than a $1 millon difference in the PMPY of that entire population.

This type of insight—that wasn't possible before—allowed the organization to build the business case for making an investment. From a care management standpoint, they knew specifically whom to reach out to, and how to think about partnering with community-based organizations that could best support their members.

Question: How can a health plan impact utilization and costs without jeopardizing quality?

If you want to impact quality, you must take social risk into account, gain insights into the challenges and risks that your members face every day, and connect them to interventions. Taking that approach, we've seen organizations make a measurable impact in terms of avoidable utilization, like emergency room visits and hospitalizations. Many times, there are increases in primary care visits, with people more engaged in their care and a positive impact in both the perceived quality of care as well as quality measures.

Question: Can you give examples of what information is known about a member before and after SocialScape is applied? Your methodology seems very comprehensive.

Healthcare is traditionally egocentric. As a practicing family physician in the past, I thought of individuals as patients, but a health plan thinks of them as members, and an employer sees them as employees. We've traditionally seen people through these different lenses. For healthcare organizations, that means they've only used healthcare data to understand somebody's healthcare journey.

If a fifty-four-year-old white male with diabetes and a cholesterol level of over 200 has been to the emergency room three times in the last year, a healthcare organization knows that information, but they don't know anything else about that person's life.

One way that healthcare has tried to close those gaps is through screening assessments related to social risk. Screening has many benefits. But the challenge can be that it's time bound and time limited, so it's related to the person in front of you and their perception at that time. There are many reasons why they may not be able to provide full information and that can leave some large gaps.

The largest challenge with screening is it disproportionately impacts people who haven't been accessing care. If you haven't been able to reach them or reach them infrequently, then you don't have any information on those people at all. That can expand inequities in healthcare and worsen healthcare outcomes.

This is why we've developed an approach that allows us to utilize data on all adult members and every community across the United States. Within days—rather than months and quarters—we're able to provide detailed information about an individual's risk, allowing the health plan or health system to proactively target those people where they know they have challenges.

Question: What is the Digital Landscape index and how did it come about?

We are continually thinking about additional domains of social risk and how we might be able to quantify them. A recent example is the Digital Landscape index that was borne out of the COVID-19 pandemic. With individuals isolating at home, not able to see their physicians and caregivers, we saw virtual care companies and tools rapidly expand. That pushed us to think about what social risk might exist in that space. We analyzed affordability, availability, and digital literacy as components of the Digital Landscape. This allowed health systems to better support the needs of their populations and mitigate those risks with resources like virtual health, virtual care, and receiving health information digitally.

Question: What is the basis for the Social Connectedness index?

We've known in healthcare for a long time that individuals who are socially isolated do not take advantage of available healthcare resources as much as people who feel socially connected. That has a real impact on their health and healthcare outcomes.

Social isolation is associated with a 50 percent increased risk of dementia, a 32 percent increased risk of stroke, a 29 percent increased risk of heart disease, and an increased risk overall in premature death.

As an industry, our goal is to understand the barriers that people face to allow them to be more engaged in their own healthcare. Social connectedness and understanding how we think about loneliness, the social network quality and a given community, and the social capital available to individuals in those communities is at the core of that. Today, we measure social connectedness at a community level but are actively working to measure at an individual level too.

Question: How is bias embedded in some SDOH programs?

The industry has been basing SDoH programs on the people we can see and not on those individuals who have the highest needs—those struggling to be able to engage with the healthcare ecosystem. We're using claims data as a proxy for challenges and risk and making assumptions based on whether somebody has been admitted to the hospital or comes into the emergency room, without understanding the broader context and the specific needs that they face every single day.

Socially Determined's opportunity has been to look at this in a holistic way, across full populations, not just those who access healthcare and have claims data within a certain calendar year. That allows us to create a more equitable approach and provide insights for everyone. It also allows plans, providers, and other organizations to think proactively about the people who have the highest needs and the highest risks, and not just on the people that have come through the front door.

Any final thoughts?

As a former family doctor, the son of a social worker, and someone who has worked in this field for more than seven years, one of the most important takeaways I have learned is that addressing social risk is a team sport. To truly make inroads, which I desperately hope that we do, we need every stakeholder thinking about this work in a coordinated way.

Earlier, I mentioned the egocentricity that exists within healthcare. Health system providers, health plans, life sciences companies, and employers all think about individuals differently, even though it's the same populations. To do this well, we need to have coordinated work across those different stakeholders and leverage the strength that each group brings. Ultimately, if you have any belief in the impact of social risk on healthcare outcomes, healthcare costs, and the quality experience for individuals, it warrants our attention and willingness to fight to do this in the right way.

Chapter 20.

Geisinger Health Plan

Introduction

Geisinger is an integrated health system led by physicians that serves 2.6 million people in forty-three counties of rural northeastern and central Pennsylvania. Its eleven hospitals generate 70,000 inpatient and 71.5 million outpatient visits each year.

Community health status indicators in the community show that predictors of health such as cholesterol levels, diabetes, heart disease, and opioid addiction call for preventive health interventions.

Geisinger's approach to population health focuses on non-clinical issues (e.g., poverty, food deserts, and environmental factors) to impact wellness and improve health status. At the same time, Geisinger is committed to developing approaches that reflect the growing diversity of its patient population to deliver culturally competent care.

Social health initiatives such as nutrition and diet exemplify Geisinger's commitment to reducing health disparities in care and closing gaps in care.

Fresh Food Farmacy

Food insecurity or lack of access to nutritionally adequate food is a significant risk factor for developing type 2 diabetes. Food-insecure adults are two to three times more likely to have diabetes than adults who have sufficient nutrition. One in eight adults and one in six children are food insecure. People with severely limited incomes often turn to inexpensive, easily accessible food that is rich in calories and poor in nutrients, which can cause and worsen diabetes.

Geisinger, as a health system, looked at Social Determinants of Health (e.g., diet and exercise) to understand why so little progress was made in treating type 2 diabetes. It developed the Fresh Food Farmacy program to determine if "food as medicine" was a viable strategy to combat diabetes.

Fresh Food Farmacy is a sustainable program designed to address the health challenges faced by patients with diabetes and food insecurity. It has four main goals: (1) provide all residents with diabetes access to quality medical care, (2) provide nutrition education, (3) provide case management, and (5) ensure access to a clinical pharmacist. These interventions help patients learn the skills they need to improve the management of the disease and make important lifestyle changes. For example:

- Ensure that people with diabetes and their families have access to at least ten meals a week of fresh, healthy food.
- Reduce the burden of diabetes in the community, including medical complications, prescription medication use, and cost of care.

- Educate students and community groups about the health effects of obesity and diabetes, and the benefits of healthy lifestyle habits on these conditions.
- Connect local farmers with local food banks to provide fresh, locally grown food to community members who might not otherwise be able to afford it.

Geisinger based its approach on two assumptions. First, eating healthfully improves health. And second, people want to eat better but may not know how to or have the means to do so.

To find out if patients were food insecure, two statements were included in the medical record of patients with type 2 diabetes.

> "Within the past twelve months, we worried whether our food would run out before we got money to buy more (Yes or No)"
> "Within the past twelve months, the food bought just didn't last and we didn't have enough money to get more (Yes or No)"

If a patient answered "yes" to either question, they were referred to Fresh Food Farmacy, which began in 2016. It provides patients with two meals worth of food a day, five days a week, if it is needed by the household.

Patients were screened for food insecurity electronically (via the patient portal), by phone, or in person during a clinic visit. Of 458 patients initially screened, 128 were found eligible for the Fresh Food Farmacy, and ninety-five patients were enrolled. It is housed in a 3,000-foot square facility that resembles a supermarket at the Geisinger hospital campus in Coal Township.

Food selection includes "diabetes appropriate" food such as fresh fruits and vegetables, mostly sourced from local food banks, and lean proteins and whole grains. The cost is $2,400 a year to feed a family of four with two meals a day or $0.65 per meal. The program provides 175,000 meals a year.

Clinical results showed a 40 percent decrease in the risk of death or serious complications. Financial results over eighteen months indicated an 80 percent reduction in costs for pilot patients (yearly cost of $240,000 per member was decreased to $48,000 per member).

Geisinger's program of providing free food as a treatment for diabetes yields improved outcomes for patients while reducing the cost of care.

To qualify for the program, participants must be eighteen years or older, diagnosed with type 2 diabetes, HbA1c of 8 percent or higher, paying for needed food is a challenge, and having a specialty or primary care patient at Geisinger. A mobile food app keeps track of food pick-ups and sends messages to the patient's care team.

Once enrolled, patients receive twenty hours of diabetes education with health coaches, receive a welcome kit that includes measuring cups and spoons, recipes, and nutritional information to use at home.

Patients begin with a "welcome class" where they meet with the care team: RN health manager, pharmacist, dietitian, wellness associate, and a community health associate. Each team member fulfills a different function that meets a specific social health need. Community Health Workers, for example, can address housing issues, heating bills in winter, and transportation barriers.

Two pilot programs subsidize the cost of transportation for clinical and non-clinical health-related activities. These services include counseling, getting food to food banks, grocery stores and pharmacies, and applying for government benefits.

Program Impact

Geisinger saves an average of $8,000-$12,000 for each percentage point reduction in patients' HbA1c level.

In addition to blood glucose changes, patients frequently experience decreases in bad cholesterol (down 15 percent to 18 percent) and blood pressure as well as decreases in ED visits. Of the 360 patients in the food program each week, blood glucose levels went down by 2 percent, and blood pressure decreased by five points.

The program's focus is nutrition, but a by-product is also weight loss. Most patients lost 10-50 pounds.

Patients attend an evidence-based weekly diabetes self-management program and can utilize an online suite of wellness programs, interactive nutrition education, grocery store tours, and cooking demonstrations. Recipes and menus are provided.

The program also shows improvements in mood, increased confidence in managing chronic conditions, improved testing, and monitoring health metrics. Healthcare gaps, such as diabetic eye exams and diabetic foot exams, are also being closed. Incentives are worked into the program to encourage participation.

Fresh Food Farmacy is funded through grants (40 percent), in-kind-contributions from Geisinger Health System (30 percent) such as administrative support and rent-free space, and private donations (30 percent).

Springboard Health

Fresh Food Farmacy is the first major project of Geisinger's Springboard Health initiative. It is a new approach designed to transform the health of a community by addressing the socioeconomic determinants of health. Fresh Food Farmacy brings a "food-as-medicine" approach to communities designed to combat high rates of obesity, pre-diabetes, and diabetes. An estimated one in three people in Lackawanna County are obese, while 11 percent have been diagnosed with diabetes.

According to the 2015 Geisinger Shamokin Area Hospital Community Health Needs Assessment, 12 percent of Shamokin residents over the age of twenty have diabetes. One in three Shamokin residents are considered food insecure.

"Nearly 50 percent of Shamokin residents are predisposed to diabetes, mostly because of obesity," said Dr. Houssam Abdul-Al, the primary care physician treating patients in the program. "If we really want to control diabetes, we need to remove obstacles for our patients. And providing free, healthy food is a lot less than the cost of treating complications from diabetes, including cardiovascular disease, nerve and foot damage, eye problems and kidney disease."

The goal is to design and implement an intervention that prevents disease and empowers participants to manage their conditions through food-related behavior and lifestyle changes. The focus on healthy eating is critical. Research finds that a healthy diet and exercise can be just as important as medication in regulating blood sugar and preventing long-term complications from diabetes. However, many people lack access to healthy food or knowledge about a healthy diet.

Economic challenges also play a major role, with some families running out of food before the end of the month or being forced to choose between buying food or buying medication.

Health Access

Geisinger Health developed a number of programs to complement diet and nutrition initiatives. The underlying theme is improving access to health for all plan members and the community at large. The following programs address social determinants of care as well as health equity.

ConnectedCare365 is a care delivery model for patients with chronic diseases like diabetes, heart failure, and hypertension. It uses remote patient care monitoring, artificial intelligence, and data analysis tools to improve patient outcomes.

By using a smartphone to monitor weight, blood pressure, and glucose, patients can take more control of their health. By analyzing patient-generated data and relevant information from the electronic medical record, the platform communicates directly with the care team. This allows clinicians to triage and prioritize care for high-risk patients to prevent unnecessary ER visits and hospitalizations.

Karen Murphy, PhD, RN, chief innovation officer and director of Geisinger's Steel Institute for health innovation, said, "using predictive analytics as well as real-time data analysis of clinical and patient-generated data, *ConnectedCare365* helps our patients achieve health goals and better manage chronic conditions. It furthers our mission to making better health easier by developing digital solutions to provide better care and drive down healthcare costs."

ConnectedCare365 works with *Noteworth*, a digital health company, that supports Geisinger's commitment to improving health outcomes, increasing patient engagement, improving access, and lowering costs. The collaboration aims to develop a fully integrated delivery model that includes additional clinical initiatives for diabetes, heart failure, history of stroke risk and post-stroke care, chronic obstructive pulmonary disease, case management, behavioral health, and substance use disorders.

Noteworth is a modular platform that fosters continuous engagement of patients and providers across ambulatory, post-acute, and transition care services. It addresses all aspects of virtual care, including condition management, remote patient monitoring, home health, behavioral health, telemedicine, and patient engagement.

65 Forward is a senior-focused facilities program dedicated to meeting all the needs for health and well-being of patients sixty-five and older.

Geisinger Primary Care Scholars provides debt-free medical school and a modernized curriculum on emerging approaches to primary care.

Mail Order Pharmacy generates a 37 percent increase in medication adherence prescription refills delivered to the home.

Neighborly platform gives Pennsylvania residents the ability to connect with organizations that provide food, housing, utility assistance, and healthcare through partnership with Aunt Bertha, a social service referral platform. It serves as an online resource hub for social, health, and human services. The program connects people with local programs and services such as food, childcare, housing, mental health services, and medical care. It also uncovers coordination gaps in care.

Neighborly opened its doors in 2020 for individuals, providers, and community-based organizations. It provides contact information for referring resources and tracking outcomes. The program relies on community help to continually update the directory with multiple forms of social assistance.

Free2BeMoms is a program for new mothers with opioid addiction. Medication-assisted treatment is available through community partners such as social service agencies, mental health providers, and the judicial system. Unlike many treatment programs, it does not take place in a hospital room and addresses the common barriers to seeking care such as stigma and shame.

Geisinger at Home brings personalized care to the sickest patients in their home. It keeps patients healthier, safer, and better connected to healthcare team members.

The program moves comprehensive care upstream and into the homes of this dependent population. Working closely with patients' primary care physicians, a team of doctors, nurses, dieticians, case managers, pharmacists, mobile paramedics, and other support staff bring care to frail, medically complex patients where they live.

Unlike hospital-at-home models, which typically provide episodic care for three to five days, Geisinger at Home is longitudinal. It starts with a comprehensive in-home assessment and care plan, coordinates with primary care, and provides ongoing clinical services as needed.

For the more than 5,000 patients enrolled in the program, there has been a 35 percent drop in emergency department visits, a 40 percent decline in hospital admissions, and an average annual reduction in spending per patient of almost $8,000. Patients report an improved quality of life as a result.

Patient Example: Chronic Care

> Jack, a seventy-nine-year-old man who suffered from heart failure and COPD, was missing his specialty care visits. His primary care team at first thought he was simply non-compliant and asked the *Geisinger at Home* staff to evaluate him for enrollment in the program. An in-home visit revealed that Jack had become so sick that his wife had moved his bed to the living room where he ate, slept, bathed, and watched TV. His breathing was labored even with using a portable oxygen unit, his appetite was dwindling, and because he could no longer walk or even stand, he had to wear a diaper.
>
> The team huddled and put a plan into action: immediately administer IV steroids, increase oxygen, and change the nebulizer to use both ipratropium bromide and albuterol. Then, using a secured communication link, the team called

Jack's pulmonary specialist from his living room to review his case. Oral antibiotics and corticosteroids were added to the plan. The team arranged for additional in-home physical therapy and nutritional guidance and got Jack to agree to a flu shot (a vaccination he had long refused).

With regular in-home visits and secure daily and weekly communications across the team, Jack made rapid progress. Soon he could walk into the kitchen and feed himself, could get to the bathroom with minimal help, and gained ten pounds thanks to his high-protein diet. Ultimately, he was able to make an in-person visit with his pulmonary specialist and primary care doctors.

Learnings

Careful patient selection is critical in order to identify those most in need of intervention. Using medical claims data, the team evaluates Medicare Advantage members by utilization and chronic medical conditions to find high-risk patients. Half of eligible patients had heart failure, 40 percent had chronic lung disease, and a third had diabetes.

Many had related complications such as kidney disease. Their median age was eighty-four with average annual costs exceeding $30,000. Many had annual costs of more than $100,000. More recently, the health plan has taken referrals directly from primary and specialty care providers, which now account for almost 50 percent of enrollment.

The program has grown to include more than 100 clinicians covering more than fifteen counties. One key to scaling has been to deploy the right skill set and "tag team," with the physicians and advanced practitioners, completing a comprehensive physical exam while the nurse or Community Health Worker assesses the patient's home—the food on hand, medications the patient is using (or failing to use), and safety issues. Sometimes simple interventions have a big impact. Community Health Workers, for example, focus on cost-effective measures such as fitting a shower rail or providing a rolling walker that can head off a debilitating hip fracture.

The program also leverages technology to gather clinical data remotely. For example, Bluetooth scales are used to allow patients to transmit their daily weights, helping the care team monitor potential fluid accumulation. And digitally transmitted wound images are allowing joint decision making with hospital-based surgical experts, eliminating transport and wait times.

Post discharge telehealth visits include a Community Health Worker visit with the patient at home and connects him or her virtually through an iPad that connects with peripherals such as a pulse oximeter, stethoscope, and blood pressure cuff.

Other examples of cost-effective technology include pharmacists doing a medication review from the office with the Community Health Worker stationed in the home instead of traveling with the patient to a clinic site. Mobile paramedics provide acute care services to free up nurses for other patients who need a more comprehensive assessment.

As volume grew to more than 1,200 patient calls a week, it was necessary to add a stationary triage staff in the office. The triage staff now frees up the mobile team to spend more time with patients with fewer interruptions.

An additional learning is that specialists prefer real-time communication using a secured messaging service. PCPs on the other hand prefer fewer text interruptions as long as they can review the visit notes in the EHR to stay on top of the care being provided.

Patient Example: End of Life

Working with Geisinger's highest needs patients has meant directly providing care to a number of dying patients. End-of-life discussions and coordinated care are as important as any other element of Geisinger services. For these critical patients, the staff engages in frequent discussions with the patient and family about the patient's prognosis, priorities, and wishes. This requires that all team members become competent and comfortable with skills needed to help patients and families make decisions regarding end of life.

Specialized training incorporates interactive sessions with role playing and case studies involving trained actors playing "standardized" patients. *Geisinger at Home* teams work with the EHR team to organize documentation and create a single location for information about the patient's wishes, goals of care, and healthcare surrogate.

> One Geisinger patient who had had surgery for bowel cancer was discharged home, but in time developed metastatic disease. Recently, the patient had developed skin breakdown due to declining health and had increasing difficulty leaving home. Her primary care case manager

called the *Geisinger at Home* team to request a visit, and the team (including a Community Health Worker) made an immediate trip to the home. The team addressed the new health issues and the CHW opened a telehealth connection with a regional medical director.

Given the patient's recent decline, the virtual conversation that followed with several family members turned to goals of care and the patient's end-of-life wishes. The medical director raised the idea of hospice and discussed its benefits, and the patient and family agreed that it would be a help. The team arranged for hospice care to begin the next day. The patient was able to spend her remaining days at home, surrounded by family, and under the watchful eyes of the hospice and *Geisinger at Home* teams

Keystone Accountable Care Organization (KACO) is a partnership between Geisinger and physicians, hospitals, and other healthcare providers. Population health is a primary focus with the objective of closing care gaps through the health navigator program. It coordinates care for 78,000 Medicare fee-for-service patients in rural areas of Pennsylvania.

The program was developed to improve patient outcomes by addressing social determinants of heath. The program helps patients navigate non-clinical areas such as:

- Housing instability and quality
- Food insecurity

- Utility needs
- Interpersonal violence
- Transportation needs (beyond medical transport)

Health assistants are embedded in primary care offices and conduct home visits to ascertain how to connect patients with community services to close care gaps. A new program enhancement is identifying patients with congestive heart failure and collecting clinical information from patients in their homes to support cardiologists' treatment plans.

The hospital provided training to community members who then became home care employees who provided diabetes management and insulin administration. The hospital also hired a certified diabetes educator and a certified insulin pump trainer.

The hospital collaborated with clinical service lines and community partners to offer nutrition screenings, childhood obesity screenings, and community health presentations.

Community Health Needs Assessment

Every three years, Geisinger conducts a formal survey to identify the specific needs of nineteen counties in northeast, central, and south-central Pennsylvania.

Geisinger Community Medical Center offered the following nutrition education programs to employees and residents:

- MyPlate Nutrition: On a budget
- MyPlate Nutrition: Food labeling

- Tips for weight management
- Healthy cooking
- Healthy gardening
- Emotional eating
- Monthly support groups for diabetics
- Cooking for older adults
- Gluten-free or vegetarian eating

The Geisinger employee wellness program, *myHealth Rewards*, is an ongoing initiative to promote physical activity, healthy eating, tobacco cessation, and other healthy lifestyle choices. Some components of the program were available to family members of employees.

Patient wellness programming was offered through Geisinger Heath in collaboration with nutrition, pulmonary, cardiovascular, and diabetes service lines.

One of the action items of the Community Health Needs Assessment was to promote community safety and injury prevention. The objectives included:

- Educate seniors on practical strategies to manage falls.
- Provide educational programming for school districts to prevent traumatic injury among students.
- Three-fold impact of preventing injuries, minimizing existing injuries, and improving injury outcomes.

The following programs support the CHINA priorities expressed by the community:

Fall Prevention is designed to reduce fear of falling and increase activity levels among older adults. Trained facilitators conduct eight two-hour sessions for participants to learn how to view falls, and fear of falling, as controllable, and set realistic goals for increasing activity. Participants also learn how they can change their environment to reduce fall risk factors and learn simple exercises to increase strength and balance.

A Matter of Balance classes for seniors. The program is designed to manage falls and increase activity level.

Car Fit that helps mature drivers find their safest fit. Car seat technician classes are also provided in conjunction with the reopening of the maternity unit.

ATV Safety teaches children eight to fifteen how to safely operate age-appropriate ATVs, reducing the risk of serious injuries such as facial fracture and spinal cord damage.

First responder courses, including *Stop the Bleed*, *Advanced Cardiac Life Support,* and EMS education.

Healthy Steps enhances early pediatric care by incorporating preventive, developmental and behavioral services into the healthcare model.

School student education includes topics on binge drinking, bullying, child abuse, concussion prevention, dating violence, distracted driving, and *Students Against Destructive Decisions.*

Firearm Safety provides education about safe firearms storage and the use of gun locks; participants receive a complimentary gun lock.

Collaborative resources for these programs include the Geisinger *myHealth Rewards* program, school districts, law enforcement, and senior centers and housing providers.

Geisinger Community Medical Center also maintains community partnerships with organizations like Lackawanna Drug & Alcohol, PA Trauma System Foundation, EMS, police departments, fire departments, PennDOT, and churches offering safety education programming. The hospital contributes to morning television and radio shows, newspaper articles, and health fairs to offer education to residents.

During the three-year cycle of the CHNA study (2019-2022), Geisinger Health developed a comprehensive Implementation Plan to guide community benefit and community health improvement activities. The three top goals and objectives of the plan are:

1. Access to Care

Goal: Ensure residents have access to quality, comprehensive healthcare close to home.

Objectives:

- Increase the number of residents who have a regular primary care provider.
- Increase access to primary and specialty care physicians practicing in Medically Underserved Areas or Health Professional Shortage Areas.

- Foster integration of behavioral and primary healthcare within Geisinger Community Medicine.
- Reduce barriers to receiving care for residents without transportation.
- Increase cultural competency among all Geisinger healthcare providers and staff.
- Foster pursuit of health careers and ongoing training of health professionals.

2. Behavioral Healthcare

Goal: Model best practices to address community behavioral healthcare needs and promote collaboration among organizations to meet the health and social needs of residents.

Objectives:

- Advance local and state dialogue to address behavioral health needs.
- Foster integration of behavioral and primary healthcare.
- Provide education to increase residents' awareness of behavioral health issues and reduce stigma associated with behavioral health conditions.
- Increase access to behavioral health services.

3. Chronic Disease Prevention and Management

Goal: Reduce risk factors and premature death attributed to chronic diseases.

Objectives:

- Encourage community initiatives that support access to and availability of healthy lifestyle choices.
- Initiate early-stage interventions for individuals at high risk for chronic disease.
- Address health literacy to improve residents' self-efficacy in disease management.

Diversity and Inclusion

Geisinger Health offers a range of programs that foster diversity and inclusion for health plan employees and members.

Regional Education Academy for Careers in Health-Higher Education Initiative (REACH-HEI) grew out of the recognition that Education is the cornerstone of a healthy community. *REACH-HEI* is an out-of-school program that provides academic enrichment opportunities, including mentoring by medical and graduate students, for 700 low-income and or first-generation-to-college students in northeastern and central Pennsylvania. The objective is to enable them to succeed in health-related professions.

In 2017, the first cohort of high school students graduated from universities, three have been admitted to medical school, two of which were admitted to Geisinger Commonwealth School of Medicine. Thirty-four of seventy-five undergraduate students have been admitted to medical schools, and the remainder completed their pursuit of health-related professions.

The program's characteristics and eligibility criteria are as follows:

- Free for selected students in grades 8-12
- An engaging health sciences curriculum
- Required community service and leadership experiences
- College and career counseling
- Mentoring by Geisinger Commonwealth Medical and graduate students
- Advanced integration of educational technology
- Exposure to state-of-the-art laboratories and simulation center
- Extensive job shadowing program
- College academic readiness skills in research, writing and reading

Eighty-eight percent attended four-year colleges or universities in Pennsylvania. Eighty percent of students are first generation to attend college and many students entered undergraduate pre-med or health-related programs. Forty percent of undergraduate students have attended medical schools. A number of employee resource groups support diversity and inclusion by providing opportunities for all Geisinger employees to build internal and exterior networks and further professional development. The program supports leadership development and career opportunities for employees at all levels through mentoring opportunities from the top-down and bottom-up (e.g., younger employees mentoring senior leaders on social media).

The program is also part of talent acquisition, talent management, and recruitment efforts expanded to engage a diverse employee base through the connections and networks of resource group members. Likewise, it enhances customer retention through culturally sensitive marketing and product development created with input from employees with expertise in specific demographics or regions.

The Geisinger brand is also enhanced by increasing visibility in the community as a diverse and inclusive employer as represented by employees who work to benefit the community.

Employee resource groups (ERG) include:

VETNET ERG offers a support network for Geisinger service members, veterans, and their families. This group forms collaborative relationships with local veteran support organizations and fosters a veteran presence throughout the Geisinger community by recruiting and retaining military talent.

G-PRIDE ERG (Geisinger—People Ready for Inclusion, Diversity and Equality) works to foster a welcoming, caring, inclusive environment for Geisinger employees of all sexual orientations, gender identities, and expressions. G-PRIDE serves functions as a source of support to LGBTQ employees in the system as well as educating and enhancing understanding around important LGBTQ issues.

G-PRIDE focuses on the following activities:

- Recruitment
- Physician advocate group
- Developing a cultural consulting service

- Professional development
- Education and training
- Sponsoring and promoting social events and community connection.

GAIN ERG (Geisinger Ability Inclusivity Network) seeks to attract, hire, engage, retain, and empower employees with disabilities to fully enrich the workforce while educating Geisinger family and community about how to best include those with disabilities and positioning Geisinger as a caring place to work. The group helps address the needs of individuals with disabilities among employees, patients, and members.

Women LEAD ERG (Legacy, Empowerment, Advocacy, Development) enhances women's recruitment, retention, promotion, and professional development across Geisinger. *Women LEAD* priorities include:

- Recruitment and networking—Support recruitment efforts and develop networks to increase the representation of female talent at all levels.
- Professional development—Offer professional development opportunities to ensure continuous learning for diverse talent.
- Community outreach—Lead and collaborate on community outreach initiatives that align with Geisinger's values and diversity mission.
- Education and engagement—Provide engagement and education opportunities to members, patients, and the

Geisinger family to support inclusion and increase cultural competence.

BOLD ERG (Black Outreach Leadership Development) is a catalyst for increasing awareness of racial issues in the workplace and provides a network that supports the development of employees who self-identify as Black, African-American, or of West Indian or of African descent. BOLD objectives include:

- Share BOLD stories that include experiences relating to diversity, inclusion, and belongingness.
- Host enterprise-wide events for Black History Month.
- Ensure all Geisinger marketing publications represent its diverse workforce.
- Support talent management in recruiting, retaining, and promoting Black/African- American talent, and serve on search committees.
- Host "meet and greet" events for new and current employees, and diversity and inclusion educational sessions for middle/high school students.
- Provide a professional, personal mentoring and sponsorship community, helping ensure a pipeline of talent for upcoming strategic leadership positions.

Summary

As the largest rural HMO in the country, Geisinger Health aligns its financial and clinical components to focus on improving community health status as well as individual patient outcomes. Twenty percent of physician salary is reserved as an incentive to achieve specific performance benchmarks.

The organization has invested in a range of social health programs that focus on preventive care, behavioral health, and economic growth to build stronger communities and healthier families. This strategy is reflected in primary care practice models that emphasize prevention and treatment to close care gaps) as well as medical homes.

Social Determinants of Health initiatives such as "food as medicine" and chronic disease prevention programs demonstrate an ongoing commitment to population health management.

Key Takeaways

- Organizational learning must be a system-wide business objective.
- Clinical team member flexibility is essential in adapting to evolving medical practice models.
- Longitudinal home-based care, rather than episodic care (e.g., 3-5 days), is especially important for seniors.
- Healthy diets and exercise can be as important as medication for certain conditions such as diabetes.

- Creating partnerships with local, community-based organizations is imperative.

Executive Comments

Andrea Feinberg, MD, was formerly Medical Director of Health and Wellness at Geisinger Health.

Healthy food is good for everyone.

When you're on a tight budget, you'll eat whatever food is filling and cheap. Unfortunately, that food tends to provide a nutritional void. The clinic's patients often experience not just temporary hunger, but food insecurity—the enormous physical and psychological impact of not knowing where your next meal is coming from. That has huge, long-term health consequences.

If you're poor, your risk of diabetes is higher. We're trying to close the food gap when it comes to social inequality. The benefits are multi-layered and far-reaching.

We know that eating habits formed by food insecurity are adopted by the whole family. And because family members often have the same inherited risk factors, those who don't currently have a diabetes diagnosis can benefit from the healthier foods their relatives bring home from the free pantry. Our hope is that the Fresh Food Pharmacy enables patients to model healthy eating habits for their children.

Eating correctly for diabetes means fresh fruits and vegetables, lean proteins, and complex carbohydrates. These very same foods prevent heart disease. They're anti-cancer.

This is about creating a healthy community for our existing patients and for generations to come. The goal is to diminish complications of diabetes as well as closing the meal gap to end hunger.

References

Feeding America USA.

Andrea Feinberg, Allison Hess, Michelle Passaretti, Stacy Coolbaugh, and Thomas Lee. "Prescribing Food as a Specialty Drug," *NEJM Catalyst*. November 19, 2018.

Andrea Feinberg, Jonathon Slotkin, Allison Hess, and Alistair Erskin. "How Geisinger Treats Diabetes by Giving Away Free, Healthy Food," *Harvard Business Review*. (updated) December 19, 2017).

"An Rx for Good Health: Geisinger Launches Fresh Food Farmacy," PRNewswire, November 10, 2016. Program quote by Dr. Abdul-Al, Geisinger Health System.

"Mail brings new benefits to prescription delivery." Times Leader. July 20, 2020. Reference by Dr. Alfred Casale, cardiothoracic surgeon, and chief medical officer for surgical services for Geisinger Health System.

"How Geisinger's home care program reduced ED visits—and saved money," Advisory Board, November 8, 2019.

Janet Tomcavage, Jaewon Rye, and Sanjay Doddamani. "Geisinger's Home Care Program Is Cutting Costs and Improving Outcomes," *Harvard Business Review*. November 6, 2019.

"Closing care gaps with Keystone ACOs health navigator program." Geisinger Heath System. November 4, 2020.

"Community Health Needs Assessment," Geisinger Health System. 2021.

"Regional Education Academy for Careers in Health—Higher Education Initiative (REACH-HEI)," Geisinger Health System.

Chapter 21.

Scan Health Plan Executive Interview: Francesca Rinaldo, MD, PhD

Francesca Rinaldo, MD, PhD, formerly Chief Clinical Innovation Officer and Corporate Medical Director

How did SCAN originate?

SCAN Health Plan is a mission-driven, not-for-profit, Medicare Advantage plan. Almost fifty years ago, a group of older adults, affectionately called the "Twelve Angry Seniors," unable to access the services they needed to age safely at home in their communities, formed the organization that became SCAN: the Senior Care Action Network.

It began as a network of services and programs that included meal delivery, home repair to medical centers, transportation, and housing support.

How are incentives structured to guide the organization?

Our financial incentives center around the beneficiary. Payments made to SCAN by CMS are directed toward high-value benefits for our members and fair compensation for our providers. Non-profit plans like SCAN are accountable to our communities, resulting in a better understanding of our members' needs, culturally compatible and sensitive care, and tangible investment in local communities.

For twelve years, SCAN has received a four-star or better rating from the Centers for Medicare & Medicaid Services.

What is the organization's approach to preventing and managing chronic disease?

When the Twelve Angry Seniors founded the Senior Care Action Network in 1977, their priorities were to manage the process of aging gracefully, keeping patients in their homes instead of in facilities, and preventing and managing chronic illnesses.

How would you sum up SCAN's mission?

Our mission is to keep members healthy and independent.

Thanks to the flexibilities in the MA program, SCAN prioritizes preventive care. For example, SCAN keeps cost-sharing rates low on services like primary care and prescription drugs that keep chronic diseases in check.

Meanwhile, our financial incentive is clear: more preventive services and more upfront interventions mean fewer expensive and unnecessary acute care services, like emergency department trips or extended hospital stays.

Beyond these structural advantages of Medicare Advantage, our benefit design and clinical interventions are designed to prevent disease.

Can you say more about benefit design?

Medicare Advantage plans can offer supplemental benefits not covered by fee-for-service Medicare. These benefits include reduced cost-sharing, health-related benefits such as transportation to doctor's appointments or in-home support to assist with activities of daily living (ADLs), and targeted benefits that address social risk factors, such as meal delivery for seniors experiencing food insecurity.

SCAN offers some combination of these three benefit types. They are appealing because of affordability and accessibility, but also because they emphasize wellness.

By focusing on preventive care, we aim to keep our members from needing costly, acute care whenever it is avoidable.

What nutritional services are provided to members?

SCAN is a strong advocate of the "Food as Medicine" concept.

We recognize that access to high-quality, culturally tailored, nutritional meals and targeted nutritional counselling are essential for managing chronic diseases. In the case of diabetes, for instance, we have engaged with meal partners to offer appropriate diabetic meals and nutritional counselling to members at no additional cost.

In 2023, SCAN delivered 41,000 meals monthly to our members under several different programs we offer. Many members qualify for more than one type of meal benefit. These programs include:

1. Post-acute meals, which enable members to receive daily meals delivered to their homes for four weeks following a hospital stay.
2. Chronic condition meals, which are tailored both nutritionally and culturally to support chronic condition management. Members receive eighty-four meals annually to support their health needs.
3. Long-Term Services and Supports meals for our Dual Special Needs Plan members.

Dual Special Needs Plan members are among the most vulnerable in the communities we serve and receive home-delivered meals regardless of their health conditions.

What about other benefits?

Supplemental benefits can also address barriers to care, like the inability to physically reach a provider. SCAN offers transportation benefits to physician appointments and to other settings where members can obtain healthcare services.

In 2023, SCAN members took 320,000 rides to access primary care, dialysis, physical therapy, and specialty medical services. SCAN also provides thousands of rides a month to grocery stores and senior centers.

For members who prefer to receive care in their homes, SCAN offers a substantial suite of supplemental benefits. For example, we provide unlimited telehealth for urgent care needs and behavioral health support through video-based therapy and psychiatry.

We also offer an online program with a series of mental activities designed to strengthen attention, memory, and other skills. To deal with inevitable technical barriers, SCAN offers a 24/7 telephone support line with experts who can answer members' health-related technology questions.

What about clinical support?

To address both clinical and social risk factors, SCAN provides fully integrated primary care to members through our Institutional Special Needs Plan, Embrace, as well as through other care delivery services that SCAN developed as strategic investments.

Embrace currently serves more than 3,000 members in southern California and Arizona, delivering care directly to seniors in their setting of choice, typically assisted living facilities. In this model, SCAN is both the provider and the payor and assumes full risk for the care of these patients, which is value-based care to its fullest extent. Embrace's team of mobile clinicians (medical directors, nurse practitioners) provide frequent visits and care to this population, coordinating all aspects of their care, including medication management, behavioral health services, and other care. The latter includes skilled nursing care, podiatry, labs, imaging, and medical specialty referrals.

SCAN's mission to keep seniors healthy and independent also provides an ethical foundation to solve some of healthcare's biggest problems. There are still many unmet needs for seniors in an increasingly complex and fragmented ecosystem. Our goal is to create services that fill these gaps across the healthcare value chain, resulting in lasting impact to older adults' health and independence. We strive to differentiate SCAN through these investments, which include:

- Homebase Medical—Home-based services serving the needs of clinically complex patients with chronic conditions. Homebase helps to navigate patients through transitions in care, assists and educates them on managing their chronic conditions, and wraps around the primary care provider with services such palliative care.
- Healthcare in Action—Serves the highly vulnerable unhoused senior population, providing fully integrated primary care and housing services for these individuals with an interdisciplinary, street-medicine care model.
- Welcome Health—Scales the best principles in geriatric care to a novel primary care model that leverages home-based, virtual, and brick-and-mortar clinic-based care for clinically and socially complex older adults.

- MyPlace Health—SCAN's Program of All Inclusive Care for the Elderly (PACE) program. It serves complex, frail older adults who are nursing home eligible, but prefer to reside in their homes and communities with an integrated care model that supports their independence. This includes a new center in downtown LA.

Can you give a further example?

Homebase Medical complements primary care providers by offering wraparound, home-based services to support managing clinically complex patients. These services facilitate smooth care transitions, streamline care coordination for effective chronic disease management, and deliver preventive care directly in the home.

> Homebase Medical example: Ninety-one-year-old patient with hypertension and congestive heart failure.
>
> This patient has experienced multiple hospitalizations and readmissions over the course of the year. Homebase stepped in to provide counseling for the patient, and to their family caregiver, on dietary changes that could prevent heart failure exacerbations. Homebase coordinated care with the treating cardiologist to closely monitor the patient's condition and adjust medications as needed.
>
> As a result of these additional layers of support, the patient has not been hospitalized in several months. For an older adult patient, whose cognitive and functional status can decline significantly with every hospital stay, this is a major victory.

How does SCAN support non-members in the communities it serves?

Independence at Home (IAH), a community service of SCAN Health Plan, supports older adults regardless of plan membership. IAH programs are provided free of charge and exemplify SCAN's commitment to its nonprofit mission by connecting underserved older adults and their caregivers to services that help them stay out of healthcare facilities and nursing homes.

Digital literacy is something many people talk about regarding older adults. What does IAH do to bridge the "digital divide"?

We have several programs designed to increase digital literacy among older adults, but one we're very excited about is the Technology, Education & Coaching (TEC) program.

Research indicates that only 21 percent of older adults in the US used telehealth services during the COVID-19 pandemic, often because they had limited access to technology and lacked digital skills. The TEC program was designed to address this problem. Originally, it paired "Digital Coaches" with clients in the Insights program, which provides no-cost therapy to individuals fifty-five and over and their caregivers.

Based on the program's success, we've expanded TEC to a wide array of IAH clients in various programs. Also, one of the interesting outcomes of the program is that it has helped senior participants access social media and other online engagement platforms, reducing social isolation.

Reference

Dr. Rinaldo's comments are based in part on testimony before the Health Subcommittee of the Ways and Means Committee of the US House of Representatives. September 18, 2024.

Chapter 22.

UPMC Center for Social Impact Case Study

Introduction

UPMC employs an integrated approach to healthcare coverage and delivery based on clinical effectiveness. It recognizes that improving health depends on more than providing healthcare services. It requires insight into disparities and action to close gaps in care.

In 2019, UPMC established the Center for Social Impact to expand social needs programs and innovation required to favorably impact health, quality, and cost. The intent is to reduce health disparities in underserved communities with a focus on housing, workforce development, and employment. To do this, the organization recognized the need to build connections to human services with a host of community partners: public agencies, nonprofits, academia, business, and financial institutions.

The effort is led by UPMC Health Plan in conjunction with the UPMC Center for High-Value Health. Health Plan leadership recognized that premiums alone cannot meet social needs that pose a barrier to better health for everyone in the community. Healthcare organizations take different approaches to remedy limitations in the social safety net. It is not clear which approaches are most important since published results to date are limited.

The Center for Social Impact is taking a more holistic look at outcomes beyond utilization and cost. It includes implementation of best practices, engagement, and member satisfaction. Evidence-based practices, which take years to document, are supplemented with qualitative feedback from the lived experience of beneficiaries to make decisions on how to increase member access to fresh food, for example, that result in health benefits.

The Center for Social Impact considers six factors in deciding to invest in a particular intervention:

- Is there a significant member need?
- Does it align with the organization's mission?
- Does it align with UPMC's business goals?
- Is there an evidence-based rationale?
- What are the outcomes the intervention is trying to impact?
- Does UPMC have the capacity to address the member need and achieve the outcome?

The Center has an evaluation strategy for each domain investment and a specific evaluation plan for each program or initiative, along with key performance indicators at the community and member level. Initiatives support three broad strategies:

- **Social Determinants of Health:** Initiatives go upstream and are aimed at the community broadly and may impact public policy. For example, housing investments that can reshape community health at a system level, but only over many years and affecting more than UPMC Health Plan members.
- **Shallow and broad social needs interventions:** Initiatives can blend and braid resources to maximize reach with a lower per member investment. For example, supporting enrollment in public programs such as SNAP have an impact at a scalable, population level, where early results show continuous enrollment correlating with lower total cost of care.
- **Deep and narrow social needs interventions:** Initiatives are focused on specific sub-populations with high levels of individual investment and higher expectations for impact. For example, supportive housing for members experiencing homelessness has shown pronounced quality improvement and cost-avoidance in far excess of the program's investment.

Tactics employed fall into five primary domains:

- **Approaching employment as a social determinant of health and building "Pathways to Work."** UPMC's Pathways to Work program primarily focuses on Medicaid members with job navigation and support. This program was inspired by a decade of programming around recruiting TANF (Temporary Assistance for Needy Families) members and a new state contract requirement to aid Medicaid recipients expressing interest in vocational training or employment. It has grown into community collaborations, workforce investment, and board partnerships.

- **Connecting members to resources that meet health-related social needs and reduce healthcare disparities.** This domain includes work to combat food insecurity and meet nutritional needs, providing permanent supportive housing to members experiencing homelessness or housing instability, a community paramedicine program to divert social care needs from the emergency room, transportation, social isolation, enrollment support for public programs such as SNAP and LIHEAP, and assessment and referral to community programs.
- **Leveraging community-based organizations and human services to connect with difficult to reach members.** Health plans are often victims of their own data, seeing only what is in a member or claims file. UPMC established a mutual data exchange with Allegheny County to identify members and use such data to build programs to better serve individual member needs (e.g., intellectual disabilities). Similarly, UPMC is building relationships with community-based organizations that can build connection and engagement with difficult to reach members.

- **Investing upstream in affordable housing.** Pittsburgh faces an affordable housing crisis with a deficit of 20,000 units that are affordable to households earning less than 50 percent of the area median income (i.e., households who qualify for Medicaid). UPMC has committed more than $40 million through charitable giving, tax credits, program-related investments, and partnerships through its *Homeward* program to tackle this issue.
- **Improving access for all.** Accessible and quality care for LGBTQ+ individuals has been a focal point through the creation of a dedicated concierge team within UPMC's member services. UPMC has also worked to build an inclusive network with an LGBTQ+ affirming designation that participating providers can earn through enrolling in training modules developed in partnership with Fenway Institute's National LGBTQIA Health Education Center. UPMC has also invested in network infrastructure to be more responsive to people with disabilities.

The UPMC Center for Social Impact uses these initiatives and community interventions in four ways: align programming related to corporate social responsibility, enhance charitable giving, demonstrate where meeting health-related social needs can show impact, and guide future business and investment opportunities.

Domains

UPMC initiatives impacting the Social Determinants of Health include the following: employment and workforce development, housing, homelessness, food insecurity, intellectual disabilities and autism, STEM (science, technology, engineering, math), behavioral health, social isolation and dementia, LGBTQ+, gun violence, health equity regarding cancer and other chronic diseases, and access to care.

1. Employment and Workforce Development

As one of Pennsylvania's largest employers, UPMC is committed to providing a path toward a rewarding career for people seeking employment assistance—especially those who may need additional support or resources to reach their goals. Many community members remain out of work, in jobs without family-sustaining wages, and encounter barriers to finding such work. As a result, UPMC started a new *Pathways to Work* program that is built on years of success in hiring individuals off TANF along with a new state Medicaid requirement to help Medicaid members find work or career readiness supports.

Pathways to Work is a comprehensive approach to workforce development and job training for UPMC *for You* (Medicaid) members and others in the community who are unemployed or underemployed.

The goal is to offer workforce development opportunities and job placement resources to UPMC *for You* members and unemployed or underemployed individuals in the community who have significant barriers to finding work. The latter includes those who lost jobs during COVID-19 or need help transferring their skills to a new career.

The approach focuses on building relationships with UPMC *for You* members and others seeking employment, and the social service organizations that support them—while using UPMC's training and recruitment resources to connect people to job opportunities and training within UPMC and other organizations.

Community and government partners help power this effort. UPMC collaborates across its own hospitals, facilities, departments, and with community-based organizations, and local workforce investment boards such as *Partner4Work* to offer the best match to the individuals participating in the program.

Highlights of the program and recent successes include the following:

- 200 UPMC *for You* members are typically hired each month into positions at UPMC. More than 60 percent of these hires reside in the City of Pittsburgh.
- As of April 2022, four cohorts of emergency medical technicians and Community Health Workers have been fully trained through Freedom House 2.0, an initiative based on the groundbreaking 1960s program. The program recruits individuals from economically disadvantaged communities, many of which have been significantly impacted by COVID-19. These cohorts were in the Hill District, Northside, and Mon Valley. Two additional cohorts in East Liberty and Wilkinsburg will be completed in late 2022. Many graduates and

trainees of Freedom House 2.0 are Black women. This program uses funds from Partner4Work, the Workforce Investment Board in Allegheny County, and represents a model that can be replicated across the Commonwealth and the country.

- The Pathways to Work "Dream Makers" were instated in 2021. These are dedicated UPMC Human Resources personnel who primarily support the UPMC Pathways to Work and Freedom House 2.0 programs. They work directly with candidates to ensure the best fit for open positions and walk them through the employment process from application to interview.
- *Pathways for Veterans* launched in 2021, and *Pathways for Students* is planned for 2022 and will follow the same job, training, and recruitment support model as a part of the larger Pathways to Work.

2. Housing & Homelessness

UPMC Health Plan has pledged $40 million through *Homeward*, an initiative aimed at improving affordability and access to housing. It supports programs that address member housing needs and partnerships that increase available homes in the Pittsburgh Area. Supporting healthy communities means supporting policies and programs that address living conditions, including access to safe and affordable housing that can have major impacts on individuals' health. The Homeward program supports this vision and lays the groundwork for the creation of affordable housing for individuals in some of Pittsburgh's most disadvantaged neighborhoods. Initiatives include subsidized rentals as well as home ownership initiatives.

Addressing Homelessness

The foundation of this work has been Cultivating Health for Success (CHFS) as the main building block for addressing homelessness. Homeless adults are two times more likely to be hospitalized than the general population and two times more likely to be hospitalized than other low-income individuals. This finding demonstrates the fundamental connection between health and housing. CHFS is an adaptive permanent supportive housing model that utilizes locally allocated housing subsidies, a community agency to navigate housing and related social needs, and UPMC clinical staff to coordinate individualized care plans for members with significant medical needs and who experience an acute or long-term housing issue.

The program started as a partnership with Community Human Services (CHS), a Pittsburgh nonprofit that provides housing and in 2010 as a part of HUD's Shelter Plus Care Initiative. The Shelter Plus Care model limited subsidies and services to a maximum of twenty-five individuals, because it relied on Allegheny County Administered HUD Continuum of Care Funding.

From 2010 through 2018, fifty-one individuals were housed and supported through Cultivating Health for Success. All individuals were disabled and homeless. These members saw decreased hospital admissions and unplanned medical care cost, which resulted in annual cost avoidance of $6,400 per member (i.e., savings from eliminating in low-value care). This resulted in a marked improvement in primary care utilization, increased engagement with specialists, and improved medication adherence.

Using expected cost avoidance as the basis for sustainable program funding, the model was restructured into a value-based purchasing agreement in 2019. Now, any subsidy source (e.g., housing choice vouchers, project based rental assistance, income restricted units) can cover housing expenses for enrolled members, and community partners (e.g., CHS) receive incentive payments for elements of the program they can influence. These factors include faster move-ins, longevity of housing placement, and member graduation (i.e., when all members of the care team agree the individual is ready to live fully independently).

Some payments are fixed such as when a member has been housed for two years consecutively or graduates. Others, like move-in bonuses, are determined by the time it takes to secure a member-approved occupancy agreement. Ninety-eight members have been enrolled in CHFS from January 2019 through March 2022. Fifty-three are still enrolled in CHFS receiving housing assistance and supports, twenty-two successfully graduated to full independence, and twenty-two left the program or died while enrolled.

Starting in 2021, the Pennsylvania Medicaid program required its contracted Managed Care Organizations (MCOs) to enter into value-based purchasing agreements that include Community-Based Organizations (non-healthcare providers). Agreements stress financial and clinical partnership models. These provisions integrate health and social support spending into MCO contracts.

CHFS has expanded to two additional counties with this change. State value-based payment requirements also permit related program expenses to be filed under Medicaid medical expenditure reporting rather than as an administrative cost. This change enables UPMC Health Plan to include CHFS costs as part of its medical costs and should enable the program to expand to all service areas. A total of 133 members have been housed since 2010, thirty-nine of whom graduated the program. Thirty-four did not complete the program due to fatality or other reasons.

Improving Affordability

Pittsburgh has an estimated affordable housing deficit of 20,000 units. Through *Homeward*, UPMC Health Plan has engaged a range of partners: local government agencies, nonprofit and community development partners, mission-driven financial intermediaries, and other civic stakeholders. They work together to identify shared priorities, advocate for solutions that combine funding sources, recognize barriers to housing, and invest in strategic collaborations that help low-income individuals achieve their housing goals.

UPMC *for You* has pledged $15 million in mission-related investments with the goal of helping to accelerate the preservation or production of 1,000 units over the next ten years. Examples of UPMC investments and partnerships in affordable housing in Allegheny County and City of Pittsburgh include:

- $5.6 million committed to housing related DCED (Department of Community & Economic Development) Neighborhood Assistance Program projects within the City of Pittsburgh during the 2020-2021 and 2021-2022 funding cycles.
- $3 million from UPMC *for You* catalyzed a $7.95 million affordable housing loan program to close care gaps in affordable housing projects. It began in 2021 in partnership with the Robert Wood Johnson Foundation, Kresge Foundation and Bridgeway Capital, who manages the program. The loans have financed 387 rental homes to with 269 units affordable to very low-income households, sixty-three affordable to low-income households, and fifty-five workforce units:
    - 122 units of Northside Properties Residences II LLC
    - Forty-three units with ACTION-Housing's Flats on Forward (a high opportunity neighborhood)
    - Fifty-four units at ACTION-Housing's Stanton-Highland Apartments
    - 105 inclusionary units as part of Mellon Orchards South in East Liberty
    - Three units in Hazelwood's Affordable Rental Preservation program

- $2.2 million invested in partnerships with nonprofit organizations that help UPMC Health Plan members stay in their current homes and neighborhoods:

    - $1 million to Rebuilding Together Pittsburgh for a home stabilization pilot program
    - $450,000 to Rising Tide Partners to renovate the Bry-Mard Apartments and develop a wellness program for all residents living there
    - $400,000 to Neighborhood Legal Services to pilot a medical-legal partnership that addresses housing issues and supports long-term community living
    - $360,000 to support ACTION Housing's emergency rental assistance and operate a housing stabilization center

- $2.2 million in donations and long-term leases of parcels to create affordable housing in Oakland and Homewood. (i.e., appraised value of parcels).
- UPMC Center for Social Impact helped to launch a Pittsburgh Preservation Work Group aimed at maintaining long-term affordability through deed restriction, Low-Income Housing Tax Credit compliance, and Housing and Urban Development project-based contracts and subsidies. Partners from this coalition engaged in state advocacy to increase funding for housing through Real Estate Transfer Taxes, and American Rescue Plan funding provided to Pennsylvania.

UPMC recognizes that the health and housing crises are interconnected and multidimensional.

John Lovelace, President of UPMC Government Products, emphasizes the critical importance of affordable and safe housing in order to improve health.

> Improving the value of healthcare in people's lives, beyond advances in current medicine, is why UPMC is focusing on how to stabilize patient treatment in a more productive way, to get better value. Just spending millions of dollars on clinical services doesn't much impact community health in the long run. We need to focus on social factors that influence outcomes and behavioral health by aligning charitable giving and tax credits to invest in affordable housing and jobs and economic opportunity.
>
> After a decade of operating supportive housing programs, we strongly believe that health and housing stability are interconnected. The condition of people's living conditions increase stress or worsen existing health conditions. Our priority is to create more equitable communities and stabilize housing circumstances for rent-burdened and housing insecure members.
>
> Health plans invest in affordable housing, but it's not necessarily tied to anything else. Housing has to be tied to outcomes to make it scalable, and that means having better metrics than good intentions to measure impact.
>
> Continuously build and update the business case. A holistic approach can improve both individual and community health.

4. Food Insecurity

Fifty-five percent of eligible older Pennsylvanians are not enrolled in Supplemental Nutrition Assistance Program (SNAP). *Community Health Choices* program, which focuses on adults who have a disability and low-income seniors (dually eligible for Medicaid and Medicare), receive assistance enrolling in the program through targeted outreach and phone-based eligibility and screening.

The UPMC Center for High-Value Health Care is evaluating health and cost outcomes when UPMC pays to enroll its dual eligible members in SNAP and other benefits. The study will assess whether it is cost-effective and practical to invest members in SNAP. There are numerous national studies[1] that support this hypothesis, but little evidence on the managed care impacts. Early results have shown significantly lower costs for members continuously enrolled from 2018-2020.

Based on these preliminary findings, UPMC began enrolling Medicaid members in SNAP, LIHEAP, state property tax and rent rebates, and other programs through Benefits Data Trust. Since 2021, more than 2,400 benefits applications have been submitted for more than 2,000 households.

This type of benefits access and enrollment has expanded beyond food and SNAP efforts. The American Rescue Plan Act made significant resources available for emergency rental assistance and utility assistance to promote economic relief from the pandemic. UPMC has employed a similar tactic by funding community partners administering funds to accelerate and ensure access to its members.

5. Intellectual Disabilities and Autism (ID/A)

Historically, ID/A care in Pennsylvania has not been a high priority for government-sponsored health insurance coverage. The system currently serves 57,000 individuals across Pennsylvania, with more than 12,000 additional individuals on a waiting list. Managed care organizations such as Medicaid, Medicare, Dual, Community Health Choices, and CHIP are not fully integrated with I/DA home and community-based waiver care programs. Many individuals with ID/A across the Commonwealth receive a comprehensive array of non-medical services and supports through a variety publicly funded and state-administered programs.

These programs and supports include state-operated centers and private intermediate care facilities for persons with intellectual disabilities (ICFs/ID), community residential and nonresidential services provided through Home and Community-Based Services (HCBS) waiver programs, and community services provided through the county-based funded program (state-only funds). The latter are managed and distributed to eligible consumers directly by counties). Located within the Department of Human Services, the Office of Developmental Programs is responsible for administering the ID/A system in Pennsylvania.

While many individuals enrolled in HCBS waiver programs, ICF/IDs, and county-base funded programs receive medical services across UPMC product lines, historically, there has been little coordination between health plans and service providers.

This partially stems from the fact that no state-wide mechanism currently exists to inform insurers that an enrolled member has ID/A, whether the member is enrolled in an I/DA HCBS waiver or other program. Insurers do not know what non-medical services the member receives, the name of the individual's service provider or supports coordinator, or other information necessary to enhance care coordination activities or create programming to address member needs and barriers to care.

After discussions and data exchange agreements with Allegheny County DHS, which now enable UPMC, Health Plan is able to identify members with ID/A in Allegheny County. The Health Plan began providing a dedicated Care Manager to an initial cohort of Allegheny County members with ID/A receiving residential services in waiver-funded Community Living Arrangements operated by three providers: ACHIEVA, Mainstay Life Services, and UPMC Western Behavioral Health at Mon Yough Community Services. The Health Plan initially approached these providers based on ther location in Allegheny County and the number of Health Plan members served, as identified through data matches.

As part of this pilot program, UPMC's Special Needs Plan care management team and medical director conduct monthly "case consults" with the three participating providers to discuss current member health needs. These include hospital transitions, HEDIS gaps in care, education, and scheduling, and obtaining updates on members with significant health needs or recently changed health status. The pilot included one hundred individuals and achieved a "closed" care gap rate of 95 percent as compared to a 67 percent rate for UPMC's Allegheny County ID/A membership. It significantly improved annual Health Assessment Survey responses for pilot versus non-pilot members (99 percent versus 21 percent, respectively), and reduced seven-day and thirty-day readmissions for pilot members by 50 percent.

UPMC's Community Team has twenty paramedics, twelve Community Health Workers, and more than sixty nurses and social workers. The team is involved in a pilot program to reach out to the most acute members on the ID/A waiting list. These members tend to have more unplanned care and lower quality outcomes than members enrolled in HCBS waiver services. UPMC's Community Paramedicine Team conducts in-home outreach and Social Determinants of Health screening for these members and connects them with Community Based Organizations and agencies capable of providing nonclinical supports such as housing, transportation, and food. Since implementing the Community Paramedicine Team, outreach services have been provided to one-hundred individuals and is working on the next cohort of one-hundred members. Individuals are prioritized based on waiting list status, which is determined by a variety of social and clinical factors.

6. Education

UPMC sponsors a free STEM program that exposes children in underserved communities to the medical and health sciences. The purpose is to plant seeds of interest in healthcare careers.

It is a pipeline education program that starts with elementary-age students and is developed and led by graduate health science students.

7. Behavioral Health

UPMC Health Plan has 4.2 million members. Its UPMC Community Care Behavioral Health Organization manages behavioral health services for more than one million members in forty-three counties. Community Care is the largest non-profit behavioral health MCO in the country.

8. Social Isolation and Dementia

UPMC's *Community Health Choices* is one of three Medicaid MCO programs in the state that provides Medicaid coverage for dually eligible Medicare/Medicaid beneficiaries, including those dual-eligible individuals residing in a nursing facility or receiving home and community-based services. It coordinates Medicaid/Medicare eligibility and long-term services and supports for 134,000 participants, 33,000 of whom are fully aligned where UPMC has responsibility for managing both medical and support services.

Service coordinators support Community Health Choices (CHC) participants and administer an evidence-based screening tool for functional needs and social supports. One aspect of the assessment identifies individuals with moderate to severe cognitive impairment who are referred for more in-depth cognitive assessments. The screening tool is part of a pilot that deploys Service Coordinators to serve as tele-presenters for UPMC clinicians who conduct virtual Montreal Cognitive Assessments in the home to establish a dementia diagnosis. Care managers engage with members and their families in making shared decisions about long-term care planning. Service coordinators also use screening tools to spot other home-based services and social support needed by members.

For members living in senior affordable housing, UPMC is piloting the use of 225 data-enabled tablets to connect CHC participants with family and friends to address issues of social isolation. The tablets contain games, puzzles, movies, and audiobooks specially designed for older adults. Service coordinators conduct video calls via the tablets to support members without access to smartphones or computers.

9. LGBTQ+ Community

Individuals who identify in LGBTQ+ communities often face heightened levels of discrimination and a host of other challenges when seeking healthcare. Sexual and Gender Minority communities often experience poorer behavioral and physical health with a range of disparities. These include higher rates of depression, anxiety, substance use, cardiovascular disease, and sometimes limited access to healthcare.

Given those realities and through community feedback, UPMC developed several initiatives designed to meet the needs of LGBTQ+ members across all lines of business. These include:

Multidisciplinary Team for Transgender Members. UPMC has a specially trained multidisciplinary team of member services representatives, health coaches, prescription drug experts, and care management professionals to help answer members' questions (appropriately and effectively) related to transgender-specific issues. These include insurance coverage details, recently expanded coverage for individuals seeking gender-affirming care, provider referrals, hormone replacement therapy, and community support groups.

LGBTQIA+-Friendly Physicians and Providers and New Designation Forthcoming. UPMC's members have access to hundreds of self-identified LGBTQIA+-friendly healthcare providers across service area, primary care physicians, endocrinologists, ob-gyns, plastic surgeons, psychiatrists, and other specialty care providers specializing in working with the LGBTQIA+ community. UPMC will soon launch a new LGBTQ+ Affirming Provider Designation, in partnership with the Fenway Institute, to identify providers that have taken specific trainings on LGBTQ+ clinical and cultural competency.

Employee Experience and Staff Training. To better understand the challenges of the LGBTQIA+ community, UPMC has partnered with several community organizations to provide ongoing training to member-focused employees. UPMC will continue to partner with additional organizations to make sure that every member receives resources to provide the best care.

Environmental Sustainability

UPMC supports a wide range of environmental sustainability initiatives and practices. An environmentally preferred purchasing process is in place at all forty hospitals. Pharmacies also participate in the US Department of Justice's National Drug Take Back Days, which collected more than 700 tons of unwanted medications in 2021, removing them from community access through environmentally sound disposal.

Food and Nutrition departments support sustainability by purchasing RGBH-free milk (recombinant bovine growth hormone), locally produced eggs, vegetables, and fruits. Vegetables and herbs are grown on campuses and cooking demonstrations are provided. Food services also reduce the use of foam-based products and make reusable beverage cups available. Hospital cafeterias signed on to Allegheny County's Living Well Initiative and earned a certification through the Sustainable Pittsburgh Restaurant program.

All UPMC campuses are smoke-free. Smoking of any tobacco, narcotic, and e-cigarettes is prohibited. Diesel-fueled delivery and transport vehicles are likewise prohibited from idling during their service UPMC offers support for multimodal transportation access to all urban facilities, especially hospital campuses. Options include public transit, bike racks, level II electric vehicle charge stations, and CHG-fueled transit shuttles for hospital employees. UPMC sponsors WalkPittsburgh that promotes transportation options such as walking.

Energy efficiency projects throughout the healthcare system are in place because of better facility design and operation. A UPMC garage lighting demonstration project contributed to a revised City of Pittsburgh parking garage lighting ordinance to align with modern energy efficient technology.

The organization's IT infrastructure is environmentally and energy efficient. Service-side technology enables patients and visitors to conserve resources by opting for e-billing, e-documentation and sign-on, and having their information managed through electronic health records, thereby reducing paper and printing demand.

Likewise, UPMC collaborates with the US Department of Energy on developing healthcare energy efficiency programs. It inserted a clean construction requirement into construction RFP contracts. UPMC East built a new LEED hospital and Children's Hospital of Pittsburgh was the first LEED Children's Hospital campus in Pennsylvania.

UPMC also collaborates with municipal and utility partners by installing a district energy-based microgrid in Uptown Pittsburgh that will benefit the community. Green spaces are incorporated in each urban campus to mitigate heat cap.

UPMC Horizon, with partial funding from the UPMC Horizon Community Health Foundation, manages the Medical Equipment Recycling Program, which provides refurbished medical equipment to people living in the hospital's catchment area who lack insurance coverage or means to buy new medical equipment. Since the program began in 1999, more than 15,000 pieces of equipment, including wheelchairs, canes, walkers, and lift equipment, have been given to more than 10,000 people. Volunteers clean and refurbish the devices before a final inspection by qualified professional staff.

Summary

Providing effective healthcare services to vulnerable populations requires much more than medical expertise and resources. The impact of healthcare services on beneficiaries, their families, and their communities is heavily influenced by social and economic factors. The best medical care accounts for an estimated 20-30 percent of health outcomes, with the majority attributed to factors such as genetics, personal lifestyle choices, and environmental factors such as adequate nutrition, housing, and disparities in access to care.

As a large regional health system and integrated health plan, UPMC recognizes the role it can and must play in impacting health outcomes not only through world-class medical care, but also by addressing the many social conditions that influence health outcomes. To accomplish this, UPMC has marshalled internal resources and established impactful partnerships with community organizations to address critical issues such as:

- Housing insecurity by committing millions of dollars of investments to finance affordable housing.
- Inadequate nutrition by developing programs to address food insecurity through insurance benefit plans,

provision of medically tailored and prepared meals, and by supporting local food banks.

- Employment for people who are under or unemployed by creating Pathways to Work programs for Medicaid recipients, people with disabilities, students, and veterans entering or reentering the work force.
- Assuring that all UPMC employees are paid a living wage and have access to necessary and affordable benefits.
- Building capacity to better serve people in communities with disproportionate health access struggles, including racial and ethnic minorities, immigrants, members of LGBTQIA+ communities, and people with disabilities.

Key Takeaways

- Evidence-based practices take years to document and must be supplemented with direct patient feedback (qualitative research) to guide project investments and funding priorities.
- Anchor institutions have a community responsibility to train local residents for jobs and careers in their organizations, and to pay living wages and benefits.
- Quality of life depends on healthy and affordable housing. That is the rationale for healthcare institutions, such as health plans, to invest in stable housing units in communities they serve.
- Housing investments to address social influences of health (by healthcare organizations) must be tied to specific

outcomes (i.e., impact measures) to be scalable. These investments cannot be made by health organizations only; they require collaborations with other community-based organizations.

- Eighty percent of health outcomes are tied not to healthcare itself but to biological and social influencers of health.
- Health disparities can be measured, and their impact can be addressed with thoughtful partnerships and better engagement with community partners. No one can do this alone from a single sector perspective.

Endnote

1. https://bdtrust.org/new-research-shows-snap-reduces-hospital-and-er-visits-lowers-medicaid-costs-by-2-360-per-person-annually/#:~:text=The%20study%20found%20that%20the,to%20those%20who%20did%20not.

Chapter 23.

Health Rosetta Executive Interview: Dave Chase

Introduction

Health Rosetta is a nonprofit firm that encourages organizations to adopt an approach to healthcare quality that improves the care experience for both the individual and clinician that naturally reduces expenses, aligns incentives, and improves outcomes. It concludes that organizations must apply financial processes to healthcare plans equivalent to the processes they apply to managing employee retirement plans.

The Health Rosetta model is based on eight components:

1. Transparent open networks (known prices, no financial penalties, outcomes focus)
2. Individual stewardship (understanding individual preferences and health profiles)
3. Advanced primary care (proper incentives)

4. Active and independent plan management (ongoing oversight)
5. Transparent pharmacy benefits (facts and data for decision making)
6. Major specialty and outlier patients (proper diagnosis)
7. High performance plan design (incentives, documentation, risk management)
8. Transparent relationships with certified benefits advisors (aligned financial incentives).

The firm contends there is no well-functioning healthcare system or health plan not built on proper primary care. The belief is that communities that focus on local primary care and prevention do a better job of managing problems that most affect employees, including substance abuse. It affirms the need for employers to champion local primary care systems in which physicians have sufficient time to develop relationships with patients.

Question: What is the role of employers in this model?

Health Rosetta understands that employers should enlist mayors and local governments in the effort to rally companies and citizens around developing a local, primary-care-based health ecosystem. Organizations that successfully manage healthcare spending often opt for self-insurance and combine it with stop-loss insurance to cover catastrophic claims. Employers who self-insure (i.e., pay their employees' health claims directly) reduce exposure to insurance carriers' exorbitant pricing, and reduce their spending by up to half.

By providing incentives for employees to visit only approved, value-based physicians and specialists (defined by adherence to appropriateness standards and fair price), companies control spending. The savings dividend can be used to address Social Determinants of Health.

By following the Health Rosetta's principles, firms create captive self-insurance consortiums so that small employers (i.e., fewer than fifty employees) can obtain local coverage. This strategy can slash healthcare costs by working with local primary care providers who bundle physicians, health coaches, nutrition experts, and wellness advice into per-patient subscriptions. The bundle of services cover visits and preventive care.

At the same time, such initiatives should discourage employee use of providers, including pharmacies, unless they are screened and approved based on excellence and low costs. This entails working with a benefits adviser, rather than a misaligned benefits broker organization, that has the financial and statistical skills like those of a retirement plan administrator (i.e., the right mindset).

Question: Can you give examples of how Health Rosetta principles and strategies have been successful?

Certainly, a number stand out that reflect our core principles.

Rosen Hotels in Florida has applied these approaches and saved more than $500 million. One of Rosen Hotels philanthropic initiatives, funded by health savings, is Tangelo Park in Orlando. Rosen's $13 million in donations to that community over twenty-five years generated a $90 million return on investment.

The Nuka system of community health services was created by the Southcentral Foundation in Alaska. It has improved life and health in villages across the state. Hospital admissions were reduced by half and specialist visits by two-thirds over ten years. Quality was significantly improved in the process. The Alaska Native population went from some of the worst health outcomes in the world to a system many consider the best in the world.

Ashtabula School District in Ohio designed a health plan to address their top priorities: improving outcomes, increasing member satisfaction, and saving money. This resulted in $2.4 million in savings, a 20 percent year-over-year savings.

Question: How are these principles demonstrated as part of an American healthcare comeback?

You can find the seeds of America's healthcare comeback story growing in a previously crime-ridden community in Florida, a living laboratory that has produced incredible gains in high school graduation rates and college degree attainment alongside a 78 percent decrease in crime rates.

The investment in Tangelo Park was just 5 percent of the savings Rosen Hotels & Resort achieved from a high-performing employee health plan benchmarked against similar employers mired in wasteful, status quo health plans.

This dividend was reinvested into a modest long-term commitment to children and education. In combination with an engaged community, they produced spectacular results. Typically, a community in the first income quartile has a mere 9 percent of its children continue their education to earn a college degree, while those in the fourth quartile have 77 percent of their kids become college graduates.

Despite being in the first income quartile, an impressive 78 percent of Tangelo Park kids who maintain residency in the community and remain in the program now earn college degrees. This is especially significant when you consider that the lifetime earnings of college graduates are more than $1 million higher than the lifetime earnings of those with only a high school degree.

It's notable that the annual financial investment enabling Tangelo Park's turnaround has shifted in recent years as the need for scholarships has decreased while they invest more in preschool education. Early scholarship recipients have grown up and become parents reading to their children, so they enter school with higher reading levels. Scholarships are now attained through other avenues due to higher academic achievements of students who attended preschool, are achieving higher grade point averages, and are college ready.

Question. How did this happen?

There's a good news, bad news angle.

The good news is that recovering currently squandered money is what we call the Health Rosetta Dividend—a $1 trillion opportunity to restore the American Dream that Tangelo Park has demonstrated is possible. Healthcare waste is having an adverse effect on schools throughout the country. With proper focus, recovering money squandered on healthcare waste is more than enough to fund a world-class healthcare system, as well as to fund the drivers of more than 80 percent of health outcomes, such as well-paying jobs, education, and public health.

The bad news is that the US wastes more than $1 trillion every year on ineffective healthcare, basically a $1 trillion "tax" by Wall Street that takes the form of price-gouging, administrative bloat, fraud, and perverse financial incentives. The focus isn't on community well-being.

The example of Rosen Hotels & Resorts, which enabled Tangelo Park, make it clear there's not only a business imperative to remove the waste rampant in the healthcare industry, but that doing so is also a community imperative. In fact, at Health Rosetta, both aspects go together.

Question: What generates the funding for such a community investment model?

The transformation of the Tangelo Park community in Florida is a successful role model for how to turn around long-term, systemic issues in predominantly African American communities. It demonstrates what any company or community can do today without any legislative changes. It's important to remember that the Tangelo Park Program was funded by money that would have been otherwise squandered on healthcare waste.

The magnitude of currently wasted money (more than $1 trillion) in the US healthcare system would make it the fifteenth largest economy in the world and using the Tangelo Park model could similarly reform so many communities throughout this country. Tangelo Park suffered many of the same issues that faced its counterparts in other urban neighborhoods with an unacceptable number of its high school students dropping out.

Just five miles from Disney resorts, this 90 percent African American community was a world apart from the millions of tourists flocking to Orlando with one sad exception: The neighborhood school was a location where tourists seeking drugs could go for their hit. Education and community leaders wanted to change the dynamic.

When Robert Allen was hired as principal of Tangelo Park Elementary, he inherited a school with a D–F classification that desired to connect with the community to create better opportunities for its youngest citizens. Many parents worked multiple jobs and didn't attend parent-teacher conferences; some families feared the walk to school because of rampant crime while some saw their children's education as the school's responsibility. Despite this, the neighborhood had a palpable sense of pride and was trying to "take back" its streets from crime, drugs, and gangs.

Question: How did the emphasis on education come about?

While Tangelo Park residents were organizing to improve their neighborhood, Harris Rosen, the president and CEO of Rosen

Hotels and Resorts, was studying what prevented Orlando's children from achieving life success. Knowing that educational success precedes life success, Rosen met with local education leaders, including an early childhood education coordinator and the principal of a nearby high school. The meeting led to a program that would provide a college scholarship to any child in the designated neighborhood who was accepted to a vocational school, community college, or state university.

A key to this scholarship was that it was inclusive of all college-related expenses, including books, room and board, travel, and tuition. In addition, they wisely understood that a critical success factor would be a preschool for disadvantaged students to start the path to success at a young age.

Understandably, Robert Allen was initially skeptical of Rosen's plan because it came from a business leader rather than an educator. Allen recommended holding a community meeting where Tangelo Park residents could hear from Rosen himself about the planned scholarship program. Tangelo Park residents were somewhat hesitant and wondered if they'd have to wait fifteen years for the promised scholarships for the early childhood students to graduate from high school. Rosen assured the community that they would begin the college scholarship the following June as a manifestation of the partnership between the community, his foundation, and the local school system.

Rosen grew up as the child of low-income, Jewish immigrant parents so he appreciated the array of obstacles faced by Tangelo Park children. He knew that it would take more than a scholarship offer to turn the community around;

therefore, Rosen invested to meet a range of economic, community, educational, and social needs through high quality childcare, parent training, and support as well as providing students access to vocational and college opportunities.

Question: What is the community strategy based on?

The Tangelo Park Program is a community-based initiative that promotes civic commitment by private, public, and community organizations to dramatically increase the chance of success. The initiative has a three-part strategy enhanced by access to vocational programs and support from scholarship program alumni.

First, ensuring that the community's children are ready for kindergarten through a combination of quality childcare and enriching preschool.

Second, supporting parents to be full partners in their children's education from birth all the way through high school.

Third, guaranteeing college and vocational scholarships. This guarantee provides not only the hope that Rosen says is key to making college a high priority, but also the practical means to make that hope a reality.

How is this program different from others?

It wraps both arms around the community and says we're here to serve you and help you become the best person you can be. A lot of other programs have only one piece here and one piece there. The Tangelo Park Program draws on a comprehensive array of partners across the neighborhood, school, community, and experts outside the community.

A combination of a legal board and a community advisory board guide the program. Community partners include a civic association, a local church, a neighborhood YMCA, as well as a state-sponsored neighborhood center that provides family counseling, pediatric care, a food pantry, as well as computer access. Outside the community, the University of Central Florida, Junior Achievement, and Cornell University are involved.

Parents of children in the preschool are required to take two parent workshops a year. The program also regularly communicates with pre-K and kindergarten teachers to identify and reduce gaps in student readiness.

Question: What are the results to date?

Since the start of the program, the Tangelo student high school graduation rate has approached 100 percent. It was unacceptably low when the program began. Full-ride college scholarships are awarded to qualifying graduates. Through 2015, there have been 224 degrees earned.

The odds of college graduation have changed from 9:1 against to 3:1 in favor. Estimates for the increase in lifetime earnings per student is $1.05 million (comparing those with only a high school degree to those with a bachelor's).

Crime has decreased 78 percent since the beginning of the program.

The average percentage of scholarship-eligible students who moved out of Tangelo Park went from 42 percent in the first five years to 7 percent in the last five years. Lower mobility rates create more stable classroom learning environments.

While 70-75 percent of graduates with bachelor's degrees have student debt, Tangelo Park grads have zero debt.

Return on investment to society: seven dollars for every one dollar spent. Approximately $13 million has been invested over the course of twenty-six years, resulting in $91 million of societal benefit.

Today, The Harris Rosen Foundation serves as a safety net, distributing fewer scholarships because Tangelo Park students are now capable of earning financial support from other sources—a direct result of their improved academic achievement.

Question: How has the program grown in the last few years?

After the initial success of the pilot neighborhood, Harris Rosen adopted another Orlando neighborhood five times larger in Parramore.

Physician leaders in other cities are learning from Tangelo Park's experience and have adopted and successfully replicated the model. In South Dallas, Catalyst Community Foundation and community leaders are co-creating a Tangelo Park-like program to address unmet needs.

The real question is what or who will provide the sustainable funding for an effort like this to reach thousands of communities around the country. Neighborhood schools are a tangible and universal unit applicable to every community. The approximate annual investment per neighborhood school such as Tangelo Park or Parramore is $500,000 for a community to cover daycare, after-school programs, and college education costs. There are several sustainable funding options available depending on the community dynamics.

Question: What is the business case for adopting this approach elsewhere?

The case for adopting a neighborhood is that there's a strong rate of return by embracing a community financially. Consider these impacts:

- Generates new public funding and has a direct economic impact.
- Expands place-based efforts in dozens of diverse communities.
- Demonstrates how public funding can be used to drive student, family, and community well-being.
- Empowers a learning community to inform and improve like-minded efforts.
- Elicits and sustains family and community participation that requires schools and universities to be more accountable and responsive to their local communities.
- Builds coalitions that effectively bring together parents and community-based organizations to address the

variety of needs and interests of their community and make positive changes.

Question: Can you give more examples of how Health Rosetta principles were applied?

Nuka Health and Ashtabula certainly stand out.

The Nuka system of community health services was created by the Southcentral Foundation in Alaska. It has improved life and health in villages across the state. Hospital admissions were reduced by half and specialist visits by two-thirds over ten years. Quality was significantly improved in the process.

Ashtabula School District in Ohio designed a health plan to address their top priorities: saving money, increasing member satisfaction, and improving outcomes. This resulted in $2.4 million in savings, a 20 percent year-over-year savings.

Question: How does Nuka reflect Health Rosetta principles?

The Nuka model is an example of successful community-driven change.

One of the guiding principles was to build trusting relationships between providers and customer-owners, who would run into each other in everyday activities outside of the hospital and clinic.

Before the Nuka model was created by the Southcentral Foundation (SCF), Alaska Natives had worse health outcomes than most developing countries.

In 1985, under CIRI's tribal authority, SCF assumed the contract with the federal government to manage dental services, optometry, community health, and accident and injury prevention education in the region. Two years later, the Alaska Native Medical Center (ANMC) opened as the largest IHS facility in the country.

In 1998, SCF assumed ownership and management of programs located in the new Anchorage Native Primary Care Center. SCF's responsibilities expanded the following year as co-owner and co-manager of all Indian Health Service programs at the Alaska Native Medical Center Hospital campus, along with the Alaska Native Tribal Health Consortium (comprised of fifteen Native organizations of Alaska).

The organization grew from zero members in 1998 to 6,447 in 1999 when SCF began. In 2021, there were 70,102 customer-owners.

Question: What was the biggest policy change?

SCF oversaw a total redesign of the healthcare system. They kept some traits of modern medicine and melded it with Alaska Native values and wisdom of the elders. They put the customer-owner (formerly known as "patients") in charge at all levels. A no-excuses model was designed to provide care in remote Alaskan villages with no medical professionals.

SCF also embodies Health Rosetta's principle of open and transparent policies, operations, and program evaluation. The model includes outlining core concepts, integrated care training, motivational interviewing, and team performance training.

Before SCF took control of primary care services, the Alaska Native people had "coverage" that was universal and with all the downsides of a bureaucratic system.

After 150 years, Alaska Native people decided that they would no longer have "things done to them." Policies and procedures would be decided upon locally rather than by a paternalistic provider-centric organization out of touch with local issues.

In the 1960s, one doctor saw more than 160 patients in a day, which is the antithesis of personalized care. SCF customer owners wanted a primary care approach where providers knew each person and tracked their families longitudinally. They wanted same day service with minimal wait times. They wanted the option of tele-visits wherever they were, as well as email and text access to their providers with quick turnarounds.

SCF's customer owners represent local control over a primary care system that is roughly the same size as Sweden. The focus of Nuka is to keep patients out of the hospital, as much as possible. By keeping the hospital and specialists separate from primary care teams (co-location), it allowed SCF to change the measurements of success. This meant developing a broader view of health and well-being, including creating better employment career opportunities in the community than just low-wage jobs.

Question: How did the power dynamic change?

However, the power dynamic was very different from other health systems around the country. Customer-owners were in charge and the role of providers was to answer to them by adhering to a core set of operating principles unlike any other healthcare institution in the US.

Getting people out of emergency rooms and into primary care offices was one of the first goals. This was one of the top priorities of the customer-owners, rather than a corporate goal of upper management. Customer-owners knew what they wanted and what was best for them (and not providers).

They wanted less waiting times and being always treated like a person, not as a number. Since taking over their healthcare system, Alaska Native people are becoming among the healthiest people in the US despite decades of poor health and discrimination.

The concept of bringing Alaska Native people into healthcare, finding their niche, and encouraging them to increase their knowledge base has provided a stable career ladder for many. In 1954, only one Alaska Native nurse and one dental aid served the Alaska Native community.

Over half of SCF's 2,300 employees are Alaska Native people. When new hires come on board, SCF encourages them to go back to school and resume further education when needed. When they earn degrees, SCF supports them to remain in the organization and progress up the corporate ladder to higher positions and higher salaries. SCF also takes high school students through a program to find their interests, advance their skill sets, and teach respect for their elders. High school graduation rates have increased as well as college education.

Question: How is access promoted in rural areas?

Relationship-based medicine is not new, but the expansion of it is important. This is critical because Alaska has more than 200 rural villages that can only be accessed by plane or boat. And if the weather is bad, they cannot be reached physically. That stimulated creative problem-solving on how to maintain contact with local villages (the "no excuses" motto) regardless of weather, distance, or time of year.

The SCF model employs health aides in every village who are trained in medical protocols that apply to most common maladies. The original two-volume bound treatment manual is now available online. The internet allows people in the most remote villages to have access to healthcare on the main campus instead of having to fly into Anchorage. Every village has equipment to allow diagnosis and treatment of common problems.

There is also a secure vending machine in villages that has been stocked by the SCF pharmacy. The doctor will prescribe, the vending machine will drop the pills, print out a label, and the pharmacist from Anchorage can watch on the monitor as the health aide attaches the label to the bottle.

These pharmacy vending machines are frequently restocked, and medicines rotated so that nothing goes out of date. The machines are also bulletproof as a further precaution in rural Alaska.

Question: What is the role of primary care in the Nuka model?

Primary care teams are a foundational building block of the SCF model. Producing better outcomes was dependent on building high-powered primary care teams, usually 7-10 people, because 5 percent of high-utilizing patients drove 50 percent of costs. Primary care teams are responsible for seeing 7-10 individuals a day (and sometimes with family members present) versus 25-35 in the typical US primary care model, and an additional 15-20 through video and telephone, and 20-30 by text and email. Each primary care panel manages about 1,200 individuals.

Only 20 percent are seen in person by implementing a virtual asynchronous treatment model. Fifty percent of encounters are text and email, which enables team members to support a longitudinal relationship with patients and their families. Half of the physicians give patients their home telephone number.

Teams are equipped to address most everyday conditions including chronic pain management, HIV, and lactation. Specialists are co-located and can be drawn into the primary care team as needed during clinic visits and televisits, usually within five minutes. Behavioralists are a key part of the team as well as coaches, pharmacists, social workers, and case managers.

Case management was found to be most effective when caregivers reflected the culture and lived experience of patients. There were often women in their fifties who came from rough life circumstances and could empathize and understand challenges faced by patients. They are successful 90 percent of the time and excel at influencing patients to consider how to improve day-to-day decisions about better health practices and making incremental lifestyle changes.

SCF also found the most effective time to educate patients and their families about lifestyle factors (e.g., sugary drinks, interpersonal violence) was during pregnancy and childbirth. Everyone was most receptive to learn what to do for the sake of the newborn, and beyond.

Question: What is the role of physicians in this model?

The chief role of physicians, as well as every other category of caregivers on the team, is unequivocal: influencing patients and recognizing that the patient is the expert in their care. The provider's role is to listen to what the patient wants and employ communication skills that reflect cultural awareness and competency in meeting patient needs.

This is a departure from the traditional medical model where physicians are expected to be the expert even though they do not have time (or have the requisite training) to understand "consumer voice," which is often through story, or how to treat patients within a family and cultural context.

At the heart of this process is changing the culture of the traditional medical model to address disparities and improve outcomes. Over a twenty-year period, patient outcomes rose from the lowest quartile of medical indices to the top quartile of indices across the board. For example:

Question: Can you cite performance metrics that stand out?

Even though SCF is not a hospital system, it had a remarkable impact on inpatient operations.

- SCF saw a 44 percent decrease in ER visits from 2000 to 2004, and ER visits are currently below the HEDIS seventy-fifth percentile (where lower is better).
- SCF saw a 63 percent decrease in inpatient discharges from 2000 to 2004, and an overall 31 percent decrease in inpatient discharges from 2000 to 2019.

Using HEDIS (Healthcare Effectiveness Data and Information Set) rankings as a national benchmark, SCF stands out (i.e., often exceeding the seventy-fifth percentile compared to other healthcare organizations).

Representative Healthcare Results:

Diabetes care from 2013-2017: above ninetieth percentile
Cardiovascular disease (annual LDL) from 2014-2017: above eightieth percentile
Depression screening: above seventy-fifth percentile
Childhood immunizations from 2018-2017: above eightieth percentile
Adult pneumococcal vaccinations from 2013-2016: above eightieth percentile

Representative Customer Results:

> Courteous and respectful staff from 2013-2-17: above seventy-fifth percentile
> Customer satisfaction from 2014-2017: above seventy-fifth percentile
> Appointment when desired from: above sixty-fifth percentile
> Involved in decisions about care from 2013-2017: above seventy-fifth percentile
> Trust in care from 2013-2017: above ninety-fifth percentile

Question: What is the role and impact on Primary Care teams?

Even though the personnel costs of SCF primary care teams are three times more than more traditional PC teams, they are more effective in treating an array of medical conditions and produce significantly lower total costs.

The SCF model builds convenience around the patient rather than the medical team. Consumer driven means that patients (customer owners) drive the system rather than the values and priorities of medical professionals, which are largely institution centric.

To support high-powered primary care teams with multiple caregiver functions and personnel, a comprehensive data analytics and technology infrastructure is required. It is expensive to build and maintain. However, it is essential to be able to track more than 1,000 metrics per business line that show how patients are doing as well as how each provider is always performing. There is complete transparency at the clinic and system level. This is a prerequisite for population health to work and requires full disclosure by everyone.

The Nuka approach and medical model can be implemented in far less challenging terrain environments and deeply rooted medical conditions than in Alaska. As a result, the cost savings represented by the Rosetta dividend can be channeled to community development initiatives such as education, food security, workforce training, and broadband access.

Question: What about the Ashtabula school system?

It's a model of how to get better care for less money.

Ashtabula Area City Schools (AACS) is in the inner city of Ashtabula, Ohio, the eighth poorest school district in the state.

When the city voted against raising taxes to fund rising healthcare and educational costs, AACS had to do something different. Change was needed because the population was aging, and a large portion of employees and families suffered from comorbidities and chronic disease. AACS's top priority was to design a health plan with three objectives:

- Save money for the school district
- Improve member satisfaction
- Improve health outcomes

The approach was to adopt Health Rosetta principles to lower healthcare costs and improve benefits, which is supported by multiple unions. A total of 385 of the 450 employees are on the plan, which covers a total of 1,000 lives. The per family deductible is $400 with a $0 deductible opportunity, while office visit copays are $20 with a primary care opportunity of $0 copayment.

With the assistance of IEN Risk Management Consultants, new strategies were introduced as the Administrative Services Only relationship with the carrier-controlled plan was phased out. In 2020, AACS adopted an open-ended, self-funded health plan based on four core Health Rosetta features: direct primary care, diabetes management solutions, Centers of Excellence, and transparent data collection and sharing.

Question: How long did it take to turn around costs?

In the first year, the new arrangement saved $2.4 million for a 20 percent year-over-year reduction in costs. By changing the infrastructure in August 2020 to offer better benefits at a lower cost, total spend went from $13 million to $12 million, thus saving employees money.

AACS took the time to educate employees and their families about the new plan's improvements (better benefits at lower cost) and upgraded support from dedicated nurses to help them improve their health. The plan believes all members received the care they needed without any claim denial grievances.

Lower costs help sustain AACS's operating budget and improve employee satisfaction. Employees have free access to a dedicated nurse team, local direct primary care, and local independent pharmacy services.

Question: What was the community's role?

In 2021-2022, AACS was short $2 million in the operating budget. Voters again declined to approve increased funding because the new health plan avoided making any staff cuts. A full-fledged educational campaign was devised to get ongoing buy-in, which involved thoroughly educating the superintendent and the union healthcare committee. They would help lead the effort and communicate to union members the value of the new Health Rosetta-style health plan.

This level of community support is an example of how a community can come together around a shared goal. It seemed risky at the beginning, but it was far riskier than staying in the traditional health plan that was unsustainable in terms of costs and mounting chronic care conditions.

Question: How would you rate the impact of the new health plan?

In terms of the Health Rosetta Plan Grades, which is a measure of high-performance health plans, AACS efforts ranked in the seventy-fourth percentile.

- Transparent adviser relationships: 100 (median is 50)
- High performance plan design, documents, and risk management: 54 (median is 56)

- Independent active plan management: 88 (median is 42)
- individual stewardship: 59 (median is 53)
- Value-based primary care: 87 (median is 51)
- Transparent open networks: 100 (median is 51)
- Major specialties and outlier patients: 45 (median is 51)
- Transparent pharmacy benefits: 47 (median is 51)

Question: Could you elaborate on Plan Grader with more details and how it came about?

Health plan costs are typically one of an organization's two or three biggest expenses. Yet, there isn't an objective way to independently assess how it's performing and—just as importantly—how it compares to others' performance.

So, we developed a way to assess plan performance based on best practices and strategies that would enable employers to look at performance in relation to key health plan components.

What are the main components?

There are eight categories critical to performance. We analyze each one according to a multipoint scale to get a 360-degree picture of where the organization's current health plan is and what to focus on going forward. Each component is compared to best practices of other health plans (median reference point).

- Transparent advisor relationship with brokers and consultants (fees, commissions).

- High-performance plan design and risk management (contracts, plan documents, stop-loss, underwriting practices, ERISA checklist)
- Independent, active plan management (ongoing oversight of plan functions and activities, three-to-five-year plan strategy, threshold for auto-adjudicating claims).
- Value-based primary care (incentives for integrated primary care practice model, same or next day appointments)
- Transparent open networks (expanded provider choice, outcomes focus, transparent pricing)
- Major specialists and outlier patients (Centers of Excellence model, early detection, and treatment)
- Transparent pharmacy benefits (mission-aligned PBM, contractual provisions alignment, specialty drug carve-out strategies)
- Individual stewardship (single point of contact support, digital tools access, ongoing member/patient education)

What have you found to date?

Health Rosetta has analyzed hundreds of plans. High performing plans are used as a median score to assess a particular employer's health plan.

Health plan scores differ according to each component, but the bottom line is that employers are not getting their money's worth, nor are patients. They are surprised to see the lack of transparency, how broker incentives contribute to higher costs, and the fact that patients are not referred to the best clinicians as a matter of course.

The more employers dig into the details of each component, they realize how little they understand about how their money is spent and what they can do to change this based on our findings.

Do performance scores tend to cluster markets or types of business?

Yes and no.

Health plan performance is uniform across most sectors, whether it's manufacturing, school districts, or hospitality services. However, scores tend to be lower in markets that do not emphasize primary care models, often in areas with a high concentration of specialty services and facilities (e.g., low level of market competition).

How quickly do employers make a change once their health plan performance is better understood.

It's usually a two-to-three-year process.

It involves education about each component and then taking corrective action on each one over a multi-year period. Many employers decide to become more actively engaged in managing this transition by working with independent benefits advisors who are certified by Health Rosetta.

The Health Rosetta advisory community is a peer-to-peer learning program with a broad array of professional experience. They are trained to adhere to our core principles with a focus on real-life best practices.

Question: Any final thoughts?

Yes, I certainly do.

Healthcare has stolen the American Dream, and it's time to take it back.

We're spending more than enough money to get the best healthcare in the world. Health doesn't have to be expensive. What's expensive is profiteering, price gouging, and constructing unnecessary edifices rather than investing in disaster readiness.

Only $0.27 of every dollar spent on healthcare goes to primary value-creation like nurses, physicians, and other clinicians.

Health Rosetta has learned the best way to slash costs and protect workers and middle-class families. It is to improve health benefits and outcomes. We've laid out a blueprint to do that.

Community-Based Organizations

Chapter 24.

Pathways Community Hub/ Pathways Community Hub Institute

Overview

There are a variety of approaches for community-based organizations to create a hub for the purpose of coordinating services. The Pathways Community HUB Institute® Model (PCHI® Model) represents a structured model with an exacting set of policies and procedures that guide implementation and operations at each step along the way. Twenty-one such organizations have been certified, including eleven in Ohio.

PCHI has a unique set of characteristics that are tightly organized around core operating principles and reimbursement mechanisms. It pays for performance based on the confirmed completion of specific outcomes and inspires collective action at the community level through its network approach. It relies on Community Health Workers to reach out to participants who are at greatest risk and connect them to medical, social, and behavioral services in the community. Individual and community risk factors are embedded in a quality improvement framework. Each Pathways Community HUB (PCH) must be certified by PCHI.

Community Health Workers (CHW) are key to PCHI's Model because they provide care coordination services and are employed by local medical clinics and social service agencies. They serve as partners and coaches who advocate for their participants.

Pathways Community HUB Development: Part 1

The PCHI Model focuses on risk reduction through an evidence-based and best-practice intervention for individuals. Outreach to the highest-risk individuals includes support for the whole family. Home visits build trust in the community and better outcomes which, in turn, lead to performance-based payment to community-based organizations employing Community Health Workers implementing the PCHI Model of community-based care coordination.

Three main elements go into becoming a Pathways Community HUB:

First, selecting a PCH organization, which is a trusted convener rather than a service provider. The organization must be based in its service area and have the capacity to meet information security requirements, negotiate and enter into contracts, and raise funds. PCHs secure funding for startup activities and funding for outcome payments, through payer contracts.

Second, selecting care coordination agencies that hire and supervise CHWs working through the PCH via a contract for outcome payments.

Third, implementation includes a PCHI-certified technology system for care coordination, training PCH staff, CHWs, and supervisors as well as addressing SDOH barriers.

Care coordination agencies (CCA) are a foundational building block for a PCH. It starts with requesting proposals from community-based organizations to serve as CCAs that hire and supervise CHWs to work through the PCH. CCAs may already employ CHWs or agree to if selected to serve as a CCA. CHWs working through the PCH should have strong supervision, training, and background checks. CHW must have an internet-enabled tablet/laptop unless the PCH uses a paper-based system.

CCAs should be interested in connecting with PCH participants to address their health-related social needs such as: food, clothing, shelter and housing, transportation, baby items, medical/addiction/tobacco cessation care, furniture, employment and job development, and education.

Pathways Community HUBs go through a certification process that outlines seven standards to guide communities. These requirements help ensure that local PCHs improve health, reduce costs, and promote health equity. The PCHI Model assures accountability, standardized tracking of risk factors and data collection, and works to remove care silos. Only one Pathways Community HUB in a community is certified.

Funding and Payment Model

A PCH uses a braided funding approach whereby contracted funds pay for outcomes realized by PCH participants while the PCH secures additional private and government funding for services such as housing assistance. This enables participants to achieve positive outcomes such as safe and stable housing.

For example, grants support PCH start-up, infrastructure, and evaluation costs. Philanthropy often supports specific health priorities and populations. Payer contracts generate outcome-financing based on member risk reduction.

Contracts are value based. This means 50 percent of payment is tied to outcomes or completed Pathways. The remaining 50 percent is tied to confirmed engagement, measured by completed visit forms documenting home visits. If a participant is not engaged and Pathways are not completed, there is no payment.

Evidenced-Based Pathways

Pathways are tools used by CHWs to identify and track individually modifiable risk factors. These include twenty-one standardized Pathways:

Adult education, developmental referral, employment, family planning, food security, health coverage, housing, immunization referral, learning, medical home, medical referral, medication adherence, medication reconciliation, medication screening, mental health, oral health, postpartum, pregnancy, social service referral, substance use, and transportation.

Three Pathways are expanded to address multiple risks. For example:

> Learning (sixty-plus evidence-based learning modules)
> Medical Referral (twenty-five types)
> Social Service Referral (twenty-eight types)
> A list of expanded Pathways is shown in Appendix 1. Representative examples of Pathways outcomes are shown in Appendix 2.

Outcome-Based Payments

The methodology includes a unique billing code and modifier assigned to each Pathway. A standard number of outcome-based units is assigned to each Pathway that represents the measure of the complexity and time needed to successfully complete the Pathway. For example, the Housing Pathway has an outcome-based unit (OBU) value of fifteen when it is confirmed that a participant has moved into safe and stable housing and is there thirty days later.

Since Care Coordination Agencies in the local PCH are reimbursed when their CHWs complete Pathways, outcomes and sustainability are assured.

Risk Mitigation

Mitigating risks follows a three-part methodology that details the level of impact.

Category 1: Identify and address modifiable risks:

- Food, clothing, housing, parenting, depression, substance use, access to a medical home, education, employment, car seat safety, safe sleep, nutrition, and compliance with medical home.

Category 2: Completed Pathways Risks Mitigated—Outcomes

- Connection to medical home
- Housing established
- Food security
- Normal birth weight baby
- School attendance
- Employment established
- Transportation established

Category 3: Large Scale Outcomes Relate to Multiple Risks Addressed

- Reduced hospitalization
- Lower ER visits
- Reduced number of adverse childhood experiences (ACE)
- Reduced cost of care
- Improved health status (i.e., healthy birth weight baby, blood pressure under control, normal A1c levels, etc.,)
- Improved school performance

- Improved employment retention
- Economic success and stability
- Behavioral health

Pathways Community HUB Institute® Model History

After more than a decade of working with Community Health Workers to improve access to care and community resources, Dr. Mark and Dr. Sarah Redding developed and refined the PCHI® Model at the first Pathways Community HUB—the Community Health Access Project (CHAP), Mansfield, Ohio—beginning in 2000 with the development of Pathways. The Pathways Community HUB was introduced in 2004. Initial efforts focused on improving birth outcomes among at-risk pregnant women. In 2005, Toledo, Ohio, adopted the PCHI® Model and began implementing what is now the Northwest Ohio Pathways HUB in 2007 initially focused on improving birth outcomes in Lucas County, Ohio.

Northwest Ohio Pathways HUB

The Northwest Ohio Pathways HUB is now a regional care coordination system that connects low-income residents to needed medical and social services. This includes insurance coverage, food, housing, transportation, medical homes, and career development. In 2022, thirty-six Community Health Workers at thirteen care coordination agencies helped 1,077 residents with a focus on pregnant women, adults with chronic diseases, and women of childbearing age.

To combat infant mortality, pregnant women were assessed for risks of poor birth outcomes at twenty-seven local OB/GYN clinics and connected to a Community Health Worker for care coordination services. Pregnant clients had an average of 5.7 risk factors such as mental illness, family crises, lack of transportation, prior poor birth outcomes, previous births in the last eighteen months, and late entry into prenatal care. Adult patients also had chronic risk factors that included diabetes and heart disease, poor nutrition, lack of physical activity, and obesity. More than half were African American and lived in one of five zip codes.

Buckeye Health Plan, a division of Centene, contracts with the Northwest Ohio Pathways HUB to serve its members. In an internal study conducted by Buckeye on at-risk pregnant women enrolled from 2013-2017, they found that the PCH reduced nonclinical barriers to care, which resulted in lower costs for baby's first year of life. In contrast, high-risk mothers without PCH care coordination were 1.55 times more likely to deliver a baby that required neonatal intensive care or specialty care.

For every dollar spent on Pathways Community HUB activities, Buckeye Health Plan found a savings of $2.36, a 236 percent ROI through improved PCH care coordination. Savings for newborns at risk for low birthweight delivery included high risk PMPM cost savings of $403, medium risk PMPB cost savings of $252, and low risk PMPM savings of $171.

In 2022, the most common client need was learning followed by social service referrals. The most frequently completed social service referral was the diaper bank and food assistance. For adults with chronic disease, transportation and food assistance were the most common completed social service referrals.

Transportation Pathway example

The Baby and Me Ride Free program was developed by the Northwest Ohio Pathways HUB in 2016 through a partnership with TARTA Bus Service for Lucas County. Pregnant women and guardians of children up to age one enrolled in any maternal and child heath visitation program can secure a free annual bus pass and access to paratransit door-to-door services through the program. In the first year, the Social Service-transportation Pathway completion rate went from 48 to 71 percent and 561 participants secured a free annual bus pass to access paratransit door-to-door services.

Housing Pathway example

The Northwest Ohio Pathways HUB partnered with Lucas Metropolitan Housing Authority in 2018 to prioritize housing choice vouchers for pregnant women. Twenty-five families secured housing as a result and Housing Pathways completed increased from 8.8 percent to 17 percent in the first year. There are now 115 housing vouchers available for PCH participants.

In 2022, funding for the Northwest Ohio Pathways HUB for pregnant and child-bearing-age women was 61 percent Medicaid managed care plans, 31 percent grants and in-kind, and 7 percent temporary cash assistance for needy families. Participants had birth outcomes better than or like the county overall despite having a high level of risk.

Pathways Community HUB Institute

The Pathways Community HUB Institute® was founded in 2015 to develop and maintain the PCHI Model designed to help communities advance health equity. PCHI established a national certification program and now licenses the model to communities to implement. PCHI provides technical assistance, education/training, certification, research, and advocacy to further community led implementation of the PCHI Model.

The Model enables CHWs to identify and code all modifiable risk factors for residents they serve and provides a structure to address and mitigate each risk. The outcomes-based payment model incentivizes organizations to serve people and families with complex medical and social needs.

Payers and funders require evidence on the efficacy of any community-based model to justify ongoing support. The PCHI Model was designed to document service outcomes for individuals and households.

The standard data collection tools and a data structure for ensuring information data capture and coding risk is at the heart of the Model. Workflows address each risk, and educational material is provided to each participant to support behavior change. Funders receive detailed reports once risks are mitigated.

The Institute monitors each certified PCH as well as their technology platforms as part of the PCHI licensing strategy to maintain PCHI Model integrity.

A summary of the PCHI Model components and licensed contents is shown below.

Component	**Purpose**
Standards	Provides guidance and requirements on how PCHs and PAs are structured, operated, and financed. Available at pchi-hub.org
PCHI Data Model	Defines field names, field definitions, and standard picklist values for data collected and risk identification in the PCHI Model. This comprises 400-plus fields collected in the PCHI Standard Forms and twenty-one Pathways.
PCHI Standard Forms • Demographic • Visit • Progress	PCHI Vendors configure these intake instruments in their platforms, using the field descriptions in the PCHI Standard Data Model. PCHs and PAs not using a vendor to support their organization will use paper, or Excel-based versions of these Standard Forms for data collection. The Demographic form ensures uniform collection of information, including race and ethnicity. The Visit Form helps CHWs identify all 170-plus possible Individually Modifiable Risk Factors (IMRFs) the participant has. The Progress Form provides an overview of a participant's care plan at a point in time.

Twenty-One Standard Pathways	These define the required tasks, information, and outcome required to validate that a specific risk has been mitigated, and a way to indicate which risks were not successfully mitigated. PCHI Vendors configure these forms in their platforms, using the field descriptions in the PCHI Standard Data Model.
Evidence-Based Learning Modules	These sixty-plus Learning Modules provide educational tools for Community Health Workers (CHWs) to use with participants to help them change behavior to address a specific IMRF.
Standard Outcome and Engagement-Based Billing Approach	This defines a structure for billing health plans and compensating Care Coordination Agencies for Pathways work. It: • Defines a specific weight (Outcome Based Unit) for each Pathway. The OBU represents the complexity/acuity of *completing* the Pathway. • Defines an Engagement Fee structure, for each month that a CHW has at least one visit with a participant. • Provides guidance through the Model's Prerequisites and Standards on how reimbursement is distributed to CCAs. • Provides standard workflows for invoice creation and billing reconciliation.
Quality Benchmark Report	This is a standard report. PCHs and PAs create the report quarterly, using the template provided by PCHI (and available through Certified Technology Vendors), and submit it to PCHI. PCHI aggregates and analyzes the data, and will, in time create PCH/PA Report Cards to show how a PCH/PA is performing compared to the PCHI Network.

Nebraska Community Pathways HUB and Executive Interview: Part 2

Pathways Community HUB

The Pathways Community HUB (PCH) plays a critical role as the connective tissue between payers and care coordination agencies that employ Community Health Workers. The PCH sees the big picture and landscape of available services and resource gaps in the community. It understands how CHWs perform their work and how Medicaid, health systems, and other funders pay for these services. It also performs a quality control function by training all CHWs providing service through the PCH to use a single risk assessment, case management protocol, and documentation schema (Twenty-One Standard Pathways). This allows for comparison across agencies of CHW interventions in three ways: reducing health and social risk factors, improving care coordination, and health outcomes.

Omaha Community Foundation

The Omaha Community Foundation (OCF) uses both established philanthropic strategies and innovative programs to address community-wide social and economic needs. OCF has impacted thousands of organizations by connecting donors to local nonprofits and helping direct resources to areas that strengthen the community.

In 2021, OCF distributed $175 million in grants to more than 3,000 nonprofits. Following the Pathways Community HUB Institute® Model, OCF is incubating a local Pathways HUB entity to address Social Determinants of Health to improve maternal health outcomes. Both issues have been identified as top community needs in The Landscape, a community-driven snapshot of the most urgent issues facing residents. OCF was selected as the Pathways HUB entity as a neutral convener with a strong history of community leadership.

Executive Comments

Ashley Carroll, Division Manager for Community Benefit & Advocacy at CHI Health, Omaha, Nebraska

Question: What were you looking for in terms of a model framework to get started?

We wanted an evidence-based methodology that would help address modifiable social risk factors of our clients. Most importantly, we wanted a certified methodology based on achievable outcomes, not just efforts.

We recognized that CHWs are the essential building block of reaching patients in the community; building trusting relationships to identify barriers to health, increase access to care, and navigate complex health and social care systems. And they need to be adequately compensated in relation to how much improvement is achieved. Otherwise, the model wouldn't be sustainable.

Whomever was paying the bill would need to know if there was documented improvement. That's just a reality. And the reporting process had to be anchored on a standard data model to support this.

Question: What was most important to reach agreement on?

It was critical early on to reach a consensus on the focus population of the HUB. The core team conducted a data analysis to identify a health disparity that each respective organization had an interest in addressing in a new way. Each organization was asked to make a recommendation for the health need area and population with the most potential for improvement with a CHW intervention. We considered several different potential focus populations: seniors experiencing social isolation, individuals with concurrent physical and behavioral health diagnoses, residents experiencing housing instability who frequent the emergency department as their ongoing source of healthcare, and low-income pregnant mothers. There was unanimous support for focusing on low-income pregnant individuals among our core team members.

The PCHI Model has been most rigorously evaluated among low-income pregnant mother/infant dyads and was also an area of focus for many years in Omaha through efforts like the Baby Blossoms Collaborative, convened by Douglas County Health Department to reduce infant mortality. The March of Dimes gave the state of Nebraska and Douglas County a grade of "D" and "F," respectively, due to our preterm birth rates.

The PCH model flips the paradigm from organizations working independently and sometimes competing with each other for funding. A HUB aligns the resources of all stakeholders involved in pursuit of a singular mission. One of the most compelling features of the PCHI model is the standard data collection, reporting, and billing element. Through uniform data collection and reporting methods, communities can see the impact their collective efforts are making on neighbors, friends, and family.

Question: How much was raised and from what sources?

One million was raised in the first six months with equal contributions from CommonSpirit Health, Healthy Blue Nebraska, Nebraska Total Care, and United Healthcare Community Plan of Nebraska.

Question: How did you go about planning the Hub implementation model?

We first learned about the PCHI Model in 2021 and the PCH was operational in early 2024.

Question: In retrospect, what factors led to adjusting the timeline?

There is an African proverb that says, "If you want to go fast, go alone. If you want to go far, go together." We intentionally and deliberately took time to design an objective HUB selection process. We have applied the same rigor to the selection of the HUB Director, which in many ways becomes the face of this initiative. And, perhaps most importantly, that director led a transparent and community-embedded process for selection of the Care Coordination Agencies who employ CHWs, as they are the most critical relationships with those we hope to serve. At each critical juncture, the core advisory team has favored method and deliberation over speed, which will position us for rapid implementation and certain success.

Question: Who are the key stakeholders supporting the Pathways Community HUB?

There were more than thirty functional relationships and affiliated partner organizations to identify, bring on board, and coordinate on behalf of the PCH organization.

Healthcare partners represented on the Core Team included United Healthcare Community Plan of Nebraska, Healthy Blue, Nebraska Total Care, CHI Health, Medica, One World Community Health Center, Charles Drew Health Center, Methodist Health System, Children's Hospital, Nebraska Medicine, and CyncHealth (statewide health information exchange).

Affiliated functional roles included Chief Medical Officer, Director of Clinical Programs, Chief of Academic Program Officer, Director of Clinical Programs (including OB/GYN and OB practice consultants), Vice President of Quality and Process Improvement,

Vice President of Strategy and Healthy Communities, Division Manager Community Benefit and Advocacy, Vice President of Population Health, Director of Dual Special Needs Plan, Planning and Performance Director, Community and Patient Engagement Director, Community Commitment Coordinator, Housing Navigator, and Marketing Director.

Additional support is provided by the CEO and President of PCHI as well as the Co-Founder. The Program Manager from CommonSpirit Heath is likewise on the team.

Question: What is the PCHI certification process and what does it consist of?

There are nine elements the HUB is accountable for in terms of compliance with PCHI guidelines.

- **Convening:** Bring the parties together as a neutral facilitator.
- **Implementation:** Utilize the PCHI workflow and data model and meet certification standards.
- **Training:** Train CHWs, supervisors, and community partners
- **Contracting:** Develop outcome-based contracts with agencies and funders.
- **Governance:** Establish the Community Advisory Council.
- **Quality improvement:** Employ uniform data sets and reporting structures to inform quality improvement efforts.

- **Technology:** Use PCHI-certified technology vendors.
- **Evaluation and research:** Continuously monitor performance with uniform analytics and reporting protocols.
- **National:** Participate in the larger PCHI network for ongoing feedback and certification activity.

Question: What were the main activities you needed to accomplish with Community Health Workers?

There were four important objectives:

1. Find individuals in our designated service area who can benefit from this type of intensive, partnership-based, care coordination model.
2. Build trusting relationships with participants through a series of outreach actions.
3. Help participants access the services they need (medical and behavioral care and social care resources).
4. Teach and continually reinforce healthier behaviors of participants.

CHWs are indispensable and our most valuable resource to accomplish PCH goals.

Question: How do CHWs fit into the PCHI model of quality outcomes?

CHWs are the major success factor in the PCHI model. They share relevant language, culture, and lived experience with the clients they serve, which facilitates trust. Patient needs are identified through a standard risk assessment and are categorized into an appropriate Pathways-based care plan. Then the patient is directed to the appropriate provider who works with CHWs to ensure follow-ups. CHWs ensure follow through on the various Pathways opened for patients and document their interactions with patients; this provides valuable information for the clinical care team.

Question: How are CHW compensated? Can you give examples of how payment is related to outcomes?

CHWs are employed by CCAs. The CCA enters a contract with the PCH to deliver specific outcomes within a defined population. The PCH and the payer negotiate the terms of the outcomes-based units (OBU). Outcome based units are assigned proportionally to each of the twenty-one Standard Pathways based on the amount of effort required to achieve each, as well as how impactful they are in achieving the desired outcome. For example, a housing pathway, which is only billable when a patient has been stably housed for thirty days, is assigned fifteen OBUs, while a social service referral pathway is assigned three OBUs. Each PCH negotiates the value of the OBU with its payers, and the contract must be structured to allow for at least 50 percent of compensation tied directly to OBUs for completed Pathways, with the balance supporting the engagement fee (home visits).

Question: How is compensation arranged for CHWs?

CHWs are not employed by the PCH, but by various CCAs that determine compensation. In general, CHWs are full-time, non-exempt, benefits-eligible employees. The CCA continues to pay CHW salary and the PCH reimburses the CCA for CHW services for completing defined outcomes plus an engagement fee for completed home visits. OBU rates must cover the cost of all the CHW/participant interactions that take place toward pathway completion, but that do not result in a completed outcome (e.g., completing an initial client intake, meeting with a client in their home for a routine check-in, scheduling appointments).

Question: What was the most important early learning?

Success is contingent on aligning stakeholder goals and financial incentives. Our early success in convening and mobilizing stakeholders was attributable to this alignment, built on the foundation of trusting relationships.

Question: What are the next steps in the PCH's evolution?

Now that the PCH Director is in place and care-coordination agencies have been recruited and contracts are being put in place, training and implementation has begun. The outcomes of the demonstration pilot will be used to plan for sustainability and expansion, including focusing on additional populations.

Question: What does the PCH's oversight role contribute to your organization's progress?

The PCH allows us to address systemic health challenges at a community-level and achieve outcomes at a scale no single organization could do on their own. The PCH also creates a sustained financing mechanism for CHWs and ensures quality control and model fidelity.

Question: Any last thoughts?

The stakes are too high, and the needs are too great not to invest in an evidence-based model with demonstrated success such as the PCHI Model. Mothers, children, and families in any community deserve it.

San Joaquin Community Foundation and Community Bank: Part 3

Background

The San Joaquin Community Foundation is a tax-exempt public charity dedicated to improving the quality of life in San Joaquin

County. In 2022, $3.8 million in grants were distributed through 249 funds. The foundation has $29 million in assets. The San Joaquin Community Foundation was selected by a group of public health advocates and funders to serve as the administrator of the Pathways Community HUB (PCH).

In the initial phase, the program focused on providing care coordination to support Black maternal and infant care with the goals of improving birth outcomes and addressing documented health disparities. Black women die from pregnancy-related causes more than three times the rate of White, Hispanic, and Asian women.

Pathways Community HUB

The purpose of the Pathways Community HUB is to create a sustainable community-based care coordination system empowered by Community Health Workers (CHWs). One of the main roles is to identify individuals with modifiable risk factors (medical, social, behavioral) and develop relationships to connect them with local services and resources, then track outcomes to reduce health disparities.

Birth outcomes are a particularly high priority because there is a critical lack of access to prenatal care and education, resulting in poorer birth outcomes of Black birthing individuals. To improve this, the Pathways Community HUB engages organizations rooted in the community to serve as care coordination agencies and give one-on-one community care coordination through CHWs trained in using the

Pathways Community HUB Institute Model. Results for the coordinated network are tracked and measured. Unmet needs (gaps in care) are addressed by the PCH through advocacy, partnership, policy, and services tailored to the needs of the populations of focus.

Care Coordination Agencies

The roles of the Care Coordination Agency are fourfold: hire and supervise Community Health Workers, outreach to community members, assign CHWs to participants, and attend PCHI Model and CHW training. CHWs are trained to accurately document visits and participant activities through various forms and tools (Demographic forms, Visit forms, Progress forms, and Pathways).

CHW forms indicate enrollment, home visits, risk factors, and open and completed Pathways. The PCH tracks open and completed Pathways (necessary for reimbursement), meeting participation, and network development.

Payment for Outcomes

The organization paying for outcomes (e.g., health plan contracts, government agency, etc.,) negotiates the rate of each outcome-based unit of service (OBU) that is involved in completing a Pathway. For example, a Family Planning Pathway may require an educational needs assessment weighted at six OBUs. A Pregnancy Pathway outcome may require members to go to required visits weighted at twenty OBU. A Post Partum Pathway could require members to attend visits weighted at seven OBUs. An example of a Post Partum Pathways is shown below:

Code	Modifier	OBU	Fee	Pathway	Definition
G9001	O	7	$210 Based on $30 per OBU	Postpartum Pathway	Confirm postpartum appointment was kept within 7-84 days and postpartum information questions answered.

Demonstration Program

The Community Foundation's PCH Demonstration Project Implementation Plan for the first twelve months drew heavily from technical assistance provided by the Pathways Community HUB Institute®.

Key milestones include:

1. Raising start-up funds.
2. PCH Director and operations manager hired.
3. Applying for Certification and securing a license from PCHI® to utilize the Model.
4. Formalizing the role of the Community Advisory Council and recruiting members.
5. Selecting a PCHI Certified Technology Vendor or using spreadsheets.

6. Selecting Care Coordination Agencies.
7. Providing CHW, PCHI Model, CLAS Standards, and technology training.
8. Implementing PCHI® Model care coordination.
9. Submitting a Certification Review Application.

Community Bank

A Community Bank is a locally controlled pool of funds that supports community health and prevention initiatives with a common goal of improving outcomes and reducing health inequities. The Community Bank was developed by CommonSpirit and creates a sustainable funding mechanism for public-private partnerships through a combination of braided and blended financing sources. By bringing diverse sectors together, the model increases the outreach and impact of the investment.

As an extension of the PCH model, the San Joaquin Community Bank incorporates three funds to draw upon for ongoing community initiatives and investments: Infrastructure Fund, Contractual Fund, and Community Capacity Fund.

The Infrastructure Fund pays for operational expenses for the first 2-3 years. It pays for a PCH Director, data and reporting requirements, legal expenses, technology development and management, and CHW training. The Fund is supported by foundations, grants, health plans, anchor institutions, and community benefits.

The Contractual Fund covers basic day-to-day PCH operations and is tied to Outcome Based Units and engagement fees that are disbursed for completed Pathways. It is supported by health plans, government agencies, and providers.

The Community Capacity Fund is a safety net for the uninsured, housing insecure, and community members experiencing vulnerability. It is supported by foundations, grants, and community benefits focused on uninsured, specific populations.

Each Funding Partner commits to contributing for at least three years toward infrastructure costs and capacity building. This is a critical step in closing gaps in access to social care services in the community.

The process of establishing a Community Bank involves a third party—such as a Pathways Community HUB—acting as a convener and a trusted fiscal agent. In this role, the convener oversees governance activity and is responsible for bringing community groups together, the best way to allocate funds, and to make sure community objectives are carried out.

Funding Partners must likewise agree on metrics that document success and follow data-driven decision making about addressing gaps in community needs. Community members are empowered to cooperatively address problems that otherwise would not have been solved by a single organization. This reduces the burden on any one community-based agency or resource.

By bringing together different partners that represent different segments of the community, the Community Bank model ensures that each partner is motivated by the responsibility and accountability for making decisions on behalf of the entire community. This shifts the power dynamics among members away from representing a particular organization's point of view to addressing community-wide issues. Community-based organizations are freed from competing for short-term grants each year. They can work together collaboratively with a much larger pool of funding to draw upon.

The Community Bank model is designed to address inequities in health access and related risk factors of underserved communities in a more collaborative way.

Appendices

Appendix A: Expanded Pathways—Social Service Referral Pathway (31+ Other) and Learning Pathway (65)

Social Service Pathway Types	
Social Service	Clothing
Social Service	Identification
Social Service	Personal Items
Social Service	Confirm that Item(s) or Service(s) Received – Household Coordinator
Social Service	Home Improvement
Social Service	Household Items
Social Service	Internet
Social Service	Lead Abatement
Social Service	Phone
Social Service	Safety Equipment
Social Service	Utilities
Social Service	Confirmed Connection to Urgent Resource or Service
Social Service	Intimate Partner Violence

Social Service	Child Abuse
Social Service	Elder Abuse
Social Service	Family Crisis Service
Social Service	Restorative Service
Social Service	Child Development
Social Service	Citizenship
Social Service	Corrections
Social Service	Daily Activities of Living
Social Service	Fatherhood
Social Service	Financial
Social Service	Legal
Social Service	Literacy
Social Service	Medical Debt
Social Service	Parenting Education
Social Service	Tax Preparation
Social Service	Translation Services and/or Interpretation
Social Service	Voter Registration
Social Service	Adult Day Care
Social Service	Childcare
Social Service	Respite Services
Social Service	Other – must specify
Learning Pathway Types	
Medical Domain	Adult Nutrition
Medical Domain	Child Nutrition
Medical Domain	Pregnant Nutrition
Medical Domain	Breastfeeding
Medical Domain	Managing Exercise & Screen Time
Medical Domain	Primary Care & Preventive Screening
Medical Domain	Oral Health: Keeping your Mouth Healthy
Medical Domain	Respiratory Viruses & Infection Prevention
Medical Domain	Medication Adherence
Medical Domain	Life Saving Vaccine (Vaccinations)
Medical Domain	Family Planning

Medical Domain	Sexually Transmitted Infections
Medical Domain	Diabetes
Medical Domain	Asthma
Medical Domain	Chronic Obstructive Pulmonary Disease (COPD)
Medical Domain	Congestive Heart Failure (CHF)
Medical Domain	Diabetes in Children
Medical Domain	COVID-19 Vaccine Hesitancy
Medical Domain	Normal Pregnancy and Warning Signs
Medical Domain	Pregnancy: Preterm Labor & Infant Mortality
Medical Domain	Pregnancy: Preeclampsia (Pregnancy Induced Hypertension
Medical Domain	Pregnancy: Progesterone
Medical Domain	Pregnancy: Gestational Diabetes
Medical Domain	Pregnancy: Infections
Medical Domain	Pregnancy: Anemia
Medical Domain	Pregnancy: Problems with the Placenta
Medical Domain	Literacy (Birth to 12 months)
Social Domain	Housing Maintenance
Social Domain	Avoiding Eviction
Social Domain	Career Development
Social Domain	Employment
Social Domain	Financial Management
Social Domain	Citizenship Assistance
Social Domain	Parent & Family Development
Safety Domain	Safe Driving
Safety Domain	Car Seats
Safety Domain	Fires and Burns
Safety Domain	Sun Exposure
Safety Domain	Gun Safety
Safety Domain	Emergency Preparedness
Safety Domain	Fall Risks
Safety Domain	Toxic Exposures
Safety Domain	Infant Safe Sleep
Safety Domain	Lead Poisoning
Safety Domain	Safety Inside the Home – Volume 1

Safety Domain	Safety Inside the Home – Volume 2
Safety Domain	Safety Outside the Home
Behavioral Domain	Stress
Behavioral Domain	Substance Use Disorders
Behavioral Domain	Positive Parenting
Behavioral Domain	Pregnancy: Stress
Behavioral Domain	Intimate Partner Violence
Behavioral Domain	Pregnancy: Mental Health
Behavioral Domain	Pregnancy: Substance Use - Alcohol/Fetal Alcohol Syndrome (FAS)
Behavioral Domain	Pregnancy: Substance Use - Nicotine
Behavioral Domain	Pregnancy: Substance Use - Marijuana
Behavioral Domain	Pregnancy: Substance Use – Illegal Drugs
Behavioral Domain	Sleep Hygiene
Behavioral Domain	Shaken Baby Syndrome
Behavioral Domain	Stimulants
Behavioral Domain	Over-the-counter medications
Behavioral Domain	Social Support
Behavioral Domain	Neonatal Abstinence
Behavioral Domain	Postpartum Depression
Behavioral Domain	Nicotine

Appendix B: Pathways Outcomes

PCHI Standard Pathway	Defined Outcome Confirmed by CHW
Adult Education	Participant completed a training program or specific course.
Developmental Referral	A developmental evaluation was completed for the individual.
Employment	Participant is still working thirty days from the date of hire.
Family Planning	Confirmed use of specific family planning approach or procedure.
Food Security	Participant reports having no problems or anxiety about consistently accessing adequate food for the past thirty days.
Healthcare Coverage	Participant has healthcare coverage.
Housing	Household member(s) have maintained safe and stable housing for thirty days from the move-in date.
Immunization Referral	Provider, pharmacist, or clinic confirms that participant's immunizations are received and up to date.
Learning	Participant demonstrates an understanding of the subject of one of PCHI's sixty-plus evidence-based Learning Modules, or other approved educational content.
Medical Home	Participant has identified a PCP, has scheduled and kept the appointment.

Medical Referral	This addresses twenty-five medical referral needs. The outcome could range from confirming participant received needed medical equipment or has scheduled and kept an appointment with the appropriate specialist.
Medication Adherence	One month after the medication reconciliation visit, the participant reports that there are no barriers, and he/she is taking medication(s) as prescribed.
Medication Reconciliation	Primary care provider and/or pharmacist and participant agree on prescribed medications.
Medication Screening	Primary care provider or pharmacist verifies that Medication Screening Tool was received.
Mental Health	Participant confinement to have kept three scheduled mental health appointments.
Oral Health	Participant has identified a dentist, has scheduled and kept the appointment.
Postpartum	Postpartum appointment was kept, and participant responded to postpartum information questions.
Pregnancy	Participant has delivered a normal birth weight baby (> 5# 8 oz/2500 grams) for singleton birth or multiple babies at the appropriate gestational age.

Social Service Referral	This addresses >32 specific needs. The outcome includes confirmation that the participant has been connected to appropriate resources and has kept appointments to meet with them or received the services needed.
Substance Use	Participant kept appointments and treatment related to substance use for thirty days.
Transportation	Household member(s) had no problems, or anxiety about, consistently using transportation for the past thirty days.

Chapter 25.

Bon Secours Baltimore Community Works Executive Interview

George Kleb is Executive Director

George formerly led Unity Properties, Bon Secours' affordable housing corporation in Baltimore, which provides 800 affordable housing units for at least 1,200 residents.

Community Works was founded in 1991 to improve the lives of West Baltimore residents and families. It now serves 4,000 community members annually with a focus on economic development, youth and family services, and housing and community development. The organization is committed to the principles of community engagement and collaboration with community leaders to establish solutions to issues that matter most to residents.

> "Our job is to co-create a heathy community with the residents we serve in the image that they see for themselves and their families."

Background

Bon Secours' commitment to West Baltimore residents is unique because the organization is continuing a relationship (ministry) that pre-dates the hospital by thirty-eight years (1881 to 1919) and is now continuing two-plus years after the sale of the hospital. It is redoubling community investment through a range of programs that are not healthcare-driven (except for a nursing assistant training program).

The organization's mission is anchored in sustained community engagement. This commitment recognizes that building community sustainability and resiliency does not depend on a hospital. Community Works and Unity Properties have taken a different approach to community building and capital absorption in low-income neighborhoods.

The emphasis of Bon Secours Baltimore is threefold:

> *Emphasis on housing* because it is place-based, impacts all aspects of health, contributes to wealth building, and is bedrock to community sustainability.
>
> *Emphasis on community sustainability* because if low-income neighborhoods cannot be stabilized, then efforts (and funding) to improve health will be marginal.
>
> *Emphasis on co-creating healthy neighborhoods* rather than correcting illness conditions (e.g., diabetes, asthma, cardiovascular, metabolic disorders).

Question: From 2010-2020, West Baltimore lost 20-30 percent of its population. What contributed to this exodus?

A variety of things. Neighborhood deterioration was due to increased vacancy, crime and safety concerns, blight, unemployment, lack of recreation spaces, and lack of infrastructure such as grocery stores. The overall effect was due to decades' long inequities regarding how private and public resources were invested and deployed.

Question: How is Community Works supporting healthy neighborhoods in West Baltimore?

Community Works is addressing a number of conditions, but we certainly can't do it alone. We need many partners. We start with an asset-based lens. And the biggest asset is the people who live in West Baltimore. An overriding question is how Community Works can address the fundamental question: "What contributes most to the resident's quality of life from the perspective of that resident?"

It certainly includes housing and real estate development, as well as creating open spaces. For example:

- Repurposing a library building that was shuttered for decades, making it into a community resource center.
- Converting vacant land into an Urban Farm for growing and distributing food to the neighborhood, as well as a connection space for the community. It was formerly a tract of fourteen homes that were vacant for years and beyond repair.

Our job is to co-create these kinds of initiatives with the community.

Question: Why did Bon Secours recently divest itself of their hospital in West Baltimore?

Bon Secours was faced with operating a small community hospital in a city with large hospital systems such as the University of Maryland and Johns Hopkins. It was economically challenging to run a small community hospital with no other affiliated facilities in the Baltimore area.

It made sense to sell the hospital to LifeBridge Health, a nonprofit that owned and operated five hospitals in the area with 12,000 employees, and an operating revenue of $1.9 billion. The financial proceeds of the acquisition will be paid over six years to Bon Secours Community Works. This includes $25 million over a six-year period.

Proceeds will be used to expand community-based programs at Bon Secours Community Works and Unity Properties, such as the acquisition of open space, ongoing operational support, and business planning to target additional investment.

Community Works continues to grow organically and can now leverage the much larger asset base of the Bon Secours Mercy Health to fund community investments. This better serves our mission.

Question: What healthcare program is offered now?

We have offered three healthcare certification training programs for residents. Nursing Assistant/Geriatric Nursing Assistant, Medical Administrative Assistant, and Patient Care-Technician.

The purpose of the training program (workforce development) is to provide a pipeline and a career ladder to a high-demand industry (healthcare). It's also a gateway to nursing as a career, which is a high-demand occupation.

Question: What is the focus of Community Works?

Community Works furthers the Bon Secours mission by focusing on three service delivery areas:

1. **Youth and Family Services:** Early Head Start, Community Schools, Youth Employment and Entrepreneurship, Women's Resource Center, and Women, Infants & Children.

2. **Economic Development:** Healthcare Training, Clean & Green Workforce Training, Returning Citizens from incarceration, Financial and Employment Services, Food Access and Urban Farming, and Safe Streets.

3. **Housing and Community Development:** Affordable Housing Services, Open Space Projects, Facilities Development (Community Resource Center).

Question: How does community engagement work?

It's a combination of engagement techniques and community organizing. Community Works has recently developed a curriculum that is based on what we have learned over the years. (See Appendix 1)

We bring people together to discuss what they want, develop priorities, and explore what's possible.

We're not the experts coming in with loads of advice; quite the contrary. There's a difference between *organizing* and *engaging*. Engagement is as much about how you show up (*presence*) as it is about what you actually do. It's about the spirit in which you serve.

We try to do four things as a way of being authentically present. The four "Ways of Being" are Asset-Based, Collaborative, Relational, and Dutiful.

- Our work is founded on asset-based community development principles, rather than a focus on addressing deficits.
- We look for possibilities to be built upon. We're in this together. It's been going on for three decades, so we're invested in the mission.
- Collaboration is based on a group design process that values neighborhood dialogue. We also raise issues that

need clarity and resolution.

- Our organization is "dutiful." That means supporting the community to take ownership of priorities. We then follow up and apply our expertise to secure funding and implement priorities.

Question: What is the timeline and funding for most projects?

Three to five years is the usual frame of reference, but some involve five and ten-year funding commitments. Let me explain. Three to five years refers to a development project rather than an investment per se. Development projects involve a host of steps that depend on several factors. Once an opportunity is identified, it can take years to put the whole project together in terms of overall site control: design, land acquisition, applying for financing, putting tax credits and loans together—all part of the capital stack. Once the financing is arranged, which can take as much as a year, then we can proceed toward closing and breaking ground.

In other words, it can take a year to just assemble the parts of the deal, another year to close, another year for construction, and another year of delays. The latter can involve regulatory delays, supply chain disruption, and changes in funding requirements. All the while, inflation is rising, adding to the cost.

Five-to-ten-year funding for a multi-year investment requires a longer break-even or payback period. For example, \$1 million investment at 1 percent interest in a CDFI could involve a ten-year housing program tied to a local neighborhood coalition's home ownership zone, like what we are doing with the Southwest Partnership.

CDFI refers to a "Community Development Financial Institution," which specializes in lending to individuals, organizations, and businesses in under-resourced communities that includes housing, small businesses, and homebuyers.

In recent years, Bon Secours Mercy committed to investing up to 1 percent of its investment portfolio to community sustainability initiatives for ten years (e.g., up to $60 million for the initial year). Since the 1 percent ceiling was already in place with Bon Secours Mercy Health prior to sale of the hospital, it was useful to continue that commitment through Bon Secours Community Works. The latter was created as a subsidiary of the hospital several years before the sale.

Keep in mind that 1 percent loans certainly bring down the cost of development, but inflation is now increasing construction costs and housing rehabilitation projects.

Community Works would like to shift from relying just on development projects as a core source of revenue and move toward investment strategies (sole or lead investor) to increase our impact in the neighborhood.

Question: Impact investing is employed by many anchor institutions and community-based organizations. How would you describe it?

It can mean almost anything, really. It's certainly more than a set of process measures or an output metric (volume of services). It should be tied to specific project goals (i.e., actual outcomes the community wants to achieve).

For example, a priority in West Baltimore was to lower the recidivism rate. Between 2015-2020, our *Returning Citizens Program* accomplished a 5.6 percent recidivism rate. In 2021, there was no recidivism.

We're only at the beginning of being able to tease out what constitutes a meaningful impact to the community being served.

Question: What about initiatives referred to as Social Determinants of Health and Population Health?

Again, those are elusive terms that mean different things to different organizations. Such strategies are driven by institutional culture and often influenced by hierarchical relationships with the community.

Community Works is very cautious about assuming that we know what's best for a community, especially as an organization with deep roots—and biases—in healthcare and clinical medicine. The latter are obviously important, but we're learning that healthcare delivery (clinical medicine) doesn't drive the health of individuals or communities.

Healthcare institutions should not assume that clinical care is more important than healthy housing, open spaces, early childhood education, safe streets, or employment opportunity.

How much do hospital-centric organizations really understand about what communities want or how to improve health status for underserved populations? We need to be more inquisitive and figure out ways to meaningfully engage the community as full partners. Our job as community-based institutions is also to serve the community's nonclinical needs and priorities by leveraging our considerable asset base.

That won't happen overnight, but community anchor institutions, especially healthcare organizations, need to be in this for the long haul.

Question: The Social ROI is also gaining prominence in community investment strategies. SROI is particularly relevant for programs administered through social enterprises like nonprofits that use market forces to generate public or community benefits. Can you say more about your healthy housing project with a social return rationale?

Housing for Health study looked at our 802 units of affordable housing across twelve sites in West Baltimore. The analysis evaluated the economic, environmental, and social impacts (triple bottom line) of the Bon Secours program in West Baltimore. The project generated a net benefit of $1.30-1.99 per dollar invested.

The inputs were housing units, on-site service coordination, and funding. The output measures were high quality affordable housing, receipt of wraparound social services, and fewer vacant properties.

The outcomes were judged to be benefits to each stakeholder group (individuals and the immediate community). By purchasing and repurposing vacant homes, the surrounding neighborhoods benefited through increased safety and increased property values. City government benefited by decreasing the burden of demolitions, and decreased use of public social services, such as less need for homelessness services, and increased tax revenues.

For hospitals investing in affordable housing programs, a broad and inclusive definition of ROI may be appropriate since community needs around housing affordability and neighborhood revitalization are reflected in Community Needs Assessments every three years.

Hospitals also benefit financially by reduced admissions and chronic comorbidities that are associated with healthy and safe homes.

Question: How did the community center come about?

Following up on a request from community leaders to do more to serve the area's youth, Bon Secours repurposed a 13,000 square foot building, the city library that was shuttered in 1998, to a community resource center.

It was purchased for $1 million and $7 million has since been raised through a variety of granting agencies and donors such as the State of Maryland, Kaiser Permanente, Bank of America, and Under Armour.

The center will bring people together. It will house programs like healthcare career training, recreation and art programs, and a recording studio. Many of our workforce and financial services are relocating there.

Our involvement and investment signals that Community Works is in this for the long haul. Bon Secours has been serving West Baltimore for 140 years.

Question: What lies ahead for Unity Properties?

New housing units are a cornerstone of Unity Properties, but preserving existing housing is just as important. It's not an either/or proposition. It's both/and.

We're working to increase our portfolio to at least a critical mass of housing units (1,200), which is important because we want to sustain our efforts through housing operations rather than be dependent on development fees generated by new projects. That means having the infrastructure in place to assume more of the management of these units and coordinating day-to-day resident services as well as community organizing.

We will also need a well-developed business plan that clearly articulates our impact. We want to approach potential funders with targets based on community needs and opportunities rather than just what funding may be available.

Question: How does Community Works incorporate social justice concerns?

We need to reinvest as well and learn from past mistakes that harmed the community.

What I mean is that our organization is still trying to undo the terrible harm wrought by the Baltimore City Council in 1917 when redlining was instituted as well as other public policies and actions of private businesses, including ourselves. We continue to bear the burden of economic and social injustice that blocked the legitimate needs and aspirations of thousands of citizens over a century ago.

A series of three-year and five-year plans will only get us through the night and buy more time. It's still just kicking the can forward for others to deal with. That's not enough.

Today, many residents will grow up with a new library, not knowing there was no library for the past twenty-five years. Nor will many remember that the new open space used to be dilapidated row houses.

My hope is that in twenty-five years or one hundred years, future generations will not be saddled with undoing policies that we didn't recognize as unwise initiatives today.

Question: Any final thoughts?

I trust we're finally at a tipping point of respecting and engaging the community about meeting their needs and priorities in a meaningful way. That's our current mission.

Appendix 1: Community Works Training Manual Excerpts

Community Works makes three assumptions about the people we engage with:

- ✓ Everyone cares about something, and that passion is their motivation to act.
- ✓ Everyone has gifts.
- ✓ Everyone has something to contribute.

Our Engagement Framework is rooted in "ways of being" which includes four core principles:

Asset-Based

We are doing asset-based community development. That means:

- Focusing on what exists within communities and individuals.
- Building on personal and group motivation.
- Respecting these attributes.
- Using assets to conquer what is lacking or not desired.

In Relationship

Partnerships are relational. We are being relational when we are living in relation to others on the recognition of an interconnectedness with others. This means:

- Relational: not for or to, but *with.*
- Learning together.
- Coming together with assets.

Collaborative

We are collaborative when we work together, especially on a goal or shared project. This means:

- Involve diverse views.
- Incorporate all types of information.
- Problem solving centered around end users and people's needs.
- Compare and constant solutions.

Dutiful

We are responsible and accountable when we have an obligation to do something, or having control over or care for someone, as part of one's job or role. Some benefits of a quality process are:

- Provide structure for collaboration around shared interest.
- Accountability and transparency.
- Fairness, predictability, and inclusion.

Engagement is a practice: repetition, habit, routine. That also requires a way of being.

Be careful of your own agenda. My worldview is not exactly like someone else's worldview. I don't know everyone else's experience. Be aware.

When struggling with a question by yourself, the most important question to always ask yourself is: "What do they want?"

Just be present, you don't always have to say something. When with people, you're just *with* them, camaraderie.

You don't have an upper hand, and you don't have to be an expert on everything.

Chapter 26.

The BUILD Health Challenge: Healthy Homes Des Moines

Overview

Healthy Homes Des Moines (HHDM) set out to change substandard housing that puts children at risk for respiratory conditions like asthma, allergies, and chronic obstructive pulmonary disease (COPD). The focus was East Bank's aging housing stock plagued with city housing code violations and in need of extensive and expensive repairs.

The area's poverty rate (28 percent) was far higher than the rest of the county (12 percent) while household income was under $24,000 compared to $59,000 for the rest of Polk County. Residents did not have the income to move out of the area or pay for necessary repairs. East Bank residents had higher rates of respiratory illness than higher income neighborhoods based on hospitalization data.

Eight organizations came together to conduct home repairs and educate families on managing asthma. The three core partners were Polk County Housing Trust Fund (the designated CBO), three non-profit hospitals, and the local health department. Homes in need of remediation were identified by each hospital and from local schools. Home inspectors assessed homes for asthma triggers like lead, mold, allergens, and pests. Home repair was coordinated between health inspectors and contractors making repairs. Most home remediation costs were covered by PCHTF.

Families received household cleaning supplies and HEPA vacuum cleaners, while Community Health Workers (CHW) specializing in asthma and nurses educated families on how to manage asthma and keep homes healthy to mitigate asthma triggers.

Collaboration

The lead partners decided to focus on pediatric asthma because the three neighborhoods of East Des Moines had the highest concentrations of asthma emergency room visits in the county and county data indicated a high concentration of poor housing conditions. At the same time, the hospital staff voiced frustration about limiting housing remediation efforts to just East Des Moines when residents through the county could benefit. As a result, referrals could be made from any part of Polk County.

The multisector partnership grew to thirteen organizations that worked toward a sustainability plan that included third parties (one health plan and Medicaid) to fund the project long-term based on ROI to the payers.

HHDM met the initial goal of the BUILD grant (i.e., grant requirement: bold, upstream, integration, local, data). It identified an out-of-the box solution to reduce the prevalence of asthma for children (Bold), by looking at housing remediation that addressed environmental factors that contributed to illness (Upstream), by bringing together partners from key sectors that influence pediatric asthma (Integration), by involving numerous residents and local organizations to lead parts of the initiative (Local), and by using data to justify upstream interventions that were cost-effective such as legal assistance for tenants and paying for CHWs (Data).

The partners realized that conducting a community needs assessments, required by non-profit hospitals every three years, would indicate the prevalence of chronic illnesses like asthma. However, it would fall short of reducing such illness if the influence of other sectors were not engaged in the solution. Multiple agencies would need to come together to impact systems-level change in Des Moines. Collaboration among different stakeholders was required to bring valuable expertise and political clout to create community change.

The project's goal of creating sustainable change led to a series of actions:

- Suggesting Des Moines develop new housing and rental codes to ensure safe and healthy homes county-wide.
- Creating and enforcing policies that include housing repairs billed to Medicaid and health plans since they receive the financial benefit of housing remediation (ROI).

- Advocacy initiatives to protect tenants' rights to demand repairs and to remain in their homes once mitigation is completed and at the same rental rate.

Sustainability required third-party funding, especially Medicaid reimbursement, to be part of the solution. The rationale was that payers received the financial benefit from making homes healthier rather than hospitals. In fact, hospitals lost revenue from reduced ER visits because of housing remediation. Landlords also realize a financial gain from steady rental income made possible when tenants would no longer have to deal with looking for alternative housing that did not make their kids sick.

Housing conditions and health outcomes were linked, and the disparities of low-income children with asthma were an obvious city-wide concern. The project was successful in getting partners to move from delivering services to a systems-level strategy. However, it necessitated changing ingrained city and county policies that impacted childhood health. Local housing policy and code enforcement had short-term and long-term consequences on the prevalence of asthma in low-income neighborhoods.

Policy Advocacy

Advocacy was initiated in the following areas: housing policy, Medicaid reimbursement, tenant representation, and community tours for local officials and civic leaders.

Housing and Rental Policy

Data clearly indicated gross inequities and harmful impacts on childhood chronic illness. A shift from current programs and policies was needed. Rental housing codes were inadequate, many families had no written lease, and legal aid was necessary to convert month-to-month leases and change landlord practices. Housing inspectors needed additional training in healthy housing and what to look for.

Medicaid and Billing Policy

Change in reimbursement was necessary even though it was outside the traditional medical model. Other states had secured Medicaid waivers to reimburse housing mitigation efforts. Institutionalizing the source of ongoing funding was an essential building block for sustainability.

Tenant Advocacy

Iowa Legal Aid became a necessary intermediary to negotiate tenant leases for a flat fee per household. Tenant protection was necessary for up to two years after repairs are complete and meeting certain standards.

Community Tours

Two bus tours were conducted to neighborhood homes to increase awareness among local officials, political representatives, and civic leaders. The effort was intended to include "the right people to tell the right story to the right people," and to understand the context for policymakers who may be unfamiliar with high-poverty neighborhoods.

The focus on policy meant that each organization had to transition from individual efforts on service delivery towards advocacy and impacting the political process to create system-level change. This was initially uncomfortable for many partners. It was far removed from their traditional mindset.

An upstream focus entailed addressing the home environment and the policy environment since both impact asthma for families living in dilapidated homes. This enabled hospitals to become more aware of countywide conditions that affected family health and to become more engaged in changing policies that involved issues beyond traditional medical care such as housing, schooling, public works, city planning, and community education. Conditions that led to asthma had to be addressed instead of waiting for kids to arrive at the emergency room.

It was necessary to embed behavior change and individual-level initiatives within the context of how and where children lived. The root causes of asthma—the Social Determinants of Health—became the new focus. Hospital leaders recognized that traditional medical intervention did not address unmet needs of their patients.

By linking home to health and health to outcomes, the CBO and hospital leaders joined together to advocate housing mitigation as a prerequisite for treating childhood asthma. At the same time, data pointed to poor mental health caused by the stress of multiple moves and the ever-present threat of eviction. These were obvious social risk factors that needed to be addressed.

This awareness led to multilevel intervention and cemented multisector partnership. By tapping into their unique skills and assets, partner organizations were able to work together in creating a common vision along with the CBO's established network of people already working on community projects, some for twenty years. For the most part, individual agendas transitioned to embracing a common project agenda.

For the partnership to work, written "rules of engagement" and decision-making were drawn up and agreed upon. Five types of Memorandums of Agreement established responsibilities, which outlined the project intentions, deliverables, and each partner's roles. The management of HHDM was given to a committee representing the three core partners, while other organizations provided direct funding. HHDM added a full-time project coordinator and program evaluator to the management team.

Community Engagement

HHMD's community coalition partner (VEB), which represents residents and other stakeholders for neighborhoods improvement efforts, provided home health visits, education activities, and outreach to families and medical providers.

However, both VEB and school-based partners experienced push back on engagement from an unanticipated source, namely, residents living in rental units. There was a marked imbalance in the power dynamics between residents and landlords. Renters were reluctant to pressure or negotiate with landlords for improvements or even asking for a lease. Many had not even met their landlords, and most were not English-proficient.

Furthermore, HHMD partners acting on behalf of residents did not match the lived experience or ethnicity of renters. HHMD representatives were mostly white, older, and male. This represented a potential barrier for successful engagement and project implementation; this issue was never fully resolved.

HHDM's way of representing community concerns was the main problem. The traditional leadership role was to inform the community about decisions rather than supporting residents through consultation and shared decision-making on project direction and priorities. There was a glaring lack of community representation in the initiative's leadership. Partners were more concerned that their efforts were effective and produced results for the community, even if the community was not thoroughly consulted. There was a lack of power sharing, which would correspond to "degrees of tokenism" on the Arnstein ladder of citizen participation.

LEVEL OF ENGAGEMENT	TYPE OF PARTICIPATION	DESCRIPTION
Nonparticipation	Manipulation	Directed by staff and tend not to be informed of issues. May be asked to "rubberstamp" decisions already taken by staff.
	Decoration	May be indirectly involved in decisions or campaigns but are not fully aware of their rights, their possible involvement, or how decisions might affect them.
	Informing	Informed of actions and changes, but their views are not actively sought.
Tokenism	Consultation	Fully informed and encouraged to express their opinions but have little or no impact on outcomes.
	Placation	Consulted and informed. Views are listened to in order to inform the decision-making process but does not guarantee changes.
	Partnership	Consulted and informed in decision-making processes. Outcomes are a result of negotiations between organizations/staff and community/residents.
Learner Empowerment	Delegated Power	Organization/staff inform agenda for action, but community/ residents have responsibility for managing aspects or all of any initiatives/programs. Decisions are shared.
	Resident/Citizen (Learner) Control	Community/residents initiate agendas and have responsibility and power for management of issues and to bring about change. Power is delegated to community/ residents, and they are active in designing their education.

Data Role

The initiative shared data to unify partners, inform activities, and measure impact and ROI. The goal was to show that the initiative could reduce ER visits, the incidence of asthma flare-ups and reduce costs. It also sought to identify gaps in service and develop a user-friendly database referral system.

Data integration was particularly important so referrals could be made through multiple partners, including providers and nonclinical services such as home remediation and asthma education information. However, data protection issues arose due to HIPAA patient privacy regulations and the project's ability to share data with the public. Bureaucratic issues regarding HIPAA releases were not resolved with the three hospitals.

Partners needed to develop data use agreements, and this involved having each of the families sign a waiver that allowed sharing information among participating organizations. Community partners collected data on pre- and post-intervention measures on asthma symptoms and hospital use.

Data collection included multiple categories:

- Patient demographic characteristics and a ten-minute telephone assessment of family needs by a medical provider
- Face-to-face interviews by CHWs on family history of asthma and awareness of asthma triggers
- Home inspection information on household asthma triggers and housing conditions

- Environmental hazards (e.g., air quality, mold and mildew, lead and radon levels, pests, toxic household cleaners)
- Repairs completed
- Referrals to organizations
- Families losing track of information after inspection.

Additional data was collected during a two-month follow-up after the home inspection to see if there was a decrease in asthma symptoms and better daily management of asthma. Children recorded asthma symptoms every day using a refrigerator-mounted chart. Hospital and medical record data was gathered on health outcomes from providers, and medical records from a Federally Qualified Health Center.

Key metrics were collected on medical history:

- Asthma diagnosis
- Symptoms and severity
- Missed school days and missed workdays
- Frequency of urgent care and ER visits
- Zip codes for disproportionately higher rates of utilization.

The hospital partner-led strategy discussions were based on collected data from all these sources. Financial date also informed decisions about referrals for housing inspection. Remediation and home repair was restricted to households earning less than 80 percent of the neighborhood median income.

Data was also used to document project impact by comparing the cost of home remediation to healthcare utilization for Medicaid reimbursement, especially savings from ER visits.

Due to incompatibility of information systems, partners were never able to develop an integrated data management system that allowed healthcare providers to collect and share both clinical and nonclinical data.

Health Equity

Health disparity issues arose through each phase of the initiative. Partners felt that equity was addressed indirectly by focusing on upstream factors (i.e., living conditions of low-income families of color). The project helped stakeholders gain a clearer perception of the impact of housing disparities on health outcomes. The initiative focused on immediate consequences of disparities in delivering services and how to change institutional and administrative policies that systematically excluded certain population segments.

Partners were committed to altering the power imbalance between landlords and tenants, especially at the individual family level. That alleviates some of the power imbalances that underlie inequity by changing housing code policy in two respects. First, putting in legal protections for families who are not able to negotiate by themselves, families would be protected for the first time. Second, including everyone in the county, so the initiative would provide a health benefit to all families in the city.

The initiate did usher in new and better ways to provide traditional medical services. Hospitals used a visiting nurse program with care coordinators with varied cultural backgrounds and bilingual fluency. Housing and public works inspectors were accompanied by translators matched to family language preferences when inspecting homes.

Health Impact

The number of symptom-free days increased because of participating in the program. Children missed school due to asthma less than one day a month versus nine days a month (10 percent of school days) prior to the program.

This represents a savings of $620 per student each year. Children averaged an additional 6.2 symptom-free days a month and fewer absences. Parents and caregivers missed half as many workdays as before (1.4 days versus 0.4 days per month). Both adults and children increased their understanding of asthma care. Overall stress level decreased for parents and caregivers. Families are better connected to community resources such as food pantry, family therapy, energy and employment assistance programs, and lead remediation programs.

Fifty-one families received in-home asthma education, and twenty-four families completed the education program.

Des Moines reported twenty-five asthma-related emergency visits for six months prior to the project at a cost of $17,500. Emergency department visits dropped from 0.44 asthma-related visits in the months before the program to zero. This represents a savings of $308 per member per month ($3,700 per child a year). For context, Iowa spends $2,200 per child enrolled in Medicaid each year.

The average cost of household cleaning supplies per family was $391 and the average repair cost of the forty-two homes was $4,416. The average project cost for each family was $2,416. The project allocated $150,000 for home repair costs and $17,000 for supplies given to each family.

"Pre-HHDSM" vs. "Post-HHDSM" Assessments	**Pre-HHDSM**	**Post-HHDSM**
Number of asthma-related emergency department visits in the previous four weeks	0.44	0
Number of symptom-free days (month)	19.29	25.13
Number of missed days of work, due to child's asthma (month)	1.39	0.40
Number of missed days of school, due to asthma (month)	2.11	0.76
Adult's rating of degree to which asthma is controlled (1 = completely, 5 = severe, persistent, out of control)	2.54	1.84
Adult's understanding of asthma care management (1 = no understanding, 5 = very strong)	3.74	4.68
Child's understanding of asthma care management (1 = no understanding, 5 = very strong)	2.76	3.36
Level of stress related to child's asthma (1 = no stress, 5 = high stress)	2.76	2.15
Level of stress related to general responsibilities as a parent (1 = no stress, 5 = high stress)	1.73	1.39
How much did the repairs to your home seem to improve your health? (1 = greatly improved, 5 = did not improve)	1.33	
How well do you feel like you can maintain your home in a way that manages your asthma (1= very well, 5 = not well)	1.56	

Lessons Learned

Over the course of the project, six lessons learned stand out. Each are critical to the success of cross-sector initiatives.

1. If health provider referral is required for program participation, make sure the health professionals have the commitment and are adequately staffed to make referrals. If not, look at multiple referral sources.
2. Ensure management committee members have the authority within their organizations to make decisions.
3. Coordinate data collection from participating hospital systems in a standardized and uniform format to allow easier comparison and data analysis. This may require agreement from hospitals to make format changes.
4. Learn how to better leverage existing resources across partnering agencies.
5. Take sufficient time to collect feedback and adjust process and workflow practices, even minor adjustments in real-time yield large dividends for success.
6. Build trust and pursue a common objective goal so that all partners are committed to achieving shared goals rather than individual or organizational gains.

Building on these findings is important as the initiative continues to expand asthma-related housing mitigation efforts in Des Moines and Polk County.

Conclusion

HHDSM continues to provide home remediation and health education to families in Polk County, albeit at a much-reduced capacity. Third-party payment for home remediation and health education remains an ongoing goal as does the hiring of additional housing inspectors. Advocacy for more aggressive housing inspection policies as well as strengthening ordinances and state laws to protect tenants remains an ongoing effort.

Key Takeaways

- Communication is a central component of successful collaboration, particularly for cross-sector initiatives.
- Personal stories are the most powerful tool for educating policy makers and agency staff as well as management committee members who are not familiar with the lived experience of project participants.
- Achieving goals and devising solutions require diverse, cross-sector partnerships.
- Families need to be equipped with physical tools (e.g., roof repairs, non-toxic cleaning supplies) and informational tools (e.g., strategies to reduce and eliminate asthma triggers).
- It is critical for management committee members, elected leaders, healthcare administrators and agency staff to understand how poor housing conditions directly impact the health and productivity of residents.

- Referral procedures must be designed around specific asthma diagnoses so that multiple sources can make referrals to the program.
- Messaging strategies must be succinct and easy to understand so that city leaders and community members understand that environmental factors put children with asthma and families at significant health risk.

Executive Comments

Eric Burmeister is Executive Director of Polk County Housing Trust Fund in Des Moines.

Timing and politics are key factors in healthy housing initiatives.

To improve the quality of the city's rental housing, the city committed to hiring more building inspectors over five years. Unfortunately, the focus of those inspectors has been the exterior cosmetics such as paint and broken windows. It was an election year. The council wanted to invest in things voters would notice.

The state's Medicaid program was contracted out to three Medicare-managed care organizations with a fee-for-service mindset. The financial incentives were structured to reward claims efficiency rather than better care. Had the MCO been interested, their claims data would have shown that expensive ER visits for asthma-related conditions for children were significantly reduced following the project's mold remediation efforts.

The timing of the pandemic affected the project. When tenants lost their job, they weren't able to make rent payments. Plus, most tenants were afraid to rock the boat and press landlords about building code violations. That could lead to eviction.

It seemed like government agencies—federal, state, local—all had different agendas that didn't line up with making rental units healthy places to live in, especially for families with asthmatic kids. Lobbyists working the state legislature and city hall represented landlord interests. Making rental units safe places to live wasn't a priority.

Here are some takeaways for organizations to consider when implementing healthy homes initiatives:

- Timing is everything! This factor is too often overlooked.
- COVID-19 was a setback and delayed hiring more building inspectors due to the city's belt tightening. The city also changed its community planning strategy about code enforcement.
- City politics was on the side of landlords, not renters. This needs to be factored into the game plan.
- Many low-income tenants are too frightened to push landlords to make necessary repairs. The power imbalance is too great. They need advocates to negotiate on their behalf.
- Trying to get HIPAA releases from hospitals on patient data (asthma visits) was too time consuming, too bureaucratic, and ultimately futile.

Despite these barriers, the project made a lot of progress. ER visits for kids with asthma were significantly reduced. The number of workdays lost by parents due to their child's asthma episodes went way down and so did the number of school days lost. That's very encouraging.

Chapter 27.

The BUILD Health Challenge: San Pablo Area Revitalization Collaboration Case Study

The BUILD Health Challenge is a national program to support partnerships between community-based organizations, health departments, and hospitals/health systems addressing important health issues. Each community collaborative focuses on root causes of chronic disease, referred to as the Social Determinants of Health, by leveraging multisector partnerships and working with their local community. Each project encompasses four driving principles: Bold, Upstream, Local, and Data-Driven (BUILD).

Introduction

The San Pablo Avenue Corridor extends a mile north of downtown Oakland and reflects decades of inequity and disinvestment in housing, schools, jobs, and health services for residents. The San Pablo Area Revitalization Collaborative (SPARC) was developed to address these issues in partnership with residents, community organizations, and public agencies.

It was important for the initiative to preserve the culture and traditions of the community to create a sense of place and buy-in. Solutions cannot be superimposed from the outside but must come from the residents themselves. Residents make up 51 percent of SPARC's Steering Committee with the rest composed of partnering organizations.

Overview

Residents in three low-income census tracts in West Oakland sought to revitalize their blighted neighborhood through a multi-pronged, cross-sector initiative. Community-based organizations, hospital systems, and Alameda County Public Health Departments came together with the goal of reducing disparities in health, housing, and economic opportunity. Health disparities were rooted in historical disinvestment, institutional racism, and physical decline.

The area was a food desert without local options for healthy food, which contributed to high rates of hypertension and diabetes. There were few sites for recreation, few stores for shopping, and the area experienced high crime rates along San Pablo Avenue, the main transit corridor. The community also had strong community connections and a small network of nonprofit organizations working in partnership with residents to support resources, referrals, and well-being.

SPARC received critical funding from BUILD to move the partners from planning to implementation. The initiative was supported by local partners and EBALDC, which served as the lead convener and community-based organization. EBALDC had previously developed affordable housing and commercial real estate along the San Pablo Avenue Corridor and was a development partner to Community Foods Market.

Organizing Framework

SPARC employed an Asset-Based Community Development strategy to mobilize local resources for sustainable development. It is founded on the premise that communities are best positioned to identify unrecognized assets that can help create local economic opportunity. Assets can be built upon, whereas deficits cannot.

SPARC recognized that local associations and networks are the best vehicles to leverage support and create ongoing participatory approaches to development. Relationships build community. As a citizen-centered organization, SPARC empowers residents to set the agenda and identify community priorities.

Each community, like the San Pablo Avenue Corridor, has a unique set of skills and capabilities to channel for community development. These include individuals, associations (informal groups with common interests), institutions (government agencies, businesses, schools, hospitals), physical assets (buildings, land), and connections (people who are connectors).

The San Pablo Avenue Corridor has numerous assets and skills to build upon that were strengthened by SPARC. The community building initiative stressed social relationships, members working together, and treating relationships as assets.

BUILD provided critical funding to move the partners from planning to implementation.

SPARC wanted to improve neighborhood health and well-being, particularly for long-time residents, in three census tracts in West Oakland. There was a fourteen-year life expectancy gap between the SPARC neighborhoods and more affluent communities just a couple of miles away in the Oakland hills.

Improving neighborhood health meant focusing on inter-related issues of affordable housing, access to healthy food and adequate nutrition, safe spaces for recreation, and economic opportunity for residents. SPARC also started with working closely with neighborhood residents to identify their priorities and ensure that they were an active part of SPARC's decision-making process. That shared realization was fundamental to organizing and sustaining a multi-partner initiative that everyone bought into.

Initiative Activities

A coordinated vision enabled SPARC partners to address systemic issues underlying poor housing and lack of economic investment. It was a multi-pronged approach that also included hypertension since residents considered it a high priority. The initiative called for an integrated approach because hypertension is closely related to housing instability and economic stress. Hypertension rates would not be reduced until housing and economic conditions were improved, and healthy food was readily available. The partnership recognized the need to act upstream and downstream simultaneously.

SPARC priorities and activities were organized around four principles:

1. *Preserving culture* by creating a sense of place and building buy-in for change by residents. The California Hotel, formerly an entertainment and jazz mecca that fell into disrepair, was renovated to provide 137 residential units of affordable housing, on-site medical and social services, and 8,000 square feet of commercial space.

   A sense of place was reinforced by Kresge Foundation's $8 million initiative focused on placemaking, which supported community development through arts and culture. Projects that supported social cohesion included creating neighborhood murals, building community gardens, and sponsoring community events.

2. *Centering community power and voice* by centering residents in governance decisions and creating diverse options to lead and engage with SPARC's work across its priorities. For example, Design Dash was a creative placemaking program that was co-created by a resident artist and EBALC to support local people to collectively envision and lead quick creative action projects such as murals, events, gardens, and advocacy campaigns. Each project receives $1,000 seed funding and in-kind support for professional designers, program managers, and capacity building training.

3. *Collaboration across sectors* brings government, business, and nonprofit partners together to invest in economic and social development initiatives such as Community Foods Market. The full-service grocery store required five years of effort that included real estate financing and expertise by EBALDC. The market is an essential resource for residents in West Oakland, a former food desert.

4. *Affordable housing* as part of mixed-use development that combines housing and critical social services. EBALDC partnered with Lifelong Medical Care to provide primary care and case management services as well as in-house resident services. The combination of support services builds community and well-being.

A further example of these principles is the Yield 4 Life project on reclaiming safe streets. It was a community-led campaign and protest over unsafe streets, with the support of EBALDC's creative community development team. Residents designed a protest and created a video urging the city to take action for safer streets. Volunteers painted a giant piano mural at the intersection, celebrating the neighborhood's long history of producing world-class musicians, while drawing attention to the blighted roadway. In 2021, the city of Oakland's Department of Transportation completed a permanent safety improvement construction project reconfiguring the intersection with ADA curb ramps, newly painted crosswalks, raised crossing islands, and extended medians.

Videos captured interviews with passers-by about the urgent need for safer streets. Murals and street art were installed at the worst intersection to draw attention to the blighted roadway. As a result, the City of Oakland Department of Transportation started construction last year on more permanent safety measures for the intersection.

Community Partnerships

The SPARC partnership involved more than 500 residents in identifying what was most important to them. Data was gathered over a one-year planning process that led to a five-year Action Plan. Four work groups were responsible for developing implementation plans to address the four biggest priorities:

1. **Heart Health:** Decrease high blood pressure.
2. **Community:** Decrease blight and increase resident leadership and connections.
3. **Housing:** Develop 175 affordable units.
4. **Economy:** Support new business development and implement job training.

The work groups were coordinated by the SPARC Steering Committee. The CBO had multiple functions, which included facilitating meetings, supporting SPARC partners to secure collaborative funding, and developing strategic partnerships.

Alameda County Public Health Department provided neighborhood-level data to determine resident health profiles and program evaluation. Alta Bates Summit Medical Center also supported SPARC on data and evaluation, and program design of Heart Health clinics.

Many of the partners had worked on community projects together for more than a decade. There was a history of collaboration and partners were mindful of the fourteen-year difference in life expectancy for West Oakland residents compared to other higher income neighborhood.

SPARC partnership intervention was **bold** because it supported neighborhood residents to address the problem of blight throughout the corridor, which had been neglected for decades. The first full-service grocery store in more than ten years was built. Drop-in heart health clinics were opened to address high rates of hypertension.

The community-wide intervention was **integrated** because it was a multi-sector partnership that included neighborhood residents, nonprofit organizations, a federally qualified health center, housing advocacy organization, senior service provider, affordable housing developers, city departments, and businesses.

The goal was **upstream** because SPARC addressed the fourteen-year life expectancy gap, and high rate of hypertension and ER visits by both preserving neighborhood culture and increasing access to neighborhood serving health assets, services, and affordable housing.

The work groups and community involvement at each phase of the initiative was **local**. It was led by neighborhood residents and community organizations located in the neighborhood. The impact of health, housing, and economic development directly benefited residents along the San Pablo Avenue Corridor.

Information on neighborhood priorities, health indicators, and housing affordability were important **data** that formed the basis of the SPARC initiative.

Project Focus

The SPARC approach focused on improving neighborhood health through a multi-pronged approach. SPARC's heart health workgroup established drop-in clinics in the neighborhood so residents could be screened for high blood pressure. SPARC's economy workgroup focused on supporting new businesses and creating jobs for neighborhood residents. SPARC's art and culture workgroup focused on supporting resident-led projects that highlighted the neighborhood's rich history and culture. SPARC's housing workgroup focused on addressing housing affordability and homelessness. The initiative was backed by all the partnering organizations. This coordinated approach eventually led to securing $6 million in grants for neighborhood development.

Opening a new grocery store was pivotal to attracting new dollars and jobs in the neighborhood as well as more affordable housing units. Community Foods Market was attracted to locate in the corridor because of SPARC's community organizing and its collective work attracted more investment for community priorities. San Pablo Avenue Corridor community members identified access to healthy food as a long-standing need. EBALDC provided real estate and financing expertise to help raise funds and secure a location. In June 2019, West Oakland opened its first full-service grocery store in more than ten years through an $11 million investment that has created thirty new jobs for residents and will attract new business to the corridor.

Successful approaches to community development combine housing and critical services, particularly through mixed use developments. Housing was seen as directly impacting health. When residents are hard-pressed to pay current rents, there is not enough disposable income left for medicines for high blood pressure or healthy food to control their high blood pressure. By framing the problem in this way, policy makers can see the connection more clearly. This leads to a shift in focus, and a shift in policy and system change.

Collaboration among partners created new ways for partners to understand the links between health, preserving culture, and economic opportunities. Most of all, it was about the priorities and actions being resident-led.

Addressing upstream approaches to health and the built environment was key to the SPARC initiative.

Collaboration Strategy

SPARC wanted to build a civic network and collaborative infrastructure that would be a vehicle for community change. Having a governance structure in place was key to coordinating the work groups and the steering committee. Members served three-year terms, decisions were made by consensus (50 percent plus one), meetings were set for every four to six weeks for ninety minutes, there were no chairs to direct attendee discussion, and members were aided by a neutral facilitator. Work groups abided by the same governance policies.

The presence of a neutral facilitator was critical to integrating the work of partners and implementing action plans. This gave power to the group to make difficult decisions collectively. The decision making of the different work groups was data driven and made possible with a shard data dashboard that tracked progress on the five action priorities. Strategy development was grounded in a range of data sources: residents, survey information, partner feedback, and public data around housing and crime.

The collaborative recognized that stronger relationships needed to be built with residents to increase their participation on the Steering Committee as well as the Work Groups.

The work groups and steering committee members were racially diverse, like the neighborhood, but were mostly female and older. It was difficult to recruit younger residents to participate in governance. However, they were much more excited to participate in creative action projects such as murals. Building neighborhood capacity in the three census tracts was an ongoing challenge, and an important ingredient of community engagement.

Community Engagement

One way to understand the level of partnership in a community initiative is to see where residents hold power according to the Ladder of Participation developed by Sherry Arnstein more than fifty years ago. Each of the eight rungs on the ladder describe the extent to which community members hold power in determining the outcome of a goal.

LADDER OF PARTICIPATION		
LEVEL OF ENGAGEMENT	**TYPE OF PARTICIPATION**	**DESCRIPTION**
Nonparticipation	Manipulation	Directed by staff and tend not to be informed of issues. May be asked to "rubberstamp" decisions already made by staff.
	Decoration	May be indirectly involved in decisions or "campaigns" but are not fully aware of their rights, their possible involvement, or how decisions might affect them.
	Informing	Informed of actions and changes, but their views are not actively sought.
Tokenism	Consultation	Fully informed and encouraged to express their opinions but have little or no impact on outcomes.
	Placation	Consulted and informed. Views are listened to inform the decision-making process, but this does not guarantee changes.
	Partnership	Consulted and informed in decision-making processes. Outcomes are a result of negotiations between organization/staff and community/residents.
Learner Empowerment	Delegated Power	Organization/staff inform agenda for action, but community/residents have responsibility for managing aspects of all initiatives/programs. Decisions are shared.
	Resident/Citizen (Learner) Control	Community/residents initiate agendas and have responsibility ad power for management of issues and to bring about change. Power is delegated to community/residents, and they are active in designing their education.

The project's activity on equity capacity, according to Hogan's Characteristic Equity Approaches, could be described as an "Equity-Add-On-Approach" as shown in the table below.

Characteristic Equity Approaches	***Description***
Institutionalized Equity Approach	Builds organizational structure from outset to consider equity in all policies, practices, procedures.
Equity-Add-On Approach	Engages in post hoc actions to graft equity considerations and approaches onto existing (usually non-equity-supporting) institutional frameworks.
Cultural-Matching Approach	Focuses on developing, implementing, and disseminating approaches, usually limited to *education and care*, that match historical, cultural, and social needs and desires of populations of color.
Diversity Approach	Focuses on including a more diverse workforce; while organization hires more people of color, it usually does not give them power or resources.
Missionary Approach	Provides evidence-based practice in traditional ways, targeted specifically to people of color, usually delivered by people of different ethnicity than population served.
"Raise-All-Boats" Approach	Focuses on improving systems of care for outcomes, with the expectation that improved systems will automatically impact all population groups and achieve equity.
Selective Approach	Chooses selectively which population or inequity to address as sole programmatic focus (e.g., income inequality but not racial inequities; Latinas but not African Americans).
Concerned, Non-Action Approach	Knows that inequities exist, but does not know how to incorporate equity into programmatic actions.
Low-Awareness Approach	Conducts professional work in absence of recognition or consideration of need to address inequities.

In this project, community engagement varied between "Partnership" and "Delegated Power" levels. Residents were quite involved in decision-making through work groups and had some responsibility for managing programs, but SPARC often relied on partner organizations with technical expertise and more experience with developing housing and health programs.

As time went on, SPARC recognized the need to modify strategies and action plans based on community input if that signaled a better approach. There was also an awareness that more support is needed for a wider range of residents to be involved and more impactful in the decision-making process of the initiative.

Data Role

SPARC relied on data collection and data sharing to bring partners and residents together as well as to guide activities. It was critical to identify upstream factors like unhealthy housing and unaffordable rental units. It provided a baseline for assessing the rate of hypertension in the community and the lack of access to treating it in a holistic way, and to providing healthy and affordable food choices.

SPARC used the centralized collaborative dashboard to share data as well as track progress of each action priority. Data helped SPARC see what was changing, what was happening in the neighborhood, the impact of the SPARC initiative, and the work of residents and organizations.

Population-level data indicators and performance measures are routinely tracked by SPARC. These include income, demographics, policing and crime data, rent, and the number of housing units in the pipeline.

Neighborhood-wide surveys were conducted every three years. Community residents developed the survey questions and helped to administer the surveys. The effort was initially focused on seniors, but the work soon transitioned to a multigenerational effort. Residents were also involved in developing new programs such as a "sanctioned graffiti wall," trash-can mosaics, neighborhood cleanup campaigns, and a blight reduction campaign. SPARC provided training and support for residents to feel comfortable participating in meetings and engage in discussions. This followed years of marginalization and exclusion from community decision-making. SPARC realized the need to reach out and communicate continuously by text, flyers, email, and newsletters through partnering organizations.

Each partner has its own set of primary and secondary data sources. Hospital partners stressed hypertension-related data as well as qualitative information from focus groups to better understand community needs and shed more insight to quantitative data.

A Community Baseline Survey was administered to document neighborhood opinion on safety, neighborhood friendliness and feelings of connectivity, satisfaction with local business service, housing and health concerns, level of community involvement and basic demographics. Secondary data was likewise collected on housing such as Section 8 voucher use, median home prices and rent fluctuations, affordability of rental prices, and blighted properties.

To facilitate data sharing among partners, data sharing agreements were drawn up by CBO attorneys and hospital legal counsel.

A basic question is whether low-income residents in three census tracts achieved better health because of the hypertension program and its range of supportive services such as healthy food options and more affordable housing units. To date, the CBO can point to correlation data but not causation.

Two major bond initiatives were passed by Alameda County, work groups were making progress on pedestrian and public safety, and local housing policies were beginning to change on a system level. These were indicators or proxies for ROI and systems change.

The challenge was documenting changes in health over time. This was further complicated by hospital HIPAA constraints in hospitals about sharing clinical data with SPARC partners. The hospital had not grappled with a community request for patient-level data beyond general summaries and zip code-level information before.

A CBO partner recommendation going forward is to use Results-Based Accountability evaluation framework at the outset. This framework can better organize the work of each organization and agency programs, including decision-making, and allocation of resources, and budgeting.

A further suggestion was to bring in additional training related to antiracism work and equity, without further stigmatizing communities that are already viewed negatively throughout the San Pablo Avenue Corridor.

Safer streets (Yield4Life) came about when the community pressured the City of Oakland based in part on video interviews of residents on the importance of safe streets throughout the San Pablo Avenue Corridor.

SPARC achieved multiple project objectives in the initial phase of the initiative. These included greater access to health food, more affordable housing units, more new businesses, and jobs for residents. Twenty-four Heart Health drop-in clinics to measure blood pressure were opened at two sites. More than 2,500 screenings were recorded. Sutter Health, a local hospital, awarded $160,000 in direct funding plus in-kind support for SPARC and the Heart Health program work.

St. Mary's Center is developing new senior affordable housing and ground floor community space. In 2022, EBALDC broke ground on veterans and family affordable housing at West Grand and Bush. Another sixty-unit project is in the pipeline at 34th and San Pablo Avenue adjacent to the California Hotel. EBALDC is financing a family affordable housing project at West Grand and Brush.

Creative Placemaking

EBALDC works with residents, collaborative partners, and culture bearers in the San Pablo Corridor to take on creative projects such as murals, community events, protests, and community gardens. The objective is to build social cohesion and resident leadership that advances system and policy change that centers equity.

EBALDC placed a priority on building community through creative actions, which then contributed to walkable streets and public spaces. The strategy encourages social relationships between neighbors and supports development of locally owned businesses. The purpose is to foster resident pride in place by celebrating local culture, neighborhood assets, and history.

This approach to community building anchors placemaking into existing work as a community developer. Creative projects are grounded in understanding resident experience and feedback to make sure diverse voices shape program decisions and priorities. Political capital is then channeled to initiate permanent infrastructure change.

Each project advances agreed-upon goals, which build resident skills and relationships. Examples of creative placemaking include:

- Blight Busters fosters fence signage projects and public murals.
- Design Dash project collaboration is open to all residents.
- Creative Action Projects throughout the community.
- SPARCitplace organizes temporary event spaces on a vacant lot along the corridor for market days with vendors and community events.

SPARC's creative community development work also includes a Crosswalk Art project for pedestrian safety as well as the Median project of neighborhood murals on San Pablo Avenue in front of the California Hotel in West Oakland. St. Andrew's Plaza was redesigned with a mural project led by local arts organization, Attitudinal Healing. SPARC and EBALDC lobbied the City of Oakland to shut down the commercial retail stores across from St. Andrew's Plaza that was a magnet for criminal activity.

Blackball Universe is a multimedia collective that includes writers, artists, directors, and editors in addition to musicians. It includes an art gallery, recording studio, and rehearsal space to support new Black artists. EBALDC partners with them and Blackball Universe is one of EBALDC's commercial tenants. They have been hosting monthly market events highlighting local businesses and celebrating arts and culture during the pandemic through their new business ("Storefront Records").

To date, sixty-five residents have led creative action projects as community leaders who connected and implemented such projects in the SPARC neighborhood. Funds have supported leadership coaching, programming funds, and technical support from EBALDC and SPARC partners. Hundreds of additional residents have been involved in these projects as volunteers, event participants, and contributors.

Summary

SPARC's agenda was to create a collaborative decision-making table that prioritized residents in deciding what community change efforts to act on in a West Oakland neighborhood. EBALDC, a long-time community developer that values collaboration, saw a need to convene partners living and working in the neighborhood to raise awareness about long-standing issues and bringing partners together to make difficult decisions about how to reduce barriers to equitable health, economic development, and housing issues.

The first phase of building community capacity laid the groundwork for follow-up investment and collaboration among residents, government agencies, community organizations, and healthcare providers with an ongoing stake in the neighborhood.

The second cohort of BUILD funding is supporting the Healthy Havenscourt Collaborative to advance place-based strategies to reduce asthma health disparities in the Havenscourt neighborhood of East Oakland.

BUILD is currently funding HHC to advance place-based strategies to reduce asthma health disparities in the Havenscourt neighborhood of East Oakland. BUILD is supporting the leadership and advocacy capacity of a team of resident Healthy Housing Champions to advocate for Oakland to adopt healthy housing policies, such as a rental inspection program.

Through a partnership with Benioff Children's Hospital Oakland (BCHO), the champions have also been trained in BCHO's FINDconnect data platform, a virtual Social Determinants of Health tool that identifies residents' SDOH needs (such as housing instability and food insecurity) and connects them to community resources. This was done by co-creating an action plan, and strengthening social supports to reduce stress and fear around residents' SDOH needs. The action plan is a collaborative initiative with La Clinica de la Raza (a local FQHC), Regional Asthma Management & Prevention (a partner of the Public Health Institute that supports policy and system changes to reduce the asthma burden focusing on health equity), EBALDC, BCHO, and Alameda County Public Health. EBALDC serves as the lead on the project, convening and facilitating the collaborative space.

At the core of the initiative is community leadership. Over the course of the past three years, with support from the HHC partners, a small team of residents has significantly increased their leadership capacity and knowledge about the link between health and housing, the policy change process, and the critical role of community voice to advocate for basic needs such as quality and affordable housing. The Healthy Housing Champions have led presentations with Oakland city council members. While the pandemic limited in-person community engagement, the champions have implemented community actions that include building residents' awareness around their rights as an Oakland tenant, and the critical link between health and housing.

The healthy housing champions are implementing FINDconnect in two of La Clinica's neighborhood pediatric clinics. This is an important systems change in the clinic's workplan because clinic providers are recognizing the important role the champions can play *in* the clinic, as well as in the community, to build trust with patients and build a more comprehensive profile of a patient's social, economic, and environmental needs that critically shape patients' health. The workplan strengthens social supports to reduce stress and fear around residents' social care needs.

Most recently, Healthy Havenscourt has played a leading role in advocating with Alameda County for an equitable allocation of the American Recovery Plan funding to be invested in Havenscourt/East Oakland.

Healthy Havenscourt's Community Health Worker/navigator model has been recognized by Alameda County as a model for large-scale investment in COVID relief and recovery efforts in Havenscourt/East Oakland over the next 3-4 years. This recognition was earned through numerous 1:1 meetings with county district leaders and presentations and comments at public meetings.

Conclusion

Community leadership is the core of the initiative. Over the course of the past two years, with support from the HHC partners, a small team of residents have built leadership capacity and knowledge regarding the link between health and housing, the policy change process, and the critical role of community voice to advocate for basic needs (e.g., quality and affordable housing).

The Healthy Housing Champions have led multiple presentations with Oakland city council members. Despite limitations imposed by the pandemic on in-person community engagement, the champions have implemented community actions such as building resident awareness around tenant rights and the critical link between health and housing. This was a major step forward in community building.

Currently, Healthy Havenscourt is playing a leading role in advocating with Alameda County for an equitable allocation of the American Recovery Plan funding to be invested in Havenscourt/ East Oakland. The collaborative is specifically advocating for the county to invest in Healthy Havenscourt's Community Health Worker/navigator model to support community-driven and equitable COVID recovery over the next three years.

Key Takeaways

- Trust must be earned in marginalized neighborhoods that have experienced entrenched disinvestment through transparency and a willingness to share power with residents. SPARC built trust and momentum by acting on resident priorities.
- Solutions must focus on social, environmental, and economic factors that most influence community health status rather than just increasing access to healthcare delivery.
- It is essential to link built environment barriers (and historical disinvestment) to root causes of poor health and under-employment in the neighborhood.
- Hiring a neutral facilitator can help center resident voices in collaborative discussions, including uncomfortable conversations about power-sharing and equity, by building trust with one another and supporting the group to move to action.
- Neighborhood health and well-being must be well-

defined and a shared goal among all partners to establish a common frame of reference and set expectations at the beginning of the project.

- Explicit data sharing agreements with hospital partners are required to navigate HIPAA compliance concerns, including Internal Review Board approval, to readily share clinical-level data at the census tract-level. It is difficult for hospitals to share data outside of their systems.

Executive Comments

Charise Fong was formerly Chief Operating Officer and Executive Vice President of Community Building, EBALDC.

SPARC's efforts to improve neighborhood health and well-being have been grounded in the core values of centering racial equity and a deeply held belief in the inherent strength and resiliency of our neighborhoods.

So much more is possible when we collaborate closely with neighborhood residents and community, and public and private partners. And most importantly, when neighborhood residents determine the priorities and are an integral to SPARC deciding what collective actions to take.

Annie Ledbury is Senior Manager, Creative Community Development for EBALDC.

Art, culture, and creativity are critical parts of building healthy neighborhoods.

My job is to connect the dots so residents can build connections and power to make change in the built environment. That often involves connecting residents with design professionals, advocacy volunteers, and the right people at City Hall.

I'm proud of the behind-the-scenes support my team gives EBALDC staff, residents, tenants, and community members to weave art into all our projects.

Our strong belief is that public art reflects the community's histories, personalities, and priorities—whether it's built environment projects like real estate development or neighborhood services.

We can learn so much about our communities by the process in which we come together with artists to express the messages that mean the most to them—like power, resilience, and health.

Community building through art and creative design has the capacity to lift up the community and enhance cultural identity. It's very important work that makes an impact.

Chapter 28.

Women, Infants, and Children Program Case Study

Introduction

The Health and Hospitals Corporation of New York City addressed the problem of why so many pregnant women, new mothers, and their babies were not using WIC, SNAP, and Medicaid benefits. The drop off rate between 2017-2019 was especially sharp in zip codes with more non-citizens than in areas with fewer non-citizens. In some areas, 30 percent of eligible women were not accessing WIC and SNAP benefits in New York City.

Background

Systemic racism contributes to maternal health inequities in New York City where Black women are more likely to die in childbirth than White women. Maternity mortality rates in Brownsville are eight times worse than outcomes in the Upper East Side (47 percent).

These health inequities are causing preventable injuries and deaths, namely, infant mortality and morbidity. The lack of a coordinated and collaborative system of care inevitably leads to poor birth outcomes and prevents women from accessing social and financial support to promote better health.

Barriers to Access: Patient Story

Ana immigrated to the US from El Salvador and was five months pregnant when she showed up at the clinic for her first prenatal appointment. In the waiting room, a Community Health Worker (CHW) sat with her and explained WIC program benefits and flipped through a pictorial guide of food products she could obtain. Ana was not familiar with Medicaid nor how to apply. The CHW helped Ana make an appointment with the hospital counselors to apply for Medicaid.

The following steps were required for Ana to finally access WIC:

- Ana stopped by the WIC office to schedule her certification appointment. WIC offices do not allow initial appointments for certification by phone.
- On her second try, Ana was turned away because she lacked one document (proof of address) even though she could have been given temporary benefits for thirty days.
- Ana then went to her rescheduled certification appointment, but the WIC office did not enroll her four-year-old because they incorrectly determined

that she could not apply the same proof of income for her son's enrollment.

- The CHW followed up with Ana and encouraged her to continue with the WIC enrollment process and supported her at each step along the way.
- At the fourth trip to the WIC office, Ana was able to enroll her son.

As this example shows, a patient's time is not valued, and mothers must prove they deserve the benefits they are entitled to. It took Ana three months and four trips to the WIC office. It took the CHW following up seven times to make sure Ana received the benefits her family was entitled to. CHW encouragement was essential to educate Ana about her rights and to empower her to speak with a supervisor or manager when she was given the runaround and to be spoken to in her preferred language.

Ana could have been enrolled in one visit had there not been bureaucratic barriers at each step.

Project Challenges

Like most benefit programs, WIC is heavily dependent on compliance with multiple regulations and reporting requirements that make it difficult for eligible mothers to access services in a timely way. WIC staff must balance compliance with supporting individual client needs. Three systemic challenges stand out in New York State.

Barrier 1: Slow adoption of updated state-level WIC policies, which can result in decreased enrollment rates due to erroneous information and unnecessary steps.

Barrier 2: Poor access to bilingual staff and translation services creates difficulties to eligible beneficiaries with low English proficiency.

Barrier 3: In-person appointment requirements create access and convenience issues for working parents and those with young children.

Barrier 4: Misconceptions of immigration status and eligibility even though WIC does not ask for immigration status although rumors to the contrary often lead women to forego benefits for fear of how it could affect their status and being reported to ICE.

CHWs were employed to accomplish two goals during the two-year pilot: support women in accessing WIC benefits and gathering detailed data on common barriers. The latter were the basis for advocating systemic changes at all levels of the system: WIC offices, policies, processes, and procedures affecting beneficiaries.

On-the-ground feedback was critical for the success of the pilot. At WIC sites, CHWs and staff met weekly to discuss client issues and improvement steps to remove barriers. The pilot team met with the State health department quarterly to review enrollment trends, review client feedback, and how to address access barriers. This included feedback on why many recipients were not interested in returning to the program.

The main premise of the pilot was that CHWs were uniquely positioned to identify and help address barriers to WIC enrollment. Equally important is that data collected by CHs is an effective channel to inform necessary changes in local hospital and WIC office practices as well as state-level policies.

Data Strategy

An emphasis was on collecting "small data" by those contributing the information because it would be the most effective way to illustrate potential changes to improve access and maternal care. Feedback channels were created between Community Health Workers and patients to collect and document relevant data and compelling stories like Ana's.

A core principle of the initiative is that data is owned and directed by those who collected (i.e., CHWs) and contributed to it (i.e., patients). CHWs track and report monthly on outreach, eligibility screening, follow-up, and enrollment at each WIC site. These data points create an enrollment funnel that flags drop-off rates of eligible WIC clients in the enrollment process. This enables State administrators to track progress and to appreciate patients' stories about the impact of barriers to WIC enrollment.

Community Health Workers identified two drop-off points in the enrollment process:

- 86 percent drop between outreach and screening for WIC eligibility.

- 46 percent drop after referrals are made for those who are interested and eligible.

These findings were then correlated with qualitative data supplied by patients on enrollment barriers.

Patients surfaced four key barriers in the first year of the pilot:

1. Uncertainty around WIC eligibility, benefits, and application processes (35 percent).
2. Amount of time required to apply (29 percent).
3. Fears related to the impact of enrollment on immigration status (22 percent).
4. Challenges with WIC or medical referral completion (14 percent).

While patients experience barriers to enrollment firsthand, seldom are their frustrations translated into feedback for clinic administrators and policy makers to learn from. This pilot demonstrates the impact and legitimacy of closing the loop between direct patient experience and recommendations for better service and better care through enrollment in WIC benefits. By "democratizing" data, the WIC pilot establishes a roadmap for improved outcomes for low income and immigrant families.

By giving voice to patients, who are already entitled to WIC benefits, CHWs provided on-the-ground examples of challenges patients faced. This facilitated changes in the attitudes of clinic staff and state-level administrators toward beneficiaries. At the same time, reducing barriers to enrollment and reenrollment chipped away at decades of structural racism (e.g., wide disparities in access and outcomes) toward immigrant populations and communities of color.

Community Health Workers Role

CHWs carry an average caseload of 30-60 clients. However, the team is not assigned a participant quota so that they have time to understand and document trends in WIC access and enrollment, and to collect patient stories that provide insight into barriers driving enrollment trends.

CHWs are key to advocating on behalf of patients at WIC sites as well as educating enrollees about their rights to government benefits. They are also the key resource in educating and motivating patients about voicing their opinions in meetings with staff, how to speak up at focus groups on what they value most, and what is most frustrating and detrimental to their health. This does not come easily for immigrant families with low English proficiency and a low sense of agency in relation to WIC programs and administrators.

In conjunction with Health Leads staff, a partner in this pilot, CHWs and community members learned how to hold their own in group meetings. Clear expectations were developed for each meeting and participants were coached on how to be an active part of cross-sector collaboration and power sharing with site staff, hospitals, and State administrators. This fundamentally changed the power dynamic in the meeting room and, as a result, many practical suggestions were made to improve the enrollment process.

Buy-in would not have been accomplished without the full participation of each stakeholder. For example, the following observations were made, and site staff were charged with coming up with solutions for each:

- Participants were overwhelmed by the sheer amount of information about the program.
- Long wait periods between hand-offs were incredibly inconvenient and discouraging.
- Documentation required for enrollment was not clearly communicated nor was how to access WIC benefits.
- Participants could not always afford to wait in line for hours on end and often left without completing enrollment.

Waiting in line is needlessly frustrating when it could be used more productively by providing access to nutritionists and breastfeeding counselors, both of which were priorities for participants. CHWs identified this need, based on patient feedback, and helped WIC implement these services for participants waiting in line.

This change was accomplished by process mapping the situation (i.e., at safety net hospital and at WIC site) with CHWs, participants, and WIC staff.

Focus Group Recommendations

Seven focus groups were conducted in year two of the pilot: five in English, one in Spanish, and one in Haitian Creole.

Participants were screened by Health Leads CHWs based on eligibility status. Fourty-two women participated, thirty-three received WIC benefits, nine discontinued the program, and four never received WIC services. Thirty spoke English, nine spoke Haitian, and seven were Spanish speakers.

Six program strengths were identified: financial assistance, nutritional education, breastfeeding support, connection to peer counseling, reduced stress, and better health. The critical role of CHWs was cited in reducing food insecurity, and four important policy recommendations were made to strengthen the program through federal action:

1. Allowing mothers to stay on WIC for as long as their children were eligible.
2. Extending benefits to children up to six years of age.
3. Updating food packages with a greater variety of healthy foods.
4. Allowing benefits to roll over from month to month.

Another strong patient preference was about nutrition education and food programs. Enrollees wanted more personalized nutrition support that respected their dietary and cultural preferences. They wanted more food choices, and this meant reeducating WIC nutritionists about food packages and having enough flexibility to swap out items that did not match patients' dietary or cultural preferences. Nutritionists then spent more time with patients to learn more about the dietary needs of their families.

It was clear to focus group participants that more of the WIC benefit should be used for purchasing fruit and vegetables, including organic selections. Many participants did not know food packages could be customized. Recommendations included the following:

- Increase the amount of money for fruits and vegetables rather than promoting baby food and juice options. *"Nine dollars for vegetables is not enough."*
- Improve communications about what changes can be made such as soy or lactose free milk. *"I didn't find out until last month that you could get the alternative."*
- Increase the number of times Farmer's market checks can be given out or increase distribution of Health Bucks *"We should receive the farmer's checks more frequently, not just annually."*
- Align food packages with participant preferences and healthy choices. *"The juice has a lot of syrup in it. That's not healthy."*

Based on focus group feedback, shopping trips for food were destigmatized by the implementing electronic benefit cards that would reduce some of the embarrassment of buying food through the WIC program. This improved the shopping experience of participants.

Program Improvement Opportunities

Other program improvements were identified through process maps devised by Health Leads to improve site flow and operations based on participant experience. For example:

- Assure that all clients receive accurate and consistent information.
- Incorporate warm hand-offs between stages of the enrollment process.
- Reduce other appointment scheduling mix-ups at the time of certification.
- Ensure clients are prepared for WIC appointments with the proper paperwork and documentation.

While these observations and improvements seem obvious, it was not until they were voiced by patients and then funneled to site staff and state administrators that changes were made. This level of data granularity led to staff adopting the recommendations to enhance participant experience and to improve enrollment rates.

Making appointments easier for working mothers to make and keep also surfaced as a dire need. Participants wanted more flexibility in appointment scheduling and rescheduling, use of proxies, and extended hours. More communication is needed around what to expect about an appointment and how long it takes, and what documents are needed. An overriding concern was how to streamline the appointment process based on participant perceptions, rather than how the WIC office protocol was originally designed.

Participants wanted the ability to schedule and reschedule appointments online using the WIC app. Multiple points of entry into WIC should be offered in planning a WIC visit. And more clarity was needed around what proxies could and could not do.

State Department of Health officials were also interested in patient-level data collected by the pilot. The improved enrollment data as well as patient stories collected by the CHW helped policy makers to implement changes to streamline the enrollment process and increase enrollment as a result.

The pilot team also suggested changes that require state or federal action:

- Client-facing electronic scheduling of appointments (assuming participants have internet access).
- WIC should meet people "where they are" (i.e., participant cultural characteristics and language preference).
- Using the most lenient state policies to accommodate client enrollment whenever possible.
- Opt-in auto-enrollment for WIC-eligible Medicaid recipients.
- Allow hospital staff access to WIC systems for referral and appointments.

These changes would go a long way to reducing enrollment barriers as well as recognizing and respecting participants' time. This is a critical element of customer service and building trust with populations that are historically marginalized by government policies and bureaucracies and often disinclined to seek financial aid due to the stigma and shame about "taking handouts."

Lessons Learned

The pilot demonstrated that patient feedback can influence and drive solutions. It also showed that the staff (CHWs) closest to clients and communities (where CHWs live) are in the best position to collect first-person data on patient experience. Stakeholders would not otherwise have access to such detail and clarity about barriers and why health disparities are so pronounced among WIC enrollees.

First person feedback is far more insightful and persuasive than ordinary enrollment trend information. Hospital leaders are far more receptive to data on what is happening on the ground than reports from program directors who are detached from patients and CHWs in the community. State administrators were similarly persuaded by first-person accounts and recommendations on practical ways to improve enrollment levels.

While administrators had heard anecdotes before, they were not aware of specific examples. The combination of qualitative data from first person feedback, alongside more quantitative data, provided a level of detail and insight that was not usually made available to program administrators.

CHWs met with WIC staff regularly to point out barriers and share patient stories to support system-level solutions. This level of communication is essential for cross-referencing referrals to better understand how and why some patients fall between the cracks. Taking the time to build trust and relationships with WIC staff is one of the most important functions of CHWs. Without trust between CHWs and site staff, it would be challenging to persuade WIC personnel to make changes that contribute to enrollment barriers (i.e., when certain documents are no longer required).

Instead of focusing on the traditional patient quota orientation, CHWs prioritized data collection as a vehicle for capturing patient experience. It was satisfying to be a respected partner in solving problems and working with site staff on implementing solutions. This empowered and energized CHWs and greatly reduced burnout.

Summary

Community Health Workers provide a wealth of indispensable services to WIC participants. Given the scope of their roles, CHWs carry an average caseload of 30-60 clients at a time. The CHW team is not assigned a particular quota, which enables them to spend the time to understand individual needs, document enrollment trends, and collect personal stories that provide insight into barriers to care.

Key Takeaways

- First-person data (qualitative) collected by Community Health Workers is critical in addition to enrollment data (quantitative).
- Compelling personal stories elicit quicker support for changes in policies and procedures from bureaucrats than standard enrollment data.
- Community Health Workers' ability to build trust with patients is the key to program success.
- When patients' time is undervalued (inconvenient scheduling, excessive paperwork), it creates an insurmountable barrier to access benefits and medical care.

- Availability of bilingual staff, at each step in the enrollment process, is instrumental in overcoming barriers to care.
- Advocating for system-level change (policies and procedures) is required to improve service delivery in community initiatives.
- Data must be owned by Community Health Workers and patients rather than government agencies and providers to safeguard and support constituent rights to eligibility and services.
- Program eligibility must be clearly communicated and easily understood from the patient's perspective, not the agency's perspective.

Chapter 29.

Hawaii Community Foundation Case Study

Hawaii Health Overview

Several studies indicate that Hawaii faces significant challenges to improve resident well-being, preserve the culture, and ensure economic opportunity for residents in the coming years. Three studies are summarized below: *U.S. News & World Report, County Health Rankings and Roadmap Report, and Community Health Needs Assessment (CHNA)*.

U.S. News & World Report

Hawaii was ranked number one in terms of (1) access to care, (2) quality of care, and (3) overall health of the population. The three categories were equally weighted. Massachusetts, Connecticut, New Jersey, and California followed in the rankings.

Access rankings measured the affordability and access to healthcare based on six factors: child wellness visits, health insurance enrollment, adult wellness visits, adult dental visits, child health visits, and healthcare affordability. Hawaii ranked first in this category.

Quality rankings referred to each state's Medicare quality, hospital quality, nursing home quality, and preventable hospital admissions. Hawaii ranked first in this category.

Public health ranking measured the health of each state's population based on six factors: mortality rate, suicide rate, smoking rate, mental health, infant mortality rate, and adult obesity rate. California was ranked first and Hawaii sixth.

In all, seventy-one metrics across eight categories were employed to show how well states serve residents on health-related categories. The average of three years of data from an annual survey was administered to 70,000 people who were asked to prioritize each measure in their state.

Despite being ranked as the top state based on selected health criteria, Hawaii faces significant challenges in terms of health equity and addressing Social Determinants of Health in the future.

County Health Rankings & Roadmap Report

Hawaii provides local data by county for communities to consider. The four categories are:

1. Health behaviors: tobacco use, diet and exercise, alcohol and drug use, and sexual activity.
2. Clinical care: access to care and quality of care.

3. Social and economic factors: education, employment and income, family and social support, and community safety.
4. Physical environment: air and water quality, housing, and transit.

The roadmap includes four additional health categories that reflect community conditions that can change to improve health and opportunity. These factors are access to quality education, living wages, quality clinical care, nutritious foods, green spaces, and secure and affordable housing.

Honolulu County was ranked first, Kauai second, Maui third, and Hawaii fourth. However, there are significant gaps between ranked counties, especially between the second and third ranked counties compared to the fourth ranked county.

Community Health Needs Assessment

The tri-annual 2021 CHNA assessment identified five overriding priorities (like the 2018 report): financial security, food security, mental and behavioral health, housing, trust, and equitable access. It also identified seven additional and significant health needs: work together for equity and justice, strengthen safe families, prepare for emergencies, restore environment and sense of place, shift kupuna (elder) care away from sick care, invest in teenagers and healthy starts, and nurture community identity and cohesiveness.

Five themes were presented with recommendations for best practices and action steps. The recalibrated findings were influenced by lessons learned from coping with the pandemic.

First, the rapid adoption of telehealth was one of the silver linings of COVID-19 that signaled new ways to improve access to care in each county.

Second, the need for resilience and building resilient citizens is one of the lessons of COVID-19.

Third, an important investment is needed now in Community Health Workers; trained people *of* the community, working *in* their same community. Community Health Workers are a backbone of public health and trusted liaison to medical services and social care coordination in local communities.

Fourth, to better prepare for future public health crises, hospitals must get out into communities and build relationships. This is key to fostering trust with caregivers and ensuring equitable access to care. Cultural competency of healthcare providers is a necessary ingredient for building trust with healthcare institutions.

Fifth, advocates and organizers around upstream determinants need the active support, collaboration, and voice of hospitals to be heard to accelerate policy changes (systems change).

These central themes underscored the fact that 2018 and 2021 CHNA priorities require more civic involvement of communities and leaders to make tangible progress on needs that are now widely recognized.

The Hawai'i Community Foundation (HCF) is the steward of more than 1,000 funds with more than 105 years of experience in community building and supporting traditional cultural knowledge in the state.

In 2021, the Foundation awarded $7 million to 194 nonprofits to address systemic inequities throughout the state. It organizes work through the CHANGE Framework, which represents six interconnected sectors: Community and Economy, Health and Wellness, Arts and Culture, Natural Environment, Government and Civics, and Education.

HCF's equity focus is supported by data to track progress on where disparities exist and where investments are being made in the community. For its 2021 CHANGE Grants Program, HCF staff spent 340 hours with 450 nonprofit applicants in virtual interviews to learn and assess where resources could make the most impact. Grantees are given wide flexibility to use awards for general operating and program expenses. The average grant was $36,000. Fifty-one percent of applicant organizations have operating budgets below $500,000.

HCF implemented trust-based philanthropy principles in the grant process. The principles incorporate transparency, equity, and collaboration to address the power imbalance between nonprofits and foundations. The objective is to advance equity objectives, shift power, and build mutual accountability and learning.

Larissa Kick, Vice President of Community Grants and Initiative at HCF, commented that:

> CHANGE Grants were a way for HCF to live its value of building on trusted partners, reducing burden to grantees, and allowing for flexibility in resources and approaches to meet specific community needs. Our team at HCF committed to designing a different kind of grantmaking program and that is now informing our community collaboration processes in each CHANGE sector.

In addition to CHANGE Framework grantees, HCF funds a number of other projects aimed at addressing complex concerns through interdisciplinary approaches in Hawaii, including those described below.

Marine 30x30 (now called the Holomua Initiative) is an initiative that began in 2016, based on the principle that local communities should have a say in how they want to manage their resources. Its objective was to manage 30 percent of Hawaii's nearshore waters by 2030. Local stakeholders who live in the area and understand traditional Hawaiian farming and fishing techniques are brought into the planning conversation and asked what sustainability practices they propose for the area they know best.

Puna Strong was initiated because of the 2018 Kilauea eruption that destroyed 700 homes and brought about food scarcity, road closures, and evacuations. Funding came from three sources: County of Hawaii ($250,000), Hawaii Strong Fund ($100,000), and Anderson Beck Fund ($30,000).

The project funded disaster readiness and community resilience efforts through twenty-six grassroots organizations. Grantees worked toward a broad spectrum of goals in Puna that include providing mental health services, distributing food to residents, and tutoring for homeless children.

Community members were asked what they needed and how foundations and nonprofits could address the real needs of the community. The grantmaking process was another example of HCF's use of trust-based philanthropy practices, which are based on mutual learning and streamlining the application process (less paperwork).

Puna Strong funding focused on capacity building to guide nonprofits and grassroots organizations to better assist and protect their community in the long-term. Puna Strong grantees were invited to self-identify what resilience looks like and their priorities were often unique compared to other outside nonprofits.

In 2020, HCF initiated ‘lole, a nonprofit place-based research center and living scientific laboratory on Hawaii Island. The mission is to develop sustainability solutions rooted in ancestral knowledge and Indigenous practices. It aims to be a global resilience hub with an emphasis on energy security, food security, and place-based learning. Solutions emerging from ‘lole will be scaled and replicated in other parts of the world. ‘lole is the result of 2,400 acres of land and assets gifted to HCF from the New Moon Foundation and the Kohala Institute.

The Federated States of Micronesia, the Marshall Islands, and Palau are signatory nations to the Compact of Free Association with the United States (COFA). COFA gives citizens of the three member nations the right to live and work in the US, but they are not eligible for many federal and state benefits and social services. COFA was established partially in response to the US nuclear testing in the South Pacific, which dispossessed many islanders from their home islands and left many with long-term health problems.

Approximately 30,000 COFA citizens reside in Hawaii. However, most of them have no health insurance or access to needed healthcare. In late 2020, the federal law changed to allow COFA citizens to enroll in Medicaid insurance. In response, HCF is supporting eleven organizations serving COFA communities to do outreach and education about this change and to help with

Medicaid enrollment. To do so, HCF and five other funders established the Fund for Health Equity in 2021 to distribute $1.2 million in grants over two years.

HCF and Aloha United Way have partnered to administer the 2022-2024 ALICE (Asset Limited, Income Constrained, Employed) Initiative Cohort. It provides support to nonprofit organizations based in O'ahu engaged in ALICE impact areas of financial stability and savings, and safe and affordable housing. seventeen projects in the initial cohort include:

> Catholic Charities Hawai'i ($85,000 for three years): financial wellness program that includes financial literacy with mental health screening and skills to build a pathway out of poverty.
>
> Council for Native Hawaiian Advancement ($85,000 per year): workforce development training for economically and socially disadvantaged communities through financial education to improve income and savings.
>
> Family Promise of Hawai'i ($100,000 per year): co-creation of individualized plans to identify educational and financial goals (financial stability) and a course of action.
>
> Feed The Hunger Funs ($100,00 per year): increase earned income and savings by providing $3.5 million in loan capital and technical assistance to 500 low-income entrepreneurs otherwise unable to access loans.
>
> Goodwill Industries of Hawai'i ($80,000 per year): evidence-based employment and training services through a collaborative model that works across disciplines with multiple partners that provide wraparound services.

Hawai'i Appleseed Center for Law and Economic Justice ($100 per year): cohort of twenty affordable housing to help develop emerging leaders from diverse backgrounds with lived experience of housing insecurity to influence policymakers to support policies to help working families.

Hawai'i Children's Action Network ($80,000 per year): strengthen family voices to advocate for policies and system changes that increase household income and reduce household expenses.

Hawai'i Home Ownership Center ($50,000 per year): classes, coaching, and post-purchase services (online and self-paced) to create sustainable home ownership for low-moderate income families, including money management and the important role of credit.

Hawaiian Community Assets ($100,000 each year): financial counseling, income support, and career coaching to improve the financial capacity of households to achieve economic self-sufficiency.

The Institute for Human Services ($80,000 per year): affordable and permanent supportive services for formerly unsheltered families with earned income, children's enrichment and education, parent skill-building on site, and building household's tenancy skills to maintain housing tenure.

Institute for Native Pacific Education and Culture ($100,000 each year): workshops and coaching on personal finances through education and culturally relevant financial workshops with trained financial coaches, as well as matched savings to increase financial standing.

Kōkua Kalihi Valley Comprehensive Family Services ($85,000): increase economic sovereignty through an array of economic supports, including an expanded public benefit enrollment team, and guidance services on finance, jobs, and educational opportunities.

Legal Aid Society of Hawai'i ($100,000): legal information and services that address barriers to increased and stable income and consumer debt.

Parents and Children Together ($100,000 each year): immediate economic improvement and advocacy for policy and systems change to address financial burdens for under-resourced individuals and families, and with an incentive to join Get Ahead cohorts (poverty prevention and workforce success).

Partners in Development Foundation ($80,00 each year): provide vulnerable youth with mentorship and vocational training opportunities, financial literacy education, and supplemental services to increase independence and financial stability, with the goal of training a new generation of farm workers, furthering food security and sustainability.

Residential Youth Services & Empowerment ($50,000 each year): continuum of support for houseless youth aged 18-24 with dignified, well-integrated spaces in the community (i.e., disenfranchised being invited back into the community).

Waikīkī Community Center ($125,000 each year): increase financial stability for seniors and families through a network of supportive holistic services to maintain stability such as an emergency fund with matched savings, access to financial services and credit after the program, and decreasing household expenses.

Project Evaluation

Groundswell Services, Inc. was retained to evaluate the CHANGE Grants Program. This included examining community feedback from an online survey as well as conducting interviews with nonprofit community leaders and HCF staff.

The initial year of grant solicitation was a learning process for both applicants and HCF staff. Some applicants were frustrated by the metrics used as not being sufficiently relevant to their organization, while others thought the expense of extensive data gathering and tracking was too high to justify applying for a $10,000 grant. A recommendation was that application materials should be clear about the criteria for assessing data-tracking capabilities.

A few applicants reported that HCF's technical assistance was especially important. This included support for advocacy, tools training for reaching better agreements with government agencies, network-building support for developing collective goals and shared measures to foster systems change, and support for technology such as telehealth for outreach activities and data tracking.

Small and medium-sized organizations were especially concerned about training and information on fund raising and organizational stability, particularly how to raise earned revenue through service contracts. Larger organizations pointed out the need for assessing and managing federal funding as well as support for strategic planning, and board training for workforce development training was also identified as a high priority.

Several organizations felt burdened by the application process while dealing with the day-to-day repercussions from the pandemic. Organizational bandwidth was a common challenge.

Applicants generally felt staff was very interested in listening to what their organization was trying to accomplish and how HCF could best support their goals. Seventy-five percent of applicants rated their experience with the grant process as above average or excellent. Eighty-two percent felt they had a better relationship with HCF staff after meeting with them, and how to apply for grants as a result. For organizations that decided not to apply for funding, 23 percent cited not having enough time or resources to apply, and 18 percent said they were not eligible.

CHANGE Framework

The Framework rests on statewide data that begins to identify gaps in equity that can be addressed by creating shared community goals and tracking progress of collective efforts. Each sector is unique and inter-related in terms of addressing comprehensive solutions for local communities and the state of Hawaii.

Common themes that emerged from the first year of CHANGE grant making indicated that many organizations did not have the capacity to address root causes because the symptom needs were so great. Government compliance was often more of a barrier than a help (slow payment, upfront capital requirements). Collecting and utilizing data was too often an end rather than a reflection of program effectiveness. Building networks is essential for system change and requires additional technical assistance and peer learning to be successful.

The CHANGE Grants Term covered April 1, 2021—July 31, 2022. It was then extended another six months with additional funds to the first round of grantees to continue the important work with flexible funds.

Sector: Community & Economy

Data Points (Source: Change Framework: Community and Economy, pages 1-9; Data Impact pages 1-3).

Hawai‘i has a growing economy driven by tourism, yet wages do not keep up with the high cost of living. The per capita income is $56,888 and 38 percent of jobs pay a living wage (twenty dollars per hour).

The median earnings for a single adult are $34,730. Half earn less than that. Among households that accumulate wealth, 57 percent own their own homes. Yet 29 percent do not have enough savings to cover three months of financial emergency.

Forty-eight percent of households do not meet the Survival Budget and struggle to afford living in Hawai‘i. Based on the Survival Budget, $28,128 is needed for a single adult and $72,336 for a family of four. Residents spend 27.4 minutes traveling to work.

A total of 56.1 percent of renters and 40.3 percent of homeowners are burdened by housing costs. The median price of a single-family home on Maui, for example, is $1,059,000. The number of housing units needed by 2025 is 13,949.

Hawai'i has a Livability Index Score of 53 out of 100. Personal safety is an issue and is reflected in violent crime data that indicates 242 offenses per 100,000 residents. Property crime indicted 2,965 offenses per 100,000 residents. This compares to the US average for violent crimes of 386 a year, and property crime as 2,451 offenses a year.

A total of 9.3 percent of students did not go to school because they felt unsafe, either at school or on their way to or from school.

Common Themes

In 2021, the Hawai'i Community Foundation awarded twenty-four CHANGE grants in the Community and Economy sector ranging from $30,000-$40,000 for a total of $900,000. Common grant making themes found that affordable housing was a major issue and getting worse each year. Collaboration was called for rather than an "us versus them mentality." Many organizations wanted to become part of a network. Few organizations had data to show progress toward equity over time.

Grants cover five areas:

- Supporting pathways to resilient, sustainable communities.
- Building capacity for disaster relief and recovery.

- Supporting unsheltered individuals and youth and helping them meet basic needs.
- Investing in Hawaii-based nonprofits and social ventures with a social or environmental return.
- Providing emergency assistance for rent and utility payments.

Highlighted Program: **House Maui Initiative** (In 2022, $5 million in funding from HCF, as well as $25 million federal grant; $2.5 million Maui County grant; and more than $50 million in state CIP funding).

In Maui County, 50.8 percent of households are cost burdened (spending 30 percent or more of their income on housing). Local families are leaving at an alarming rate. One of the initiative's objectives is to increase the pipeline of qualified homebuyers and renters through the Maui Financial Opportunity Center (FOC).

The FOC is a program of Hawaiian Community Assets and funded by HCF and the County of Maui. It helps residents qualify for stable and affordable housing through workshops and financial counseling. The housing affordability crisis is particularly difficult in Maui where more than 50 percent of households are cost burdened. This means they spend 30 percent or more of their income on housing, the highest in the state.

Income of Maui residents is often limited by the local job market, childcare expenses, and debt (e.g., car payments and student loans). A Maui Now survey of residents found that residential rental prices spiking at 41 percent in 2022. Persistent drought conditions affected Maui's water supply with a projected 20 percent rise in electric bills. The Department of Water Supply prohibited Upcounty and West Maui water consumers from using water for irrigation, watering lawns, and washing vehicles.

The House Maui strategy rests on three pillars: (1) align resources to lower the cost of housing, (2) educate and empower prospective resident buyers and renters, and (3) organize and advocate for policy and administrative changes needed to address Maui's housing crisis. Civic engagement is central to the initiative's success. This means bringing together local, state, and federal resources to support the $5 million social impact investment in Maui housing.

Wes Lo, member of the House Maui Advisory Council, cautioned that the initiative is not just about affordable housing (a key component).

> It's part of a more comprehensive strategy that includes income, community development, financial education, self-sufficiency, food sustainability, and civic engagement—all of which support a better Hawai'i.

He also pointed out that HCF initiated the multi-pillared initiative and is a key catalyst in supporting and sustaining cross-sector collaboration.

Hawaiian Community Assets' counselors provide free individualized counseling to assist Maui residents in creating a financial action plan to build savings, pay down debt, and improve credit scores. The nonprofit organization builds the capacity of low- and moderate-income residents to achieve economic self-sufficiency, especially for Native Hawaiians.

Central Maui was identified as the starting point of the housing strategy with 4,000-6,000 downtown rental housing units, followed by South Maui. The program's emphasis is providing tools to activate residents.

Micah Kāne, Chief Executive Officer and President of the Hawaiʻi Community Foundation, stressed that:

> Employers have a stake in House Maui since 50 percent of employees are burdened by housing costs. More affordable rental units and new houses are needed for employees closer to work. And employers must be part of the collective impact to sustain the initiative.

He believes that House Maui could be a model for improving our housing system across all Hawaiʻi.

Sector: Health & Wellness

Despite being ranked as the top state based on selected health criteria, Hawaii faces significant challenges in terms of health equity and addressing Social Determinants of Health in the future.

Data Points

Improvements in social determinants of care will be necessary to meet the growing needs of the population. Food insecurity was experienced by 11.3 percent of residents. Homelessness is reflected in 2,668 persons being sheltered while 3,683 remain unsheltered. A total of 2,597 children are in foster care.

Overall, 45.4 percent of adults with a serious mental or behavioral condition did not receive needed treatment or counseling, 23 percent of children who received or needed mental healthcare had a problem obtaining it, and 29.5 percent of high school students experienced depression in the past twelve months. At present, there is one mental health professional for every 430 individuals in Hawaii.

Currently, 14.7 percent of a worker's income was spent on healthcare premiums. There is a 23 percent physician shortage for the population, which translates into a need for an additional 797 full-time physicians. By 2030, 37,930 seniors will need long-term care. This means 4,318 beds in nursing homes will be required and 5,200 spaces in assisted living and residential care facilities for seniors.

Common Themes

Hawai'i Community Foundation's CHANGE Grants Program awarded fifty-four grants in the Health and Wellness sector ranging from $30,000-$50,000 for a total of $2,029,000. Common grant making themes found that many organizations focused their strategies on Social Determinants of Health as a basis for healthcare. Access to healthcare is a critical issue in rural, immigrant, and non-English speaking populations, as well as for people with mental and behavioral health needs. Health and wellness organizations vary in size and scope of services.

Some have strong data capability, measure impact, and make system change while others have more limited capacity to embrace change. Others focus on prevention, specific diseases, or provide wrap-around services to complement medical care.

Grants covered eight areas:

- Spreading awareness against tobacco consumption.
- Connecting those in need with healthy, local food.
- Offering childcare and afterschool programs to essential workers.
- Providing mental health support for children.
- Reducing barriers to care and food to grandparents and elders.
- Preventing child abuse and neglect.
- Increasing access to healthcare providers, especially for rural and vulnerable populations.
- Delivering fresh produce and food to vulnerable people.

Highlighted Program: **Promising Minds**

The Promising Minds Initiative was developed by HCF and other funders in 2019 to increase the healthy development of vulnerable children ages 0-5. Its purpose is to build resilience in children and families who have already experienced the effects of trauma by focusing on trauma-informed professional development approaches for the early childhood workforce. These disciplines include social work, therapy, counseling, behavioral health support, pediatricians, and nurses.

The three-year Promising Minds Initiative has awarded $3 million, which included an evaluation component, conducted by Engage R+D. The assessment addressed how Promising Minds shaped practitioners' lives and professional practice, increasing their capacity to engage in trauma-informed dialogue, and supporting staff through their own trauma to be effective when working with families. Prioritizing self-care was an important part of the curriculum and practitioners recognized the need for more specialists trained in trauma-informed care practices within the health and educational system.

Thirty-one percent of Hawaii's children are at risk for developmental or behavioral issues or delays compared to 26 percent nationally. Forty-six percent experience one Adverse Childhood Experience (ACE) and 20 percent experience two or more. Native Hawaiians and Pacific Islander experience ACEs at an even higher rate.

Increasing early access to appropriate, trauma-informed services and support can mitigate the effects of exposure to trauma. Without such screening and treatment, late diagnosis of mental health problems leads to high costs in special education, mental health interventions, juvenile justice, and incarceration.

Promising Minds aims to equip early childhood educators, practitioners, and service providers with trauma-informed strategies, tools, and support.

Year 1 activity focused on developing relationships between HCF, grantees, and stakeholders. It was especially important to involve the professional practice community and to learn from their lived experience. Year 2 focused on better understanding what systems changes were necessary to improve trauma-informed practices, including the Infant and Early Childhood Mental Health Fellows Program. Year 3 assessed program impact and how to scale and grow the initiative. This effort included developing learning tools to further best practices for wider adoption. Current work includes advocating for policy and systems change and increased public investment in child and family well-being.

Among the most important systems change issues is identifying what factors contribute to a more coherent system that support early healthy development and mental health within four constituency groups: mental health professionals, early childhood educators, families, and children 0-5.

Justina Acevedo-Cross, program director of Promising Minds stated that:

> Recently new research has been coming out about the effects of adversity and toxic stress on early childhood below the age of six, and so there was a realization that this would be an important area to focus on to make an impact in Hawaiʻi. It was also clear many settings needed to be included in the solution because caring for and supporting young children doesn't only happen in clinical settings. The places where families are can be some of the most transformative spaces. When we work with people in home-visiting programs, when we work with people in childcare settings or peer parent support groups, they will have daily, weekly contact

with families. It is really powerful to have workers know how to recognize issues and make referrals. It is a many hands approach to helping our children grow and develop on track.

HCF learned that domestic violence (52 percent) and emotional abuse (48 percent) were reported as most relevant according to fifty-four program participants.

- Exposure to domestic violence: 51.9 percent
- Emotional abuse: 48.1 percent
- Homelessness: 44.4 percent
- Historical trauma: 42.6 percent
- Neglect: 42.6 percent
- Death or displacement of a family member: 40.7 percent
- Neighborhood violence: 44.0 percent
- Physical abuse or violence: 37.0 percent
- Sexual abuse: 29.6 percent
- Unsure: 29.6 percent
- Serious illness: 27.8 percent
- Serious accidents: 25.9 percent
- Other: 18.5 percent

There were regional differences as well. In East Hawaii and Oahu, homelessness and historical trauma were higher. In Maui, emotional abuse and homelessness were prevalent. Kauai noted absent fathers contributed to risk, while military deployment on bases in Hawaii commonly experienced early childhood trauma.

Participants likewise found that the need for trauma-informed approaches is increasing for families because of the pandemic, particularly for families experiencing job loss, homelessness, and individuals considered undocumented. Many families are also experiencing depression and are at risk for intimate partner violence.

Sector: Arts & Culture

Nurturing and cultivating Hawaii's diverse culture depends on supporting arts education, particularly for youth. This includes access to spaces and opportunities to practice and participate in arts and different cultures.

Data Points (Source: "Change Framework: Access to Arts Education for Youth," pages 1-2)

Twenty-nine percent of Native Hawaiians and 18 percent of non-Hawaiians participate in Native Hawaiian cultural activities. There are 18,610 Hawaiian speakers in the islands.

Three percent of individual charitable giving ($25 million) supports the arts. The total economic activity generated by the arts and culture sector is $205.5 million each year, which supports 5,968 full-time jobs.

Common Themes

Hawai'i Community Foundation awarded thirty-three CHANGE grants in the Arts and Culture sector ranging from $10,000-$50,000 for a total of $1,068,560. Common grant making themes indicated that arts and culture advances equity and justice as well as preserves and perpetuates traditional cultural knowledge. The arts and culture sector demonstrated great resilience (through collective action) in responding to hardships caused by the pandemic.

Arts organizations have difficulty leveraging data to illustrate the impact of their work overtime, but many are interested in improving data collection and evaluation practices. Broader networks based on shared interests can influence systems and policies.

The Artists in the Schools program provides residency grants for artists to integrate their art form with other core curriculum areas such as language arts, math, social studies, and science. A residency includes at least five secondary and eight elementary sessions by the teaching artist with the same core group of students. Grants range from $7,000 plus an additional $500 (optional) for professional development for classroom teachers.

Grants covered three areas:

- Expanding arts education to children in schools.
- Supporting the perpetuation of Hawaiian traditions and culture.
- Increasing educators' skills through the integration of fine arts.
- Providing opportunities for local artists to engage with the public.

Highlighted Program: **Donkey Mill Art Center** ($40,000 HCF CHANGE Grant award).

Holualoa Foundation for Arts and Culture, dba Donkey Mill Art Center, is a nonprofit arts and culture education program on Hawaii Island.

Maia Grajski, who was the center's executive director in 2022, acknowledged that:

> We live in a world of competing urgencies, but the arts are at-risk as the proverbial canary in the coal mine of community well-being. The arts provide "keiki" and the kid-at-heart in each of us with a safe space to connect through our imaginations at a deeper level with ourselves, each other, or diverse community and the environment.

The youth education program is recognized as a regional resource by weaving together literature, performing arts, environmental studies, and health. In the last five years, 972 youths and teens attended workshops and classes. At the local elementary school 1,465 were educated through artists, and 25 free classes were offered to youths and their families in west Hawaii. A total of $27,000 in scholarships were awarded for programs at the Mill.

Donkey Mill offers classes, free exhibitions, and special events that highlight histories and cultures from across the Pacific to reflect the island's diverse community of 202,906 people. A total of 46,000 live in Kailua-Kona and Holualoa zip codes adjacent to the center. Twenty-five percent are Asian or Asian/Pacific Islander, 18 percent Native Hawaiian, and 69 percent are economically disadvantaged elementary school students in the area.

Five thousand attended cultural festivals at the center, 230 students learned about Japanese and Marshallese cultural traditions in hands-on workshops, 350 students participated in classes and workshops on Hawaiian history and culture, and thirteen cultural practitioners helped to perpetuate ancestral knowledge through workshops in fibers and print.

In 2021, 142 artists showed work at the center, $14,000 was paid to artists through acquisition of five works and $82,000 for contract teaching artists. Local artists were paid $35,000 through the retail shop and online store.

In the last five years, 11,500 people visited Donkey Mill, 640 artists exhibited their work, and 400 classes were taught. Grants totaled $890,000.

Sector: Natural Environment

Climate resilience is a top priority for Hawaii. The American Society of Civilian Engineers gave Hawaii a D+ rating on the state of its infrastructure.

Data Points

Hawaii generates 27.6 percent of renewable energy through electricity. Sustainable agriculture, fisheries, and food systems are also priorities. Since 2016, 11 million gallons per day of fresh water has been added to Hawaii's existing supply through conservation, reuse, and recharge efforts.

A total of 11.6 percent of Hawaii's food supply is from local sources while 88.4 percent is from imported sources. Each year, 104 million pounds of food is produced locally. Oahu currently gets 90 percent of its water from groundwater. Statewide it is 60 percent.

Hawaii's Ocean Health index score is 74 out of 100, which represents a healthy ocean that provides maximum benefits in terms of food provision, coastal protection, biodiversity, economies and livelihoods, sustainable tourism, and sense of place.

Seventeen percent of native watershed forest (140,000 acres) is under high-level protection. Fifty-five percent of the 150 action items in Hawaii's Statewide Biodiversity Plan for invasive species are being implemented.

Common Themes

The Hawaii Foundation awarded twenty-four CHANGE grants ranging from $30,000-$40,000 for a total of $900,000. Common grant making themes noted a groundswell of community organizations involved in grassroots restoration of Hawaii's natural environment. Some organizations are forming stronger networks to leverage knowledge and expertise to influence systems change through collective action. The agriculture sector lacks access to sufficient capital to stem the impact of accelerating climate change. Infrastructure is needed to help greater food independence for community sustainability. The sector appreciates the value of data to measure impact but often lacks the capacity and know-how to collect and analyze it.

Grants covered four areas:

- Coordinated outreach and capacity building to ensure clean, fresh water in the future
- Expanding conservation education
- Supporting nonprofits working to restore oceans
- Protecting watershed areas and forests

Highlighted Program: **Fresh Water Initiative (Wai Maoli)**

For centuries, Hawaii has maintained a tradition of fresh water supply being held in trust for citizens, compared to water held as a private property right as it is in much of the US Hawaii's long-term water supply faces an uncertain future.

Micah Kāne, Chief Executive Officer and President of the Hawaiʻi Community Foundation, says:

> Hawaii recognizes that water is wealth, and that the community is only as strong as the wealth it has. And water is such a critical element so that the community can thrive.

In 2030, Hawaii is projected to receive only three quarters of the rain that fell in 1985. Expected demand in water use is expected to increase by 79 million gallons a day by 2030. Water conservation is the least expensive and most efficient way to increase available water supply. Dana Okano, Program Director of Natural Environment, states that:

> Water is foundational to everything in life. Hawaii clearly values sustainability. We've been demanding more action on sustainability from our leaders and practicing it more ourselves as people of Hawaii.

In the face of increased demand and supply uncertainly, the Fresh Water Council developed eighteen policy and implementation recommendations for the Hawaii Fresh Water Initiative. The Council established a goal to create an additional 100 million gallons of fresh water per day by 2030.

HCF and other foundations began the Initiative in 2013 to address looming water shortages due to climate change. The Fresh Water Council identified several critical environmental issues. These include reduced rainfall, increased drought, land use changes, increased evaporation, increasing population pressure, and an aging infrastructure.

These factors guided the development of a Blueprint for Change. Blueprint for Action was created to guide the investments and actions of HCF and the Council.

Three water strategy areas were proposed: conservation, recharge, and reuse.

> *Conservation* related to improved efficiency in the population's daily fresh groundwater use rate by 8 percent from 330 gallons per day per person to 305

gallons per day per person. This goal would provide 40 million gallons per day in increased water availability.

Recharge would increase Hawaii's ability to capture rainwater in key aquifer areas by improving storm water capture by doubling the size of protected watershed areas by 2030. This would provide 30 million gallons in increased water supply.

Reuse would double the amount of wastewater being reused by 50 million gallons per day by 2030, thus increasing water availability by 30 million gallons per day.

In anticipation of increased demand and water supply uncertainty, the Fresh Water Council advocated (1) a reduction in potable water use on landscape areas (with incentives and rebates), since 50 percent of potable residential water is for landscape watering, (2) encouraged leak detection systems, and (3) improving agricultural water efficiency since a quarter of all pumped groundwater is used for irrigation. Total conservation water savings by 2030 would meet the 40 million gallons a day goal.

The Council emphasized that guiding principles be forged through shared consensus. There is a recognition that water is a complex issue that demands a comprehensive set of solutions that will come from different sectors, and a good solution in one geographic area may not be appropriate for another area. A flexible and adaptive framework is required as well as better information and access to accurate data for good decision making.

The Council's guiding principles included additional recommendations:

- Solutions should focus on financial sustainability and cost effectiveness.
- Targeted education efforts are more effective that general outreach and awareness campaigns.
- Water is as important to the economy and culture as it is to ecology.
- Water supply solutions must provide for a broad spectrum of water uses.
- The current price of water does not reflect its true costs.
- Native Hawaiian cultural traditions place a high value on water and can provide guidance on how best to steward water.
- There is an urgency to the freshwater supply issue that is not widely evident to the public.
- Costs to fresh water supply will rise with each year of delay.
- The nexus between water and energy is clear and compelling.

The Council believes that investments made now (i.e., installing green infrastructure and protecting watershed capture area through fencing, fire control, and removing invasive species) will incur much less financial hardship than trying to restore dysfunctional capture opportunities after the fact. Council members advocate for reliable and consistent public funding as the most important and challenging part of watershed protection and storm water capture.

As water resource consultant Dr. Bahman Sheikh observed:

> We take water for granted. We have enough today but won't in a few decades when it runs out. There will be a deficit of 100 million gallons a day. Without water we will be nothing. Water is life.

Sector: Government & Civics

HCF's philosophy is that cross-sector collective action and shared values can create the most impact.

Common Themes

HCF's CHANGE Grants Program awarded nine grants ranging from $30,000-$50,000 for a total of $300,000. Common themes in grant making showed that few organizations applied for funding, but those that applied were strongly aligned with the criteria. Many organizations focused on specific subjects and policy issues, yet few addressed the overall sector. Volunteerism is seen by some as a direct form of civic engagement.

The strongest organizations in this sector are a resource to develop broader networks and collective action to achieve system and policy changes across all sectors. Tracking impact through data is a slow process in this sector that takes years to demonstrate results. Schools have great potential to increase civic engagement among Hawaii's youth.

Highlighted Program: **The Kaua'i Resilience Project (KRP)**

KRP is a movement to reduce suicide attempts by increasing community connection, resilience, and life skills in Kauai youth. Each month, KRP brings together a diverse group of stakeholders that includes county council members, Department of Health, Department of Education, family-business owners, major funders, mental health professionals, and civic groups to collectively support Kauai's children.

Suicide prevention for youth extends beyond mental health and incorporates gaining skills and social support networks for addressing adversities in life. The project sets goals such as creating safe places for youth and increased access to afterschool programs, social emotional learning curriculum in schools, and a community awareness campaign.

In 2019, KRP began the Kauai Kids are Your Kids campaign to encourage adults to support young people and the YouGotThis campaign. It offers tips on healthy behavior and monthly challenges for young people to support connection to community.

Sector: Education

Data Points

Hawaii has long recognized the need to improve access to early childhood education. A total of 54 percent (20,000) of three- and four-year olds are not in nursery school, preschool, or kindergarten, and 10.7 percent of kindergarten classes display ready-for-school characteristics.

Success in school as measured by high school completion rates show that 83 percent of public high school students graduate and 73 percent feel positively about their school. At the same time, 15 percent are chronically absent. Fifty-five percent enroll at a post-secondary institution following graduation. At the same time, 15 percent are chronically absent.

Sixty-seven percent of University of Hawaii graduates have a job one year after graduation. Five years later, UH graduates working in Hawaii earn $72,000 (doctor or professional degree), $47,000 (master's or graduate certificate), and $6,000 (bachelor or post-baccalaureate certificate).

Highlighted Program: **Stronger Together Hawaii**

The Stronger Together Hawaii Scholarship program is a $2.4 million fund started by HCF and First Hawaiian Bank as an emergency response during the pandemic. It ensures that Hawaii youth can achieve college and career goals regardless of changes in their academic journey. In 2020, 360 students received an average of $6,200 in scholarships to be used for tuition and educational costs. Thirty-five percent of students are from neighbor islands other than Oahu. Many students are the first in their family to attend college.

Highlighted Program: **Roots of Empathy**

Roots of Empathy is a social and emotional learning (SEL) program for elementary school children that uses an infant and parent to help children develop empathy. The program covers nine curriculum themes (with three sessions per theme) over a series of twenty-seven classroom visits. The second visit for each theme involves bringing babies and their parent(s) into the classroom. Having the baby as a living teaching tool with an instructor helps students better understand human emotions and needs including their own.

Highlighted Program: **Choose Love**

This program was developed by a mother who lost her young son in the Sandy Hook Elementary School shooting. The curriculum uses evidence-based neuroscience and positive psychology lessons to teach children four-character values: courage, gratitude, forgiveness, and compassion in action. The program is used in more than fifty-two schools and eighty-nine afterschool programs and is offered at no cost to schools.

Common Themes

Hawai'i Community Foundation's CHANGE Grants Program awarded 194 grants ranging from $30,000-$50,000 for a total of $7,055,027. The funds awarded were for general operating and program expenses to the extent possible, giving nonprofits the flexibility to meet their organization's needs. Common grant-making themes indicated that applicants had the advantage of working in the sector for many years to build a strong continuum of knowledge and relationships. Measuring long-term impact is commonplace and well-developed. Social and emotional learning and trauma-informed approaches to education are strongly supported.

Many applicant organizations are stepping up to address immediate needs of students and families facing financial hardship, food insecurity, job loss, and access to distance learning technology. Professional development for educators is commonplace for distance learning, virtual programming, and training on mental health support. However, few applicants participate in formal networks with shared goals, common data, and collective action.

Grants were awarded to organizations that:

1. Gathered data that tracks impact and progress.
2. Committed to advancing equity in Hawai'i and addressing the greatest disparities in Hawai'i.
3. Collaborated with others to fulfill an organizational mission or participated in a network of partners to foster systems change.

4. Addressed community needs in response to COVID-19 and is working toward recovery, stabilization, and resilience for the community.

Summary

The Hawai'i Community Foundation is committed to a new philanthropy approach that builds more equitable relationships with nonprofits in the state. Trust-based philanthropy aims to advance equity through multi-year, unrestricted funding that gives flexibility and freedom for nonprofits to carry out their mission in the best way. Paperwork is simplified to reduce the time and labor burden on nonprofits. Only four questions are asked.

The online interview process makes space for applicants to ask HCF team questions, which leads to constructive feedback, two-way conversations, and an appreciation of personal stories about what is most important to applicant organizations. This approach enables HCF to open new funding opportunities to nonprofits.

In addition to funding, attention is given to leadership skills, capacity building, and organizational growth. Feedback is solicited and acted upon throughout the grant-making process.

Key Takeaways

- Transparency, trust, and collaboration are necessary to achieve equity objectives, shift power, and build mutual accountability with diverse partners.

- By building reciprocal relationships with partners from all sectors, more capacity is developed to address complex challenges and nimbly address challenges (like the COVID-19 pandemic). The networks that pivoted fastest and provided aid in communities were ones previously established and with high trust.
- Cultural competency of providers is necessary to build community trust with healthcare institutions.
- Community leaders need the active support and political leverage of anchor institutions such as well-established foundations, healthcare institutions, financial institutions, and hospitals to accelerate local and statewide policy changes.

Executive Comments

Justina Acevedo-Cross is Program Director of Promising Minds Initiative.

Hawaiʻi Community Foundation is committed to understanding what young people need to thrive and grow. New research documents the effects of adversity and toxic stress on early childhood, below the age of six. There's a growing realization this is an important area to focus on because it impacts so many children in Hawaiʻi.

It's essential to improve education and health systems because families interact with each other so often. Right now, these two systems are very separate or siloed from each other.

If there was a common system of shared data, it would make things so much better.

There's often a wait-and-see approach to treatment because so few specialized clinical providers are available to refer young patients to. For example, referrals to a licensed social worker with specialized infant/early childhood behavioral health experience or a child psychologist. Part of the goal of Promising Minds is to address this workforce shortage in the state.

So much can be done at a young age through brief interventions, or positive interactions that wouldn't be recognized or documented in a typical category of clinical treatment without a visible or widely recognized medical condition. Many babies and toddlers fall through the cracks of the healthcare system as a result during such a critical developmental period.

Addressing developmental issues at an early age could have huge benefits in so many areas from schools through adult work life.

Everyone can play a positive role in the lives of young kids as demonstrated through Positive Childhood Experiences (PCEs). This encompasses a list of very simple actions that have been thoroughly vetted and tested. They make a difference. Such as having a caring adult in a child's life who takes a real interest in them. Anyone could be that caring adult role. It could be a family member or someone in the family circle of friends who could reach out to that child and help them have a better day.

Reference

Positive Childhood Experiences resources: Tufts University HOPE Framework https://positiveexperience.org/research/transforming-practice-with-hope/and National Child Traumatic Stress Network https://www.nctsn.org/.

www.ingramcontent.com/pod-product-compliance
Lightning Source LLC
LaVergne TN
LVHW052207200926
848481LV00001B/46